T0206100

Fieldwork Educator's Guide to Guide to

Level I

Fieldwork

Fieldwork Educator's Guide to Level I Fieldwork

Editors

Debra Hanson, PhD, OTR/L, FAOTA
Professor
St. Gianna School of Health Sciences
Department of Occupational Therapy
University of Mary
Bismarck/Fargo, North Dakota

Elizabeth D. DeIuliis, OTD, MOT, OTR/L, CLA
Clinical Associate Professor
John G. Rangos Sr. School of Health Sciences
Department of Occupational Therapy
Duquesne University
Pittsburgh, Pennsylvania

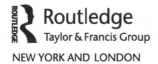

Routledge
Taylor & Francis Group

NEW YORK AND LONDON

First published 2023 by SLACK Incorporated

Published 2024 by Routledge
605 Third Avenue, New York, NY 10158

and by Routledge
4 Park Square, Milton Park, Abingdon, Oxon, OX14 4RN

Routledge is an imprint of the Taylor & Francis Group, an informa business

Library of Congress Cataloging-in-Publication Data

Names: Hanson, Debra (Professor of occupational therapy) editor. |
  DeIuliis, Elizabeth D., 1981- editor.
Title: Fieldwork educator's guide to level I fieldwork / editors, Debra
  Hanson, Elizabeth D. DeIuliis.
Description: Thorofare, NJ : SLACK Incorporated, [2023] | Includes
  bibliographical references and index.
Identifiers: LCCN 2022038015 | ISBN 9781630919627 (paperback)
Subjects: MESH: Occupational Therapy--education | Preceptorship--methods |
  Mentoring--methods | Occupational Therapists--education
Classification: LCC RM735.3 | NLM WB 18 | DDC 615.8/515--dc23/eng/20220919
LC record available at https://lccn.loc.gov/2022038015

Cover: Tinhouse Design

ISBN: 9781630919627 (pbk)
ISBN: 9781003524168 (ebk)

DOI: 10.4324/9781003524168

DEDICATION

We would like to dedicate this book and Level II to academic fieldwork coordinators, who are often serving in this essential role within occupational education without a lot of training and resources, but serve with ingenuity, dedication, and resourcefulness.

We would also be remiss without a formal dedication to fieldwork educators, who essentially volunteer their time, expertise, and energy, which makes a significant contribution to occupational therapy student learning and the future of the profession.

CONTENTS

ABOUT THE EDITORS

Debra Hanson, PhD, OTR/L, FAOTA, is currently a professor at the University of Mary, which maintains dually accredited doctoral programs at Bismarck, North Dakota and Fargo, North Dakota campuses, and an affiliated doctoral program in Billings, Montana. Dr. Hanson previously served as faculty and academic fieldwork coordinator (AFWC) at the University of North Dakota in Grand Forks, North Dakota for more than 30 years, transitioning to the University of Mary, Fargo, North Dakota campus in 2019. Dr. Hanson completed her bachelor's degrees in Occupational Therapy (1980) and Psychology (1979) and a master's degree in Counseling (1990), all at the University of North Dakota, and a PhD in Adult Education in 2009 from North Dakota State University in Fargo, North Dakota. Dr. Hanson served as the American Occupational Therapy Association (AOTA) Commission on Education AFWC representative from 2010 to 2013 and was recognized in 2014 as a Fellow in the AOTA related to her leadership in fieldwork education. She has served as a content expert and reviewer on the topic of fieldwork education for various academic journals and coordinated the Fieldwork Issues column for *OT Practice* from 2010 to 2017. She has published several book chapters and numerous peer-reviewed publications and has presented at state, national, and international conferences on topics related to fieldwork education, student clinical reasoning development, evolution of occupational therapy practice, professional identity, considerations for rural practice, spirituality, and integration of occupational therapy theory in practice and various teaching methods.

Elizabeth D. DeIuliis, OTD, MOT, OTR/L, CLA, is a clinical associate professor at Duquesne University, which maintains dually accredited occupational therapy programs at the master's-level and the entry-level occupational therapy doctorate level in Pittsburgh, Pennsylvania. Dr. DeIuliis served as the AFWC at Duquesne University for more than 11 years and assumed the role of program director in 2021. Dr. DeIuliis received a bachelor's degree in Health Sciences and a master's degree in Occupational Therapy from Duquesne University. She completed a Post-Professional Occupational Therapy Doctorate Program at Chatham University. Dr. DeIuliis also earned the credential Academic Leader via successful completion of the AOTA's Academic Leadership Institute in 2018. Dr. DeIuliis has had various leadership roles within academia and the occupational therapy profession, such as serving on the Board of Directors within the Pennsylvania Occupational Therapy Association and as a subject matter expert and volunteer within the National Board for Certification in Occupational Therapy. She has published several textbooks, numerous peer-reviewed publications, and has presented at state, national, and international conferences on topics related to fieldwork education, doctorate capstone, professionalism, interprofessional education, and teaching methodologies.

CONTRIBUTING AUTHORS

Becki Cohill, OTD, OTR/L (Chapter 4)
Clinical Associate Professor
Doctoral Capstone Coordinator
Division of Occupational Therapy
Binghamton University
Binghamton, New York

Marsena W. Devoto, MSOT, OTD, OTR/L (Chapter 8)
Associate Professor and Academic
Fieldwork Coordinator
School of Occupational Therapy
Brenau University
Norcross, Georgia

Anna Domina, OTD, OTR/L (Chapter 10)
Associate Professor and Vice Chair of
Education and Clinical Practice
Capstone Coordinator
Department of Occupational Therapy
Creighton University
Omaha, Nebraska

Nancy R. Dooley, MA, PhD, OTR/L (Chapter 2)
Associate Professor and Director
Occupational Therapy Doctorate Program
College of Health and Wellness
Johnson & Wales University
Providence, Rhode Island

Cherie Graves, PhD, OTR/L (Chapter 3)
Assistant Professor and Academic
Fieldwork Coordinator
University of North Dakota
Grand Forks, North Dakota

Jeanette Koski, OTD, OTR/L (Chapter 12)
Associate Professor and Academic Fieldwork
Coordinator
Department of Occupational and Recreational
Therapies
University of Utah
Salt Lake City, Utah

Angela M. Lampe, OTD, OTR/L (Chapter 10)
Associate Professor and Director
Post-Professional Occupational
Therapy Doctoral Program
Department of Occupational Therapy
School of Pharmacy and Health Professions
Creighton University
Omaha, Nebraska

Jason C. Lawson, PhD, MS, OTR/L (Chapter 6)
Assistant Professor
Occupational Therapy Doctorate Program
Saint Gianna School of Health Sciences
University of Mary
Bismarck, North Dakota

Amy Mattila, PhD, OTR/L (Chapter 5)
Assistant Professor and Department Chair
Department of Occupational Therapy
Duquesne University
Pittsburgh, Pennsylvania

Hannah Oldenburg, EdD, OTR/L, BCPR (Chapter 3)
Assistant Professor and Academic
Fieldwork Coordinator
St. Catherine University
St. Paul, Minnesota
Mayo Clinic
Rochester, Minnesota

Julia Shin, EdD, OTR/L (Chapter 10)
Assistant Professor
Creighton University
Omaha, Nebraska

*Rebecca L. Simon, EdD, OTR/L, FAOTA
(Chapter 9)*
Associate Professor and Academic Fieldwork
Coordinator
Occupational Therapy Doctorate Program
College of Health and Wellness
Johnson & Wales University
Providence, Rhode Island

Lacey Spark, OTD, MOT, OTR (Chapter 4)
Assistant Professor
University of St. Augustine for Health Sciences
Austin, Texas

Jaynee Taguchi Meyer, OTD, OTR/L (Chapter 4)
Assistant Professor and Academic Fieldwork
Coordinator
Occupational Therapy Program
University of St. Augustine for Health Sciences
San Marcos, California

*Joscelyn Varland, OTD, OTR/L, CLT
(Chapter 11)*
Associate Professor
Academic Fieldwork Coordinator
Occupational Therapy Doctorate Program
Saint Gianna School of Health Sciences
University of Mary
Bismarck, North Dakota

Jayson Zeigler, DHSc, MS, OTR (Chapter 13)
Clinical Assistant Professor and Academic
Fieldwork Coordinator
Indiana University
Indianapolis, Indiana

PREFACE

An intended outcome after reading this book is to consciously link the philosophy of occupational therapy to the philosophy of education. There are clear synergies that exist between occupational therapy and teaching and learning best practices that might not be fully grasped by practitioners that serve in essential roles such as fieldwork educators (FWeds).

As occupational therapy practitioners, we are trained to become experts in understanding fit between people, occupations, and environments. We understand the significance of adaptation and person-centered philosophies. We study how to be astute observers and to perform activity analyses and grade tasks and demands to influence performance. We place value in ensuring a just-right challenge. These essential ingredients also make up a good teacher, instructor, or educator. As paradigms in health care and clinical practice transform and change, so does the landscape of education. We need to adapt. Although fieldwork education has existed in occupational therapy for nearly 100 years, there are limited resources that exclusively focus on best practice and skill development specific to the FWed role and, more importantly, how best to promote student learning in fieldwork.

New models for clinical learning have emerged in the occupational therapy profession and in the broader arena of health care education. Today's learners and current health professional students have changed, and generational differences in learning need consideration. One should not have a one-size-fits-all or cookie-cutter approach as a FWed. While you do want to give your student experience in working with a client population and an appreciation for the role of occupational therapy during the Level I fieldwork experience, this book will challenge you to shift your mindset to facilitating skill acquisition (learning). You will be more conscious of adjusting your teaching approach to match your fieldwork students' needs and developmental level. *The nuts and bolts of the matter is that there is a skill of teaching skills and, more specifically, a skill to teaching clinical skills.*

This book is designed to complement *Fieldwork Educator's Guide to Level II Fieldwork*. Although the books can be utilized separately, they are designed to be used sequentially and in tandem to holistically develop service competency as a FWed in both Level I and II fieldwork experiences. Both of these books align with the American Occupational Therapy Association's (AOTA's) Vision 2025, which provides a distinct call for the profession to *inform*, *educate*, and *activate* occupational therapy practitioners (AOTA, 2017). Fieldwork education by tradition has been integral to occupational therapy education and central to our profession. This book is designed to *inform* and *educate* occupational therapy practitioners on best practice teaching and learning approaches in order to enhance their effectiveness and identity as FWeds. Finally, it is the hope of the contributing authors that this book *activates* practitioners to link arms with and serve alongside occupational therapy educators and academic fieldwork coordinators (AFWCs) as partners in fieldwork education to propel the occupational therapy profession forward together. As former AFWCs, we can confidently say that we cannot do what we do without the dedication and commitment of our FWeds.

Quality Fieldwork Is Key to Quality Occupational Therapists

This book introduces the Level I FWed to practical tools and resources that will provide a solid foundation in the FWed role. In occupational therapy, fieldwork is organized by levels to include an introductory competence level (Level I) and progressive entry level (Level II) to develop the generalist occupational therapy practitioner (Accreditation Council for Occupational Therapy Education [ACOTE], 2018). As a desired outcome of Level I fieldwork is to provide an introduction to occupational therapy practice, the role and expectations of the Level I FWed are not exclusive to only being an instructor or evaluator of student performance but also act as a facilitator of professionalism, mentor, resource curator, and clinical reasoning guide. Evolving contextual factors, such as cultural and generational changes in occupational therapy students, new accreditation requirements impacting the preparation in the classroom, and the dynamic nature of health care, require Level I

Figure I-1. Purpose of the book.

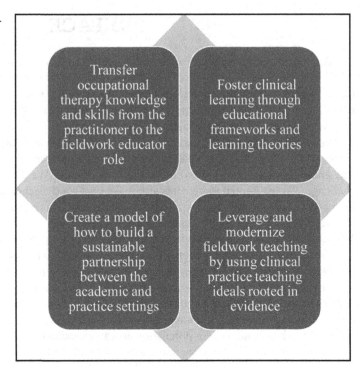

FWeds to have a widening skill set compared to the past. This book is the first of its kind to serve as a practical working guide for all Level I fieldwork types and for situating pedagogy of learning in Level I fieldwork. As editors, our overall ambitions can be summarized in Figure I-1.

We are so grateful to have partnered with an all-star cast of contributing authors to actualize a big, hairy, audacious goal that has been on our vision boards as AFWCs for some time. One of the remarkable aspects of the book sequence is the wealth of knowledge and experience behind the contributing authors. Across both books, the authors have a combined sum of more than 463 years of experience as occupational therapy practitioners and a combined sum of more than 150 years of experience as AFWCs. The authors represent occupational therapy programs at different degree levels and from different geographical regions across the United States, as represented in Figure I-2.

Our authors have directly supervised or placed thousands of occupational therapy fieldwork students throughout their careers. They are recognized leaders in their field, as evidenced by their attainment of service leadership within the AOTA, ACOTE, National Board for Certification in Occupational Therapy (NBCOT), and state occupational therapy organizations. The contributing authors have served on AOTA AFWC-Capstone Coodinator Research Committees and task forces, served as trainers in the AOTA Fieldwork Educator Certificate Workshop, engaged as mentors and mentees in AOTA's Academic Education Special Interest Section new AFWC mentorship program, been a representative on the Roster of Accreditation Evaluation Committee, and appointed as committee members on AOTA's Commission of Education. We are so thankful to have garnered occupational therapy scholars and leaders that epitomize bona fide experts in occupational therapy fieldwork education to share their wisdom and guidance.

Frequently in occupational therapy literature, fieldwork is referred to as a bridge. Each chapter in this book is intentionally designed to serve as a building block in order to create a robust infra-structure (a bridge) to connect the occupational therapy classroom to practice.

A bridge, by definition, requires support, span, and foundation to be functional and ultimately serve its purpose. Fieldwork is intended to serve as the conduit between the classroom and the clinic (Figure I-3), yet often FWeds are underprepared or unsure of how to be effective in this role.

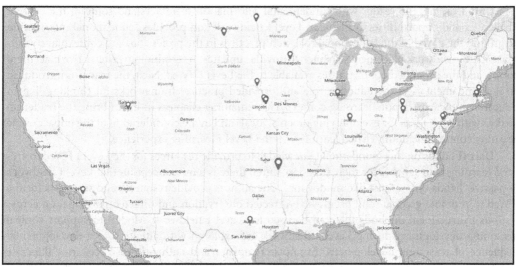

Figure I-2. Geographical locations of contributing authors.

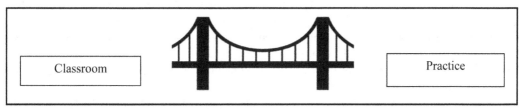

Figure I-3. Fieldwork as a bridge metaphor schematic.

Sometimes this bridge, this infrastructure, is not sound nor stable, lacks connection, and, therefore, does not provide a solid learning experience for the occupational therapy student. As clinicians, occupational therapists are expected to be lifelong learners and engage in continued competency to support their individual clinical practice and the future of the occupational therapy profession. Practitioners that are called to serve as FWeds should embody this same professional responsibility to enhance their performance and skill set as FWeds. This is referred to as *service competency*; engaging in learning and training to develop a specific level of knowledge and skill. Each chapter in this book contributes to a comprehensive blueprint on how to develop service competency as a FWed. This next section will provide a general overview of the book as a whole and the unique features of each chapter.

Book at a Glance

There are two distinct characteristics evident in this book. Throughout the text, best practices in teaching and learning are showcased and applied to various Level I fieldwork situations so that the FWed can readily apply authentic education to work with students. There is a similar emphasis on integrating best practice ideals of the occupational therapy profession, which include person-centeredness, inclusivity, ethics and professionalism, and occupation-based practice. Using these best practice ideals as a foundation not only enhances the professional identity of the FWed but ultimately the occupational therapy profession as a whole. As experts in the field, the authors thoughtfully respond to common pitfalls and challenges prevalent in Level I fieldwork today and outline a framework of action steps to address them. Vision 2025 calls upon the occupational therapy profession to be solutions oriented, influential, effective, and responsive (AOTA, 2017). Each chapter in this book serves as an essential stepping stone to realize Vision 2025.

Unit I orients the reader with fundamental information to understand some of the current challenges and opportunities available in Level I fieldwork and provides foundational information to ground the FWed in the educational role, best practices in the profession, and contextual considerations for fieldwork placement. Chapter 1 provides updates in terminology, alternative placement forms, and the expanded opportunities available to the Level I FWed. Next, the reader is introduced to the fundamentals of the educator role and provided practical frameworks for thinking like an educator in the experiential learning context. The remaining chapters in Unit I bring the reader up to date with fresh ideas for exemplifying practice ideals and invite consideration of the impact of the learning context, including virtual learning, on the Level I learning experience.

Unit II builds on this foundational knowledge to provide resources for the Level I FWed to create a learning plan suitable for their situation. Often there is a misconception that Level I fieldwork is passive, hands off, or "just like shadowing." The authors provide resources and strategies for the FWed to promote gradual- and progressive-directed observation and directed participation across various instructional methods that can be used for Level I fieldwork. Models to support clinical reasoning development during Level I fieldwork are explored with attention to a developmental sequence of reasoning development. Exemplar templates and authentic case scenarios illustrate practical strategies for engaging the student in the learning process. Occupation-focused models are discussed as a tool to anchor student reasoning development. Through case scenarios and templates illustrating practical strategies, the reader will be introduced to reciprocal learning strategies for learning with and from students to think with theory in practice. Mechanisms to foster student professional development and communication skills are explored through case examples and exemplar strategies. The unit culminates with resources and a step-by-step framework for developing a Level I fieldwork learning plan suitable for the fieldwork setting, the cooperating academic institution, and the type of experiential learning offered.

Unit III explores topics that emerge in Level I learning that are more likely to be situational in nature or in-the-moment learning experiences. The authors put emphasis on the generational make-up of today's occupational therapy student, as awareness and understanding of these factors can help the student and the educator have a better experience. Through extensive use of realistic case scenarios, practical tips for taking advantage of new and emerging learning opportunities onsite are reviewed. Current legislation as well as practical aspects of working with students with disabilities, considerations for placement, and reasonable accommodations are discussed. Scenarios are provided to illustrate best practice approaches and respectful attention to student learning needs. Current psychosocial factors impacting student success during experiential learning are identified, as well as practical strategies that might be taken by the student, FWed, and AFWC for proactively addressing anxiety and student stress management.

The focus of **Unit IV** is the formative and summative assessment of student learning during Level I fieldwork. Strategies for formative assessment including current models and considerations for providing effective student feedback are explored in relationship to student goal setting and reflection. Through case scenarios, templates, and helpful figures, the reader is introduced to best practices and guidelines for avoiding common pitfalls and biases in the evaluation of student performance during Level I fieldwork.

As occupational therapists, we know that learning occurs through doing, which is the quintessential methodology behind experiential learning such as fieldwork education. Readers are encouraged to *do* and *reflect* throughout the book. Each chapter provides opportunities for reflection, meaningful resources, and learning activities that empower the reader to translate key knowledge and skills learned to their own practice site or experience.

In Closing

Though the primary intended audience is practitioners as FWeds, these books will be meaningful to other stakeholders. For instance, occupational therapy doctoral students who are interested in exploring education as a focus area for the doctoral capstone (ACOTE, 2018) will benefit from the pedagogical groundwork and frameworks of learning threaded throughout the book sequence. To that end, serving as a FWed is often an opportunity for some practitioners to test the waters as an educator within the occupational therapy classroom. After experiencing the educator role in a fieldwork context, a practitioner might contemplate teaching opportunities to serve as a lab assistant, adjunct instructor, part-time instructor, or even pursue a full-time core faculty member role in academia. Those practitioners who are hypothesizing a potential career move from the clinic to higher education will find value in learning how to connect the dots between their capacity and skill sets as a FWed to pedagogical guideposts that can be used to foster didactic teaching and adult learning in the classroom. Finally, AFWCs will benefit from learning about best practices in teaching and learning as they are in a unique position to strengthen the skill set of their own network of FWeds and to develop innovative and unique fieldwork experiences in their program. Essentially, we have provided a blueprint for AFWCs to design, implement, and manage fieldwork programs in diverse settings and with diverse instructional methods.

This book uniquely puts together learning frameworks, educational theories, and clinical instructional techniques within and outside of occupational therapy to uniquely equip FWeds for the future of fieldwork education. In addition to infusing these new practices into everyday fieldwork practice, it is hoped that FWeds and AFWCs feel inspired to continue to innovate and expand upon these fieldwork education pedagogies. What is next in the realm of occupational therapy fieldwork education? We challenge our readers to question, hypothesize, trial, reflect, learn from, and then repeat.

Do you have questions about your practice as a Level I FWed? For instance, have you ever wondered …

- *Is what I am doing with my students working?*
- *What is my students' experience with particular teaching approaches I use? Are they effective?*
- *Do students understand what they are expected to learn during this Level I experience? How can we make best use of available opportunities?*
- *Do students appreciate having site-specific learning objectives and a weekly schedule? In what ways does it help them?*
- *How did trialing a different supervision model work in my setting?*
- *Do my students like to have weekly check-ins to discuss performance and feedback?*
- *How do I introduce my students to clinical reasoning during Level I fieldwork?*
- *How do diverse feedback models impact my students' learning and performance?*
- *In what ways do fieldwork students create value to my clients, work site, and my own professional development?*
- *Are the comments I provide during evaluations meaningful to the student's growth and development?*

Questions likes these are important ones to have and even more important to act upon and to study. Did you know that the scholarship surrounding fieldwork education in the United States falls behind other countries (Roberts et al., 2014)? Examining and expanding instructional methods and educator development resources are critical research priorities set forth by the Occupational Therapy Research Agenda, designed to propel the occupational therapy profession forward (AOTA, 2018). Armed with a stronger pedagogical foundation and deeper appreciation for the FWed role, FWeds and AFWCs truly have the power to transform the future of the occupational therapy profession. Quality fieldwork is key to quality occupational therapists.

We are truly grateful for your commitment to expand and intensify your knowledge and skill set as a FWed. We hope you enjoy the books!

Warm regards,
Liz and Deb

References

Accreditation Council for Occupational Therapy Education. (2018). 2018 Accreditation Council for Occupational Therapy Education standards and interpretative guide. *American Journal of Occupational Therapy, 72*(Suppl. 2), 721241005p1-7212410005p83.

American Occupational Therapy Association. (2017). Vision 2025. *American Journal of Occupational Therapy, 71*(3), 7103420010p1. https://doi.org/10.5014/ajot.2017.713002

American Occupational Therapy Association. (2018). Occupational therapy education research agenda—revised. *American Journal of Occupational Therapy, 72*(Suppl. 2), 7212420070p1-7212420070p5. https://doi.org/10.5014/ajot.2018.72S218

Roberts, M. E., Hooper, B. R., Wood, W. H., & King, R. M. (2014). An international systematic mapping review of fieldwork education in occupational therapy. *Canadian Journal of Occupational Therapy, 82*(2), 106-118. https://doi.org/10.1177/0008417414552187

Unit I

Building a Foundation to Support Level I Fieldwork Learning

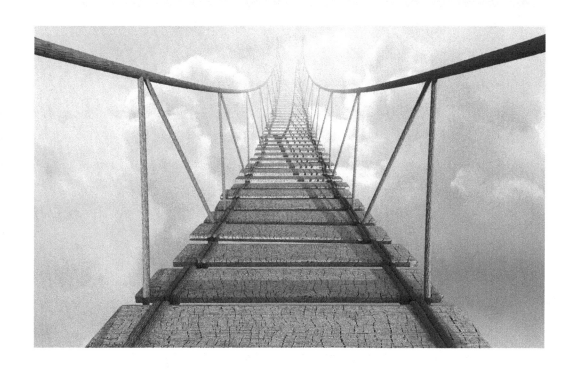

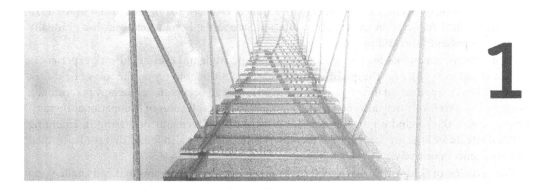

Overview of Level I Fieldwork

Debra Hanson, PhD, OTR/L, FAOTA
and Elizabeth D. DeIuliis, OTD, MOT, OTR/L, CLA

The Level I fieldwork experience plays an important role in the student's overall learning and is an important component within the curriculum design of the academic program. The goal of Level I fieldwork is to "introduce students to fieldwork, apply knowledge to practice, and develop understanding of the needs of clients" (Accreditation Council for Occupational Therapy Education [ACOTE], 2018, p. 41). The ACOTE standards further mandate that "Level I fieldwork enriches didactic coursework through directed observation and participation in selected aspects of the occupational therapy process" (2018, p. 41). As a result of the broad guidelines for Level I fieldwork, and the alignment of the fieldwork experience with the design of each curriculum, there is a great deal of variation in regard to how fieldwork experiences are designed and implemented across the United States. Variation in types of sites used, instructional methods, scheduling, intensity as well as the course objectives and types of supervision provided are common (American Occupational Therapy Association [AOTA], 2015; Haynes, 2011; Johnson et al., 2006; Keptner & Klein, 2019).

Level I fieldwork is often the first opportunity of the occupational therapy student to apply theoretical knowledge to practice, to gain first-hand experience as to the occupational needs of clients and the opportunity for directed observation and participation (ACOTE, 2018). It also sets the tone for future, more progressive learning such as in Level II fieldwork. Level I fieldwork also offers an opportunity for the student to "try on" the role of the occupational therapist and to gain confirmation of their vocational choice. Level I fieldwork is unique to the United States and is not a form of experiential education in the profession of occupational therapy in other countries nor

Hanson, D., & DeIuliis, E. D. (Eds.).
Fieldwork Educator's Guide to Level I Fieldwork (pp. 3-25).
© 2023 Taylor and Francis Group.

is it replicated in other health care professions (DeIuliis & Hanson, 2023). Introduced in the 1973 American Medical Association (AMA) Accreditation Standards, Level I fieldwork has gradually evolved to its present form and purpose.

As it is transformational for the occupational therapy student, Level I fieldwork experiences also provide opportunities for the qualified health care practitioner to try on the role of fieldwork educator (FWed). Since the qualified practitioner need not be an occupational therapy practitioner, serving in the FWed role may also be an introduction to the profession of occupational therapy. Johnson et al. (2006) found a growing number of fieldwork placements occurring in emerging practice contexts without an occupational therapy practitioner, but also found that students rated those experiences positively.

The variation of fieldwork learning objectives across academic programs makes it challenging for the Level I FWed to master expectations for the role. Programmatic learning objectives and integration into the curriculum based on the curriculum design of the academic program will vary program to program (ACOTE, 2018). Although there is collaboration between the academic fieldwork coordinator (AFWC) and fieldwork site, this may or may not include a training component for the FWed. While there are requirements for the role of Level II FWed, there are no specific requirements for the Level I FWed role beyond the designation of practicing professional. For example, a newly licensed/credentialed graduate would meet the general role requirements to serve as a Level I FWed. Little is known as to how the Level I FWed is exactly trained for the role, and little information is available that specifically prepares the fieldwork with theoretical frameworks to think like and approach this important role as an educator. Some occupational therapy practitioners only have their own experiences as a fieldwork student to guide their attitudes and actions as a FWed. This book is designed to be a blueprint to develop competency in the Level I FWed role and a guide to develop the habits of thinking and practice that lead to quality student learning. This text coincides with the *Fieldwork Educator's Guide to Level II Fieldwork* book, which builds upon these best practice principles to be used within progressive Level II fieldwork experiences.

This chapter will set the stage for the remainder of this book, providing information as to how Level I fieldwork has evolved in the history of the occupational therapy profession and the challenges and opportunities that have accompanied that process. The value of the Level I fieldwork experience to student learning will be explored, and the benefits and challenges to stepping into the Level I FWed role will be reviewed.

LEARNING OBJECTIVES

By the end of reading this chapter and completing the learning activities, the reader should be able to:

1. Identify health care and profession-specific trends that have influenced the development of the Level I fieldwork structure in the United States.

2. Describe the alternative forms of the Level I experience from its inception to present.

3. Understand the value of the Level I fieldwork learning experience for students.

4. Appreciate the benefits and challenges associated with the Level I FWed role.

THE EVOLUTION OF LEVEL I FIELDWORK IN THE UNITED STATES

The expectation that "field experience" would be a part of the education of the occupational therapy practitioner extends back to the very beginning of the profession. For example, the very first accreditation standards adopted in 1923 indicate that at least 3 months of supervised hospital practice training was required, in addition to at least 8 months of theoretical or practical work (AOTA, 1924). This was quickly revised in 1927 from 3 months to 6 months and from there has ranged up to 9 months before returning back to the present standard of 24 weeks (Evenson & Hanson, 2019). Initially, Level II fieldwork was conceptualized as focused on practice areas such as physical and psychiatric conditions to general medicine and surgery, psychosocial dysfunction, tuberculosis sanatoriums, and children's hospitals. Level II fieldwork generally occurred near the conclusion of the curriculum, to offer students opportunity to apply theory, refine their skills, and enter into practice.

The Level I fieldwork experience was not introduced until 1973, in order to offer practical experiences to occupational therapy students that were integrated throughout their academic curriculum (AMA & AOTA, 1973). The intent was that the Level I experience would emphasize "directed observation and participation in various field settings" (AMA & AOTA, 1973, p. 486), while the Level II experience would provide a more in depth experience. The designation of participation in "various field settings" was consistent with the requirements for Level II fieldwork during that era, as Level II fieldwork no longer was expected to include 3 months in physical disabilities and 3 months in psychosocial dysfunction as specified in the previous standards (AMA & ACOTE, 1965), but each program was free to choose their practice focus areas for fieldwork. Right from the start, the Level I experience was considered to be an integral part of the educational program. Initially, the focus was on fieldwork settings that would provide learning experiences that would reflect academic coursework, but in later standards (AOTA, 1983), this association is strengthened as Level I fieldwork is considered a part of didactic coursework. It is further clarified that Level I experience is not intended to emphasize independent performance. Although identified as a part of didactic coursework, it was expected that there would be cooperation between academic and FWeds in identifying appropriate learning experiences. This was especially important since Level I students could be supervised by personnel outside of the profession, including teachers, social workers, public health nurses, and physical therapists from the time it was first introduced in 1973 (AMA & AOTA, 1973).

Expectations for collaboration between the academic program and the fieldwork site were evident from the inception of the Level I fieldwork experience. A review of fieldwork articles published from 1966 to 1986 revealed that seven articles had been published about Level I fieldwork, and two of them included both Level I and II fieldwork (Leonardelli & Caruso, 1986). Three of the articles discussed how to develop student empathy, factors impacting student performance, and the potential role of computers impacting the student placement process. The remaining articles written on Level I fieldwork provide evidence of the creative learning structures representing the Level I experience. Three of the articles published were descriptions of "innovative" programs occurring in a federal prison, a camp for diabetic children, and community service. See a summary of articles published in Table 1-1.

Collaboration was not mandated until the 1998 accreditation standards (ACOTE, 1998), when the plan to ensure collaboration was required to be documented, along with evidence that the experience took place and formal evaluation of student performance occurred. The impetus behind the need for closer communication between academic programs and fieldwork sites may have been concerns expressed by FWeds and administrators who felt that Level I fieldwork

TABLE 1-1

FIRST CREATIVE LEVEL I FIELDWORK EXPERIENCES

NAME OF STUDY	STUDY AUTHORS AND DATE	FOCUS OF STUDY
Level I placement at a federal correctional institution	Platt et al. (1977)	Students worked at a federal correctional institution in programming developed by occupational therapy faculty members and staffed by students working under faculty supervision. Students showed gains in the areas of personal resourcefulness, group leadership skills, and ability to identify clients' needs. They also learned to identify the role of occupational therapy within the context of the institution.
A student practicum experience	Gill et al. (1974)	Working at a camp for children with diabetes, students were able to apply their knowledge of growth and development, define the role of occupational therapy in a nontraditional setting, and learn about childhood diabetes.
An educational strategy for occupational therapy community service	Cromwell & Kielhofner (1976)	Students worked within human services programs that did not provide occupational therapy services. Students gathered data about the agency and used it to design an activity-focused program that met health needs. Supervision was shared by members of the academic faculty and agency personnel.

placement was neither cost nor time effective for them. They called for maximum flexibility in curriculum design and fieldwork education, suggesting that fieldwork placement could most feasibly occur on evenings, weekends, and without direct supervision from an occupational therapist (Leonardelli & Caruso, 1986).

The cost-effectiveness of Level I fieldwork was identified as a concern for FWeds as early as 1982, as administrators and FWeds expressed concern about the time commitment for student supervision and the suitability of students completing short-term placements in higher acuity medical settings. Snow and Mitchell (1982) completed a study exploring professional and administrative relationships between hospitals and academic programs and noted discontentment among FWeds and a perception that educational programs were "taking advantage of them" (p. 254). Related to this perception, Teske and Spelbring (1983) noted changes in financial support for public agencies that were leading to reduction and elimination of student programs. Presseller (1983) confirmed the prevalence of issues for fieldwork related to cost-effectiveness and potential cutbacks in student programs. Leonardelli and Caruso (1986) conducted a national survey of FWeds and directors of academic occupational therapy and occupational therapy assistant programs to explore and identify issues and concerns related to Level I fieldwork. Their respondents represented 35 occupational therapy programs, 34 occupational therapy assistance programs, and 99

TABLE 1-2

LEVEL I FIELDWORK EDUCATORS, REGISTERED OCCUPATIONAL THERAPY PROGRAM, AND OCCUPATIONAL THERAPY ASSISTANT PROGRAM RANKINGS OF 14 VALUED LEVEL I FIELDWORK EXPERIENCES

VARIABLE	CLINICS (FIELDWORK EDUCATORS)	REGISTERED OCCUPATIONAL THERAPY ACADEMIC PROGRAM	OCCUPATIONAL THERAPY ASSISTANT ACADEMIC PROGRAM
Hands-on experience with patients	6	4	10
Develop basic communication skills	8	10	5
Provide exposure to variety of disease/disabilities	7	11	8
Receive feedback on professional behavior	5	6	6
Develop beginning writing skills and treatment planning skills	9	8	11
Opportunity to use evaluation and treatment techniques	12	7	12

Adapted from Leonardelli, C. A., & Caruso, L. A. (1986). Level I fieldwork: Issues and needs. *American Journal of Occupational Therapy, 40*(4), 258–264. https://doi.org/10.5014/ajot.40.4.258

clinical settings representing acute, rehab, and long-term care settings. A summary of the ratings of occupational therapy and occupational therapy assistant faculty, FWeds, and fieldwork students in regard to the factors important to Level I fieldwork are provided in Table 1-2.

It is notable that occupational therapy programs rated hands-on experience and opportunity to use evaluation and treatment techniques more highly than did FWeds or occupational therapy assistant programs whose role might suggest a higher ranking of those items. It is logical that the development of writing and treatment planning skills would be more highly valued by FWeds and registered occupational therapist programs than occupational therapy assistant programs, due to the differences in professional role. It is interesting to note that FWeds and occupational therapy assistant programs were more cognizant of the need for students to develop basic communication skills than the registered occupational therapist educators. This may be related to the maturity level expected of students in a 4-year vs. 2-year program. FWeds in this study expressed that they would like more structure for Level I fieldwork provided by the schools so that there was less time required for their planning, yet the majority (74%) also felt FWeds should design the learning experiences. Another large difference was in the area of the development of learning objectives: 73% of clinicians felt that uniform objectives developed by AOTA would be best, while only 39%

TABLE 1-3
ACADEMIC FACULTY, LEVEL I FIELDWORK EDUCATOR, AND STUDENT RANKING (1 TO 10) OF VALUED LEVEL I FIELDWORK EXPERIENCES

VARIABLE	CLINICS (FIELDWORK EDUCATORS)	REGISTERED OCCUPATIONAL THERAPY ACADEMIC PROGRAM	OCCUPATIONAL THERAPY ASSISTANT ACADEMIC PROGRAM
Hands-on experience with patients	1	5	1
Awareness of occupational therapy service delivery systems	7	6	< 10
Student observing problem solving in practice	9	< 10	5
Receive feedback on professional behavior	6	10	4
Practice writing skills	< 10	< 10	7
Develop a treatment plan	< 10	< 10	9

Adapted from Kautzmann, L. N. (1987). Perceptions of the purpose of level I fieldwork. *American Journal of Occupational Therapy, 41*(9), 595-600. https://doi.org/10.5014/ajot.41.9.595

of occupational therapy programs and 52% of occupational therapy assistant programs agreed. The study authors suggested there was a need to clarify the purpose and structures required for implementation of Level I fieldwork (Leonardelli & Caruso, 1986).

Kautzmann (1987) conducted a study to examine academic faculty members, FWeds and students as to their perceptions of the purpose of Level I fieldwork. She found a diversity of perspectives and statistically significant differences between the rankings of academic and FWeds and students. For example, fieldwork and academic educators differed on their perceptions of the need for students to receive feedback on beginning strengths and weaknesses in professional behavior and the opportunity to develop a treatment plan. Other categories where perceptions differed are listed in Table 1-3.

It is notable that occupational therapy academic faculty and students rated hands-on learning experiences as the most important learning objective of Level I placement while FWeds rated it fifth on their list. Although academic and FWeds valued learning about service delivery systems, it is clear that students valued more practice-based experiences and individualized feedback about their abilities.

As a response to concern about consistency in Level I fieldwork, various fieldwork councils nationwide begin to collaborate and share resources so as to develop some consistency in expectations for student performance for their Level I fieldwork sites. For example, the Wisconsin Council on Education (Wiscouncil), a combined council of three technical schools and three professional programs, formed a task group in 1982 to design a uniform student performance evaluation for Level I fieldwork to be used by its six-member schools (Leonardelli & Caruso, 1986).

Although the supervision standards for Level I fieldwork allowed for creativity in learning structures from the very beginning, a nationwide study conducted in 1990 by Shalik found that the majority of Level I FWeds (95%) were occupational therapists and most placements were located in hospitals (98%). Further, the survey revealed that 43% of Level I placements occurred in physical dysfunction settings in the late 1980s, and 20% reflected psychosocial practice. At that time, about 20% of Level I placements occurred in pediatric settings. FWeds reported that they were not required to structure learning experiences for students but simply to follow the normal clinical routine. Most supervised students reported being a passive observer and seldom involved in patients' treatment.

By the early 1990s, there was a declining number of available fieldwork sites in medical settings due to higher acuity of patient illness and shorter hospital stays (Shalik, 1990), which led to an increased emphasis on creation of alternative Level I fieldwork placement models. There was a renewed emphasis on fieldwork in emerging practice environments where students could be supervised by occupational therapy faculty or nonoccupational therapists (Drake, 1992; Rydeen et al., 1995) and alternative supervision models, such as collaborative and group supervision (Yanoshek et al., 1997). At this same time, there was a shift of emphasis in professional practice, with leaders such as Cohn and Crist (1995) calling on academic programs to "provide practice experiences addressing emerging issues such as quality of life, client self-determination, advocacy, health promotion, and disease prevention" (p. 104) to better prepare students for emerging health care services in the community.

At the dawn of the new century, other changes were brewing in the profession as a whole. In 2002, the *Occupational Therapy Practice Framework* was introduced, which outlined not only the domain of the profession, but also the process for care delivery to result in client-centered and occupation-based practice (AOTA, 2002a). The use of occupation-focused theory was increasingly emphasized in the academic context both with the new ACOTE standards (ACOTE, 1998) and the new AOTA Fieldwork Performance Evaluation for Level II fieldwork (AOTA, 2002b, 2002c). However, there was little evidence in the literature of students having opportunity to observe theory in practice or to experience occupation-based practice. To the contrary, students continued "to report observations of patients stacking cones and placing pegs in holes" (Johnson et al., 2006, p. 278). Johnson and colleagues (2006) conducted a study of Level I fieldwork to identify types of settings, supervisory qualifications, and student perceptions of the value of their experience and the learning opportunities available to them. Student evaluations of fieldwork (1,002) were collected over a 2-year period of time representing five local occupational therapy programs in the northeastern region of the United States. The research team found that nearly 20% of Level I placements took place in emerging practice settings, while the frequency of supervision by nonoccupational therapy personnel was at 11.6%. Students reported that they were most commonly able to practice observation and communication skills while other skill practice varied with practice setting. See Table 1-4 for a summary of key skills practiced during Level I fieldwork.

For example, range of motion was the most frequently practiced skill in physical disabilities, and manual muscle testing and splinting were practiced in 53% or less settings. Similarly, students in pediatric settings were able to practice transfers, splinting, feeding, and activities of daily living (ADLs) in less than 50% of their experiences.

The authors (Johnson et al., 2006) expressed concern about the limited opportunities for students to practice skills during their Level I placement and suggested this may impact student preparedness for their Level II placement. Haynes (2011) further investigated FWed and occupational therapy student perceptions of active participation in Level I fieldwork. She found that students reported their most meaningful learning experiences as practice of clinical skills and engagement in clinical reasoning, but their most common learning experiences were observation. Furthermore, Haynes found that FWeds reported more opportunities for active participation than students, suggesting that students wanted more active involvement than was thought appropriate by the FWeds. She suggested that academic programs take a proactive role in providing fieldwork

TABLE 1-4

PERCENTAGE OF SKILLS PRACTICED DURING LEVEL I FIELDWORK

SKILL	PEDIATRIC SETTING	PHYSICAL DISABILITIES SETTING	MENTAL HEALTH SETTING	EMERGING PRACTICE SETTING
Observation	97	99	98	94
Communication	94	95	98	96
Documentation	72	80	63	38
Wellness	23	47	59	52
Transfers	7	66	17	24
Manual muscle testing	14	53	5	7
Splinting	16	37	6	4
Activities of daily living	47	72	40	34
Behavior management	64	19	73	47
Feeding	27	24	22	24
Interviewing	45	74	63	77

Adapted from Johnson, C. R., Koenig, K. P., Piersol, C. V., Santalucia, S. E., & Wachter-Schutz, W. (2006). Level I fieldwork today: A study of contexts and perceptions. *American Journal of Occupational Therapy, 60*(3), 275-287.

sites with suggestions for active student involvement during Level I fieldwork and recording available learning experiences to ensure student opportunities for active learning. Coker (2010) further validated the benefits of active involvement during experiential learning and the impact on the development and refinement of clinical reasoning skills. She evaluated the clinical reasoning and critical thinking skills of occupational therapy students before and after week-long participation in a hands-on experimental learning program for children with cerebral palsy. She found significant changes in pre- and posttest scores of critical thinking and clinical reasoning ($p < .05$) when students had high expectations for active engagement in the learning process.

Another subtle shift occurring in the 2006 accreditation standards was the expectation that AFWCs should serve as the link between curriculum and communication with FWeds. This effectively brought accountability to expectations for communication between the academic and fieldwork sector. The role of the AFWC in ensuring collaboration was further solidified with the 2011 standards, as the AFWC was expected to ensure that at least one fieldwork (either Level I or Level II) in a curriculum was focused on social or psychosocial factors. This mandate was made in response to declining representation of occupational therapists working in mental health and a concern that occupational therapy should retain its identity as a holistic profession. The decline in availability of Level I fieldwork sites continued in the early part of the new century (Roberts & Simon, 2012), exacerbated by the continued development of new occupational therapy and occupational therapy assistant programs.

TABLE 1-5
TYPES OF EXPERIENTIAL LEARNING IN LEVEL I FIELDWORK

LEARNING TYPE	DEFINITION	SAMPLE
Simulation	A setting that provides an experience similar to a real world setting in order to allow clients to practice specific occupations (e.g., driving simulation center, bathroom or kitchen centers in a rehabilitation unit, work hardening units or centers).	The use of equipment, mannequins (e.g., a medical simulation center), or computer software (e.g., Simucase) that generates a realistic situation calling for a student response.
Standardized patient	An individual who has been trained to portray in a consistent, standardized manner, a patient/client with occupational needs.	An actor plays the role of a client who has recently acquired a spinal cord injury and the student directs the client in a dressing evaluation.
Faculty practice	Service provision by faculty members to persons, groups, and/or population.	An occupational therapy faculty member provides programming in a primary care center. Students observe and participate in selective aspects of the assessment process with focus on developing clients' functional skills, daily habits, and routines to promote health. Students also assist to facilitate coordination services with families, physicians, and nurses.
Faculty-led site visits	Faculty-facilitated experiences in which students will be able to participate in, observe, and/or study clinical practice first-hand.	An occupational therapy faculty member arranges to provide weekly health and wellness programming to a local assistive care center. The faculty member models leadership of a wellness group for two sessions, after which students lead the group in pairs, under the supervision of the faculty member, for eight more sessions.

(continued)

In the meantime, the research evidence for the effectiveness of many alternative forms of experiential learning, such as student-run clinics, faculty-led experiences, simulation, and standardized patient encounters, increased (Benson et al., 2013; Falk-Kessler et al., 2007; Giles et al., 2014; Goldbach & Stella, 2017; Nielsen et al., 2017). In response to a declining number of fieldwork placements, and increased evidence of the effectiveness of a number of forms of experiential learning, the 2018 ACOTE standards expanded opportunities for Level I fieldwork, indicating that requirements could be met through simulated environments, standardized patients, faculty practice, faculty-led site visits, or supervision by a FWed in a practice environment. Table 1-5 provides a definition and sample of each learning type.

TABLE 1-5 (CONTINUED)
TYPES OF EXPERIENTIAL LEARNING IN LEVEL I FIELDWORK

LEARNING TYPE	DEFINITION	SAMPLE
Supervision by FWed in a practice environment	A FWed is an individual, typically a clinician, who works collaboratively with the program and is informed of the curriculum and fieldwork program design. This individual supports the fieldwork experience, serves as a role model, and holds the requisite qualifications to provide the student with the opportunity to carry out professional responsibilities during the experiential portion of their education. Supervision is provided through two-way communication that occurs in real time in the practice environment of the FWed and offers both audio and visual capabilities to ensure opportunities for timely feedback.	A student completes a Level I fieldwork in an inpatient rehabilitation center for a 1-week placement, supervised by a clinician who is employed there. The student observes the FWed in a one-handed dressing technique on two occasions, and then directs the client in the technique under the direct supervision of the FWed. Following the session, the student receives direct feedback about professional communication and skills performance.

Adapted from definitions provided by Accreditation Council for Occupational Therapy Education. (2018). *2018 accreditation council for occupational therapy education standards and interpretative guide.* https://acoteonline.org/wp-content/uploads/2020/10/2018-ACOTE-Standards.pdf

THE EVOLVING NATURE OF THE LEVEL I FIELDWORK EDUCATOR ROLE

The history of Level I fieldwork shows the progressive nature of the purpose and the structure and intended outcome of the Level I fieldwork placement. Each change also influenced the focus and emphasis of the FWed role. See Table 1-6 for a review of changes in Level I fieldwork accreditation standards from 1973 (AMA & AOTA, 1973) to the present.

There have been many changes in the occupational therapy profession in the United States, as well as changes in Level I fieldwork across the past 50 years. As a result, there are many avenues for misconceptions and miscommunications about the present standards and expectations for the Level I FWed role.

The mandate in the original standards (AMA & AOTA, 1973) for directed observation and participation in various field settings opened up placement possibilities beyond those of psychosocial and physical dysfunction. However, it perpetuated an older concept from Level II fieldwork that the primary means of connecting the curriculum and fieldwork was through identification of practice focus areas. In fact, this concept is evident in later research undertaken by Shalik (1990) when she found that 43% of Level I placements occurred in physical dysfunction settings in the late 1980s and 20% reflected psychosocial and pediatric practice respectively. Although there was an expectation as early as 1983 that Level I fieldwork should be considered part of the didactic coursework, there did not appear to be research or other tracking mechanisms that connected Level I fieldwork with didactic coursework but rather with practice areas. The Shalik (1990) study further

TABLE 1-6

A REVIEW OF LEVEL I FIELDWORK ACCREDITATION STANDARDS FROM 1973 TO PRESENT

DATE	TITLE	SIGNIFICANT CHANGE	SOURCE
1973	Essentials and Guidelines of an Accredited Educational Program for the Occupational Therapist	**First time the term fieldwork experience is used and divided by descriptions of Level I and Level II** • Level I: initial experiences in directed observation and participation in various field settings • Level II: supervised fieldwork placement with focus on application to provide an in-depth experience Fieldwork experience is integral part of the educational program	AMA & AOTA, 1973
1983	Essentials of an Accredited Educational Program for the Occupational Therapist	**FWed as term to describe the supervisor is introduced** Collaboration between academic and FWeds **Level I: part of didactic courses; not expected to emphasize independent performance** • Supervised by qualified personnel (teachers, social workers, public health nurses, physical therapists)	AOTA, 1983
1991	Essentials and Guidelines for an Accredited Educational Program for the Occupational Therapist	**Fieldwork center must be documented as a formal affiliation** Fieldwork to be conducted in settings equipped to provide application of principles learned in the classroom **Advising is collaborative process between faculty and FWed** Level I: supervised by qualified personnel (occupational therapist, occupational therapy assistant, teachers, social workers, nurses, physical therapists)	AOTA, 1991

(continued)

TABLE 1-6 (CONTINUED)

A REVIEW OF LEVEL I FIELDWORK ACCREDITATION STANDARDS FROM 1973 TO PRESENT

DATE	TITLE	SIGNIFICANT CHANGE	SOURCE
1998	Standards for an Accredited Educational Program for the Occupational Therapist and Standards for an Accredited Educational Program for the Occupational Therapist Assistant	Plan is documented to ensure collaboration between academic and fieldwork representatives with agreed upon student objectives Level I: goal is to provide introduction to fieldwork to have basic comfort level of client needs • Supervised by qualified personnel (occupational therapist, psychologists, physician assistants, teachers, social workers, nurses, physical therapists) • **Experience must be documented** • **Formal evaluation of student performance documented**	ACOTE, 1998
2006	ACOTE Standards for an Accredited Educational Program for the Occupational Therapist or Occupational Therapy Assistant	**The term: "academic fieldwork coordinator" is introduced** • **Responsible for advocating for links between curriculum and communication to FWed** Level I fieldwork: no changes from previous standards	ACOTE, 2006
2011	ACOTE Standards and Interpretive Guide	**Academic fieldwork coordinator responsible for ensuring at least one fieldwork experience has focus on psychosocial or social factors** Level I fieldwork: no changes from previous standards	ACOTE, 2011
2018	ACOTE Standards and Interpretive Guide	**Level I fieldwork: requirements can be met through simulated environments, standardized patients, faculty practice, faculty-led site visits, or supervision by a FWed in a practice environment**	ACOTE, 2018

revealed that most FWeds were not structuring learning experiences for students but simply following their normal clinical routine. This would be expected when the emphasis for learning was focused on introduction to specific practice areas rather than a connection to didactic coursework. The misconception of Level I fieldwork as an introduction to a practice area continues today. It is most evident when students are placed in a setting with no expectation for structuring of learning experiences that connect with didactic coursework but simply allowed to "follow along" with the usual clinical processes or procedures.

A second misunderstanding related to Level I fieldwork is the level of active participation required beyond observation. Most students have already completed extensive observation as a part of their preoccupational therapy curriculum and are ready for both "directed observation and [directed] participation" (ACOTE, 2018, p. 41) in select aspects of the occupational therapy process. Of course, expectations for student involvement during Level I fieldwork might also be stretched beyond the student's capacity, and that is why the 1983 standards clarified that the expectation is not independent performance. Unfortunately, whether related to higher patient acuity, less therapist time, or inadequate communication between the academic program and fieldwork site, there seem to be many missed opportunities during Level I fieldwork (Hanson, 2011). For example, most students in the Shalik (1990) study reported being a passive observer and seldom involved in patients' treatment.

The designation of Level I fieldwork as "directed observation and participation" (ACOTE, 2018, p. 41) carries with it the assumption that directed observation will play a key role in student learning, implying that modeling on the part of the Level I FWed would be expected. Although there was never an expectation that the FWed would automatically be an occupational therapy practitioner, the expectation for role modeling on the part of the FWed may have influenced the practice of placing students primarily in role established settings (Shalik, 1990). The term "directed observation" (ACOTE, 2018, p. 41) would also imply that the lead FWed, whether an occupational therapy practitioner or not, could collaborate with the academic program to identify key observation experiences that would enhance student learning and connect with the didactic coursework. The same is true for "directed participation." Haynes (2011) provides a number of ideas for directing the participation of students even when they are not able to participate in some of the more complex tasks undertaken in the practice setting. Select examples of her suggestions are provided in Table 1-7.

The broad directives provided by the initial Level I fieldwork accreditation standards also led to confusion as to what the overall goals and learning objectives should be for the Level I learning experience. This was evident in the work of Kautzmann (1987) who noted many areas of disagreement between FWeds and academic educators as to what goals and learning objectives should be accomplished. Her recommendation was a call for consistency in the assessment process and expected learning experiences across academic programs (Kautzmann, 1987). This finding would not be surprising given the prevailing accreditation standards at the time (AOTA, 1983), which associated Level I fieldwork as part of each curriculum's didactic coursework. However, it is a continuing myth that the objectives for Level I fieldwork are or should be the same across academic programs. In fact, the FWed should instead find that each program has unique didactic coursework and would therefore have a unique emphasis for their fieldwork learning objectives. Although it has always been expected that academic programs would communicate about their curriculum to their fieldwork partners, the depth of communication was not carefully defined until the 1998 accreditation standards when it was required that a plan be documented to ensure collaboration between academic and fieldwork representatives with agreed-upon student objectives. The 2006 standards further clarified the process for communication by designating the AFWC as the link between the curriculum and communication with FWeds. The role of the FWed, then, is to communicate with each affiliated program to find out learning objectives and collaborate with the AFWC as to learning activities available at the site that would meet students at their level of skill and meet the required learning objectives. Although some academic programs

TABLE 1-7

IDEAS FOR STUDENT DIRECTED OBSERVATION AND PARTICIPATION ON LEVEL I FIELDWORK

TASK	DIRECTED OBSERVATION	DIRECTED PARTICIPATION
Conducting an evaluation	Follow along with test administration using separate handbook, identify modifications made in response to client behaviors, and discuss reasoning for choices with FWed	Get background information from the chart; list abbreviations you do not understand and look them up Introduce yourself and the role of occupational therapy to the client
Attending a team meeting	Write a summary of the results or decisions made and implications for occupational therapy intervention	Report at a team meeting on one specific area of evaluation results Report on client progress in one goal, with written summary of progress prepared in advance
Helping a client with dressing task	Observe client in dressing task, noting impact of underlying components (sensory, motor, etc.) identified in initial evaluation on the dressing task	Practice using assistive dressing device (e.g., button hook) in advance and explain and demonstrate to patient how to use it
Making an orthosis	Explain to the client what the therapist is going to do Review the steps of making the orthosis in advance and make notes regarding specific techniques used by therapist to accomplish each step	Gather the materials and set up the work area for the client and the therapist Assist therapist as needed in measurement of the orthosis on client
Planning and conducting an intervention session on feeding	Identify assistance levels used throughout the session Review client goals in advance of session and write a subjective, objective, assessment, and plan note on the session	Identify and describe one intervention to support occupation, activity-based or occupation-based activity, that may address feeding concerns and provide ideas to FWed in advance of session FWed directs student to assist in select aspects of one preparatory activity for feeding session
Conducting a patient education session	Identify the cultures represented by the client population and determine if there are any modifications that should be made based on this information	Identify and teach caregiver/aide a skill to practice with the client

Adapted from Haynes, C. J. (2011). Active participation in fieldwork Level I: Fieldwork educator and student perceptions. *Occupational Therapy In Health Care, 25*(4), 257-269. https://doi.org/10.3109/07380577.2011.595477

provide suggestions for learning activities (Haynes, 2011), the FWed must determine the learning activities appropriate for their unique fieldwork environment. This is an important aspect of the Level I fieldwork education process. Further information and examples of learning activities and sequenced plans are provided in Chapter 8.

Evaluation of student performance during Level I fieldwork was not initially required but was first mandated in the 1991 accreditation standards. The role of evaluation of student performance may be new to many FWeds who may not be supervising other personnel as a part of their practice role. A *Level I Fieldwork Competency Evaluation for OT and OTA Students* was introduced in 2017 (AOTA, 2017) and identifies specific performance skills that might be required by occupational therapy students in relation to fundamentals of practice, foundations for occupational therapy, professional behaviors, screening, evaluation, and intervention. Although it is a tool developed at the national level and endorsed by the profession, its use is not required. Instead, programs often modify the tool or develop an assessment tool to reflect their unique learning objectives. Evaluation responsibilities are a very important aspect of the Level I FWed role, as the student gains a perspective of their strengths and areas of challenge in the profession, which can be built upon in subsequent fieldwork and didactic coursework in preparation for a successful Level II placement. Chapter 13 will provide further perspective on the evaluation role, as well as helpful tools for the process.

Given the breadth of focus for the Level I FWed role, the relatively brief time frame given (as compared to Level II fieldwork), and the diversity of focus given the unique emphasis of each academic program, it is hardly surprising that FWeds are tempted to simply revert to what is traditionally been done at the site, or what they experienced as a student during Level I fieldwork. For example, if the experience of the FWed as a student was passive observation during their Level I placement (Johnson et al., 2006), they might also have that expectation for their students. If they participated in learning experiences beyond the usual clinical routine, the FWed might be more inclined to take initiative to introduce new learning experiences for their student. It is very important that the objectives for Level I fieldwork, as outlined by the academic program, be clearly understood, as there is a tendency otherwise to blur expectations and simply view it as "my week-long student"…or my student assigned this semester. The expectations for two students coming for a block placement from two academic programs might be remarkably different, and this needs to be taken into account by the assigned FWed. Further information is provided in Chapter 4 about the impact of the placement context on student learning, and Chapter 8 provides a roadmap to individualizing student learning experiences to fit the academic curriculum.

Changes in the make-up of the occupational therapy student population have compelled the FWed to address student psychosocial variables that impact student learning. Student professional behaviors, such as time management, responsiveness to feedback, and verbal/nonverbal communication skills, have been identified as concerns for FWeds (Rodger et al., 2011; Varland et al., 2017). Derdall et al. (2002) found that the clinical self-efficacy of occupational therapy students evolves during early fieldwork and clinical practice experiences, affecting the development of clinical decision-making skills, as well as student self-appraisal. In a study of Level II fieldwork students, Andonian (2013) found a link between emotional intelligence, work performance, and self-efficacy of occupational therapy students, noting that "understanding one's own and another's emotions was related to the intervention section of performance skills on the fieldwork performance evaluation" (p. 211). In addition, college students experience adverse health concerns related to stress; these concerns include increased anxiety, depression, and other factors that negatively affect physical, mental, and social health and the student's ability to learn (Almhdawi et al., 2018; American College Health Association, 2019). Helpful information is provided in Chapters 10 and 11 of this text for working with students with disabilities, as well as helping students to navigate psychosocial stressors during fieldwork. Chapter 7 provides helpful resources for addressing the development of student professional skills during Level I fieldwork.

Changes in the profession have also influenced the FWed role. At the time that Level I field-work was introduced, the profession was primarily anchored in a reductionistic paradigm, as the majority of practice occurred in settings where the medical model was primary. Since that time, there has been an emergence of focus on occupation as the central contribution of the occupational therapy profession through the contributions of occupation-focused models, such as the Model of Human Occupation introduced in the early 1980s. The emphasis on occupation as a focal point in treatment continued with many other models being developed throughout the 1990s and the first edition of the *Occupational Therapy Practice Framework* developed in 2002 (AOTA, 2002a). Models were designed to articulate the unique contribution of occupational therapy representing the big picture of attention to the whole person, the occupations of value to the person, the impact of occupations, and a tool to organize the clinical reasoning of the therapist. Given these changes in the profession, it is expected that the education of the student not only include attention to the various clinical skills expected in the occupational therapist role, but also the thinking behind those skills and how the occupational therapist uses the various skills and tools to promote the occupational performance of the individual. With these changes in the profession, it was an expec-tation that students would be able to experience occupation-focused practice during their Level I fieldwork that would be modeled by their FWed and site. Furthermore, there was an expectation that students would be introduced to the use of an occupation-focused model to direct their rea-soning process. However, this is not always realized, due to the disparities between the emphasis of occupational therapy education for FWeds and the clash of the holistic values of the profession and the more reductionistic emphasis of many medical practice settings. Ideas for bringing best prac-tice ideals into the students learning experience are explored in Chapter 3 and expanded upon in Chapter 6 with suggestions for application of occupation-focused models during Level I fieldwork.

Another challenge in the FWed role expectations is the range of focus areas for the Level I experience. Since the expectations for Level I fieldwork are determined by the design of the curriculum, the Level I experience might involve focus on any or all aspects of the occupational therapy process from assessment to treatment planning, to choosing and implementing therapy, to documentation and discharge planning. Other aspects of the occupational therapist role might be emphasized, such as education, consultancy, or advocacy. The context might be actual or simulat-ed. If actual, the population could vary from children to older adults, from an inpatient or outpa-tient medical setting, to a community mental health center or school to name a few. The experience might be dosed over several weeks or occur in a focused "blocked" time frame of 1 or 2 weeks. The length of the experience could vary, although all Level I experiences in one academic program are expected to demonstrate equal rigor. See Table 1-8 for a representation of some of the common contexts for Level I fieldwork placement. In Chapter 4, you will be provided additional information regarding the various contexts of Level I fieldwork and unique opportunities for learning in each.

There has been a documented shortage of both Level I and Level II fieldwork placement oppor-tunities for students over the past 20 years and more recently given the traumatic impact of the global pandemic. This has pushed many occupational therapy and occupational therapy assistant programs to develop emerging practice settings and alternative supervision models (Johnson et al., 2006). The range of focus areas could be conceptualized as both a challenge and an opportunity for expansion of the FWed role, depending on whether supervision was provided by an occupa-tional therapy practitioner or another licensed professional. FWeds who are occupational therapy practitioners are most competent to oversee the Level I fieldwork placement that is focused on the occupational therapy process, such as assessment, treatment planning, provision of skilled occu-pational therapy intervention, and documentation of client progress/outcomes. FWeds who are not occupational therapy practitioners are able to introduce to students a broader understanding of the occupational therapy process in comparison with other professional practice areas. Johnson et al. (2006) found in their review of more than 1,000 Level I placements that the community-based Level I fieldwork provided more broad opportunity for students to develop professional behaviors

TABLE 1-8
CONTEXTS FOR LEVEL I FIELDWORK PLACEMENT

PEDIATRIC	MENTAL HEALTH	PHYSICAL DISABILITIES	NONTRADITIONAL	EMERGING PRACTICE
Schools: charter, public, private	Hospital	General	Senior centers	Therapeutic riding, hippotherapy
Hospital	Community	Rehabilitation	International	Homeless shelters
Early intervention	Group settings	Outpatient-orthopedic-neurologic	Simulated environments	Assisted living
Outpatient clinic		Home health	Standardized patients	Telehealth
Community-based head start: Preschool		Skilled nursing facility	Faculty practice	After school programs
			Faculty-led site visits	At-risk youth

and targeted skills within the mission and philosophy of the setting, such as increased abilities in interviewing skills. Further tools to promote student clinical reasoning development during Level I fieldwork are provided in Chapter 5, while Chapter 9 provides a helpful framework for taking advantage of emerging learning opportunities onsite.

Collaboration between AFWCs, faculty, and FWeds is essential to the development of learning objectives for the occupational therapist, occupational therapy student, and the Level I fieldwork setting. Choosing the type of experiential learning desired for Level I placement is considered by the academic program during curriculum design, and the choices made are then built upon in further collaboration between the academic program, the Level I fieldwork site, and the AFWC. The myriad of focal points for collaboration are represented in Table 1-9.

THE VALUE OF THE LEVEL I FIELDWORK TO STUDENT LEARNING

The overall quality of the supervision provided influences student perceptions of the value of their fieldwork learning experiences. Generally, students appreciate university preparation for their learning experience, as well as a detailed orientation, welcoming environment, and clear expectations by the fieldwork site (Rodger et al., 2011). The availability of quality modeling coupled with a graded program of learning is appreciated by students, along with quality feedback provided by skilled and experienced supervisors within the context of a positive relationship (Koski et al., 2013; Rodger et al., 2011; Thomas et al., 2007). Chapter 8 provides helpful guidance for the development of a Level I fieldwork learning plan.

TABLE 1-9

SUMMARY OF COLLABORATION DURING LEVEL I FIELDWORK

FOCAL POINTS FOR COLLABORATION	OCCUPATIONAL THERAPY ACADEMIC INSTITUTION (FACULTY, ADMINISTRATION)	LEVEL I FIELDWORK SITE	ACADEMIC FIELDWORK COORDINATOR
Identify course content areas to be enhanced by Level I fieldwork experiences	X		X
Develop goals that reflect the purpose of the experience and the level of performance to be achieved	X		X
Sequence objectives from concrete to conceptual (simple to complex)	X		X
Identify settings that may be able to provide necessary learning experiences	X	X	X
Collaborate with FWeds to determine if objectives can be met at the site		X	X
Coordinate administrative issues (memorandum of understanding, scheduling, deadlines, evaluation of student, number of students)		X	X
Collaborate with Level I fieldwork site about the curriculum, skill level of students, and expectations of active participation		X	X
Determine if administrative aspects of Level I fieldwork will impact effectiveness and quality of experiential learning		X	X
Identify learning activities at the Level I fieldwork site that will meet objectives	X	X	X

Johnson et al. (2006) found that students highly value their Level I fieldwork experiences as helpful to their learning but more highly value supervision by occupational therapy practitioners than by Level II students or nonoccupational therapy personnel. Further study results revealed that students reported less opportunity for participation in occupation-based practice and clinical skills in physical disabilities or emerging practice settings than mental health or pediatric practice settings even though the majority of their experiences (41%) occurred in physical disabilities settings. The authors speculated, based on National Board for Certification in Occupational Therapy (NBCOT) that students placed a higher value on valued learning experiences in physical disabilities and pediatric practice settings due to anticipated employment in those settings (NBCOT, 2004).

The value placed on the Level I fieldwork by students is not only dependent on the type of fieldwork site but also on the opportunities available for active participation on the part of the student and the type of supervision models used. Learning models that use limited supervision or collaborative peer learning have the potential to enhance active learning and client centeredness (Keptner & Klein, 2019; Nielsen et al., 2017). Opportunities to participate in simulation provided students with practice experience without the safety risks of the clinical practice environment (DeIuliis et al., 2021; Mattila et al., 2020).

Keptner and Klein (2019) investigated the experience of students during a faculty-led Level I fieldwork using the collaborative learning model. Students were assigned partners and participated in learning activities divided into three phases: preparation, onsite, and follow-up reflection. Students reported learning to recognize issues and become more independent in decision making. They solidified their understanding of the role of occupational therapy. Although at times they desired more supervision, uncertainty propelled them toward independence and confidence. Specifically, they felt their communication skills had improved, both with other professionals and their peer group. Nielsen et al. (2017) similarly explored the perceptions of students participating in a nontraditional Level I fieldwork involving classroom preparation for working with refugee populations under the supervision of a faculty mentor who met with students weekly to apply the theoretical framework of the Person-Environment-Occupation Model to reflect, problem solve, and plan weekly interventions. Students reported learning communication skills, specifically, to be direct and to clarify understanding. They reported learning several methods to identify meaningful occupations and learning how to shift their therapeutic modes as needed to benefit their clients. They felt their skills in activity analysis improved as they learned to identify and then sequence their intervention activities so that their clients were able to learn foundational skills first, which enabled development of more complex skills for activity completion in later intervention sessions. They also gained confidence and problem-solving skills and learned to be flexible in addressing organizational aspects of the experience.

Students participating in clinical simulation report benefits to practicing clinical skills such as assessment, identification of interventions, documentation, and clinical reasoning in a safe environment (Mattila et al., 2020). In addition, students spoke of the positive impact of debriefing and reflecting on their learning. Group discussions provided multiple perspectives on reasoning choices, which helped students feel more prepared for their Level II fieldwork experience.

BENEFITS TO MENTORING A LEVEL I FIELDWORK STUDENT

As the gateway to serving as a FWed for longer term Level II students, supervising Level I students introduces the practitioner to the benefits of student mentoring. The altruistic benefit of mentoring students is mentioned often in the literature (Hanson, 2011; Rodger et al., 2011). Evenson et al. (2015) found, in a national survey of FWeds, that *the personal satisfaction gained through supporting the development of others* was one of the highest incentives for practitioners to undertake student supervision. When teaching others, the mentor has the opportunity to reflect upon one's own practice. This benefit will help the practitioner to recognize their own thinking process as they reflect it on to students (Delany & Golding, 2014). In return, students are able to not only share the knowledge that they have learned in the academic sector but also the newest textbooks and resources they have obtained with the FWed, thereby offering reciprocity of exchange (Johnson et al., 2006). Opportunity to maintain and demonstrate competency in practice is also supported through Level I fieldwork supervision, as supervising students is recognized by the NBCOT and many state regulatory boards as a venue for achieving continuing education and professional development credits (NBCOT, 2020). Those who have mentored students report that the process has enhanced their job satisfaction and has helped to reenergize their career (Rodger et al., 2011).

Supervision of Level I students also provides benefits to the fieldwork site. Through responsibilities completed over a period of time, the employer has the opportunity to view first-hand the skills of the student and access their "fit" for employment with the agency and congruence of student professional goals with agency objectives (Hanson, 2011; Thomas et al., 2007). In addition, those agencies that take the initiative to partner with local academic programs not only gain access to resources and incentives provided by the academic program but also project a progressive and state-of-the-art image to their consumers and to the professional community and other external audiences due to their commitment to academic and community partnerships. Beyond the benefits to the FWed and site, supervision of Level I students offers occupational therapy practitioners the opportunity to give back to the profession the opportunities that were provided to them while students (Hanson, 2011; Swinth, 2016).

Giving back to the profession is not only an opportunity but it is also a professional responsibility that each practitioner should not take lightly. Building on the work of the Centennial Vision (AOTA, 2017), the AOTA has adopted Vision 2025 to guide the occupational therapy profession forward in the future: "Occupational therapy maximizes health, well-being, and quality of life for all people, populations, and communities through effective solutions that facilitate participation in everyday living" (AOTA, 2017, p. 1). It is our hope that this book will provide you with the skills to help accomplish this reality through the preparation of occupational therapy students. Quality fieldwork is key to quality occupational therapists!

SUMMARY

The history of Level I fieldwork in the United States illustrates the ongoing development of the learning structures, accreditation expectations, and pedagogy associated with student learning during introductory experiential learning, such as the Level I fieldwork. The evolving health care environment coupled with changes within the profession of occupational therapy have altered the landscape of student learning and the expectations of the FWed role. Newly revised accreditation standards, as well as emerging research related to the potential impact of experiential learning on student clinical reasoning, have introduced new opportunities for student growth during the Level I learning experience. This book is designed to orient new and experienced FWeds to the opportunities, as well as resources available to navigate the changing terrain, beginning with an orientation to best practices in the profession and an introduction to educational theories associated with experiential learning. Subsequent chapters will help you to manage practical challenges you may experience as a Level I FWed, AFWC, or student, and to take advantage of available learning opportunities.

LEARNING ACTIVITIES

1. Identify how health care trends, such as shortened hospital stays and higher acuity of patient illness, have influenced the development of Level I fieldwork structure in the United States. How have these trends influenced your own work with Level I fieldwork students?

2. How have profession-specific trends, such as increased emphasis on occupation-based, evidence-driven, and client-centered practices, influenced the development of Level I fieldwork in the United States? How have these trends influenced your own work with Level I fieldwork students?

3. Contrast the role of the Level I FWed 30 years ago (in the early 1990s) as compared to today (as illustrated in Table 1-6). What differences do you see?

4. On a scale of 1 to 7 (with 1 being very proficient, 4 neutral, and 7 very proficient), rate your level of proficiency with the various tasks identified that are associated with your role in setting up and carrying out the Level I fieldwork process in Table 1-9. Where are you feeling most confident? What tasks seem most intimidating or confusing?

5. As you review aspects of Level I fieldwork most valued by students, what aspects would you like to develop or refine at your site?

REFERENCES

Accreditation Council for Occupational Therapy Education. (1998). Standards for an accredited educational program for the occupational therapist. *American Journal of Occupational Therapy, 53*(6), 575-582. https://doi.org/10.5014/ajot.53.6.575

Accreditation Council for Occupational Therapy Education. (2006). *2006 accreditation council for occupational therapy standards and interpretative guide.* https://fdocuments.net/document/2006-standards-and-interpretive-guide-aota-2006-accreditation-standards-for-a.html?page=1

Accreditation Council for Occupational Therapy Education. (2011). *2011 accreditation council for occupational therapy education standards and interpretative guide.* https://acoteonline.org/accreditation-explained/standards/

Accreditation Council for Occupational Therapy Education. (2018). *2018 accreditation council for occupational therapy education standards and interpretative guide.* https://acoteonline.org/wp-content/uploads/2020/10/2018-ACOTE-Standards.pdf

Almhdawi, K. A., Kanaan, S. F., Khader, Y., Al-Hourani, Z., Almomani, F., & Nazzal, M. (2018). Study-related mental health symptoms and their correlates among allied health professions students. *Work, 61*(3), 391-401. https://doi.org/10.3233/wor-182815

American College Health Association. (2019). *National College Health Assessment II: Reference Group Executive Summary.* https://www.acha.org/documents/ncha/NCHA-II_SPRING_2019_US_REFERENCE_GROUP_EXECUTIVE_SUMMARY.pdf

American Medical Association & American Occupational Therapy Association. (1965). Essentials of an accredited curriculum in occupational therapy. *American Journal of Occupational Therapy.*

American Medical Association & American Occupational Therapy Association. (1973). Essentials of an accredited educational program for the occupational therapist. *American Journal of Occupational Therapy, 29,* 485-496.

American Occupational Therapy Association. (1924). Minimum standards for courses of training in occupational therapy. *Archives of Occupational Therapy, 3*(4), 295-298.

American Occupational Therapy Association. (1983). Essentials of an accredited educational program for the occupational therapist. *American Journal of Occupational Therapy, 37,* 817-823.

American Occupational Therapy Association. (1991). Essentials and guidelines for an accredited educational program for the occupational therapist. *American Journal of Occupational Therapy, 45*, 1077-1084.

American Occupational Therapy Association. (2002a). Occupational therapy practice framework: Domain and process. *American Journal of Occupational Therapy, 56*(6), 609–639. https://doi.org/10.5014/ajot.56.6.609

American Occupational Therapy Association. (2002b). *Fieldwork performance evaluation for the occupational therapy assistant student.* American Occupational Therapy Association.

American Occupational Therapy Association. (2002c). *Fieldwork performance evaluation for the occupational therapy student.* American Occupational Therapy Association.

American Occupational Therapy Association. (2015). Philosophy of occupational therapy education. *American Journal of Occupational Therapy, 69*(Suppl. 3), 6913410052. http://doi.org/10.5014/ajot.2015.696S17

American Occupational Therapy Association. (2017). Vision 2025. *American Journal of Occupational Therapy, 71*(3), 7103420010p7103420011-7103420010p7103420011. https://doi.org/10.5014/ajot.2017.713002

Andonian, L. (2013). Emotional intelligence, self-efficacy, and occupational therapy students' fieldwork performance. *Occupational Therapy In Health Care, 27*(3), 201–215. https://doi.org/10.3109/07380577.2012.763199

Benson, J. D., Provident, I. & Szucs, K. A. (2013). An experiential learning lab embedded in a didactic course: Outcomes from a pediatric intervention course. *Occupational Therapy in Health Care, 27*(1), 46–57. https://doi.org/10.3109/07380577.2012.756599

Cohn, E. S., & Crist, P. (1995). Nationally speaking—back to the future: New approaches to fieldwork education. *American Journal of Occupational Therapy, 49*, 103–106.

Coker, P. (2010). Effects of an experiential learning program on the clinical reasoning and critical thinking skills of occupational therapy students. *Journal of Allied Health, 39*(4),280-286.

Cromwell, F. S., & Kielhofner, G. W. (1976). An educational strategy for occupational therapy community service. *American Journal of Occupational Therapy, 30*, 629-633.

DeIuliis, E. D., & Hanson, D. (2023). *Fieldwork educator's guide to Level II fieldwork.* SLACK Incorporated.

DeIuliis, E., Mattila, A., & Martin, R. (2021). Level I fieldwork in a simulated environment: A blueprint on how to use simucase. *Journal of Occupational Therapy Education, 5*(2).

Delany, C., & Golding, C. (2014). Teaching clinical reasoning by making thinking visible: An action research project with allied health clinical educators. *BMC Medical Education, 14*(20), 2-10.

Derdall, M., Olson, P., Janzen, W., & Warren, S. (2002). Development of a questionnaire to examine confidence of occupational therapy students during fieldwork experiences. *Canadian Journal of Occupational Therapy, 69*(1), 49-56.

Drake, M. (1992). Level I fieldwork in a daycare for homeless children. *Occupational Therapy in Health Care, 8*(2-3), 215-224. https://doi.org/10.1080/J003v08n02_11

Evenson, M. E. & Hanson, D. J. (2019). Fieldwork, practice education, and professional entry. In *Willard and Spackman's Occupational Therapy* (13th ed.). Wolters-Kluwer

Evenson, M. E., Roberts, M., Kaldenberg, J., Barnes, M. A., & Ozelie, R. (2015). National survey of fieldwork educators: Implications for occupational therapy education. *American Journal of Occupational Therapy, 69*(Suppl. 2), 1-5. https://doi.org/10.5014/ajot.2015.019265

Falk-Kessler, J., Benson, J. D., & Witchger Hansen, A. M. (2007). Moving the classroom to the clinic: The experiences of occupational therapy students during a "living lab." *Occupational Therapy in Health Care, 21*(3), 79-91. https://doi.org/10.1080/J003v21n03_05

Giles, A. K., Carson, N. E., Breland, H. L., Coker-Bolt, P., & Bowman, P. J. (2014). Conference proceedings—Use of simulated patients and reflective video analysis to assess occupational therapy students' preparedness for fieldwork. *American Journal of Occupational Therapy, 68*, S57–S66. http://dx.doi.org/10.5014/ajot.2014.685S03

Gill, A. A., Clark, J. A., Hendrickson, F. R. & Mason, C. I. (1974). A student practicum experience. *American Journal of Occupational Therapy, 128*, 284–287

Goldbach, W. P., & Stella, T. C. (2017). Experiential learning to advance student readiness for Level II fieldwork. *Journal of Occupational Therapy Education, 1*(1). https://doi.org/10.26681/jote.2017.010103

Hanson, D. J. (2011). The perspectives of fieldwork educators regarding Level II fieldwork students. *Occupational Therapy in Health Care, 25*(2-3), 164-177. https://doi.org/10.3109/07380577.2011.561420

Haynes, C. J. (2011). Active participation in fieldwork Level I: Fieldwork educator and student perceptions. *Occupational Therapy In Health Care, 25*(4), 257-269. https://doi.org/10.3109/07380577.2011.595477

Johnson, C. R., Koenig, K. P., Piersol, C. V., Santalucia, S. E., & Wachter-Schutz, W. (2006). Level I fieldwork today: A study of contexts and perceptions. *American Journal of Occupational Therapy, 60*(3), 275-287.

Kautzmann, L. N. (1987). Perceptions of the purpose of Level I fieldwork. *American Journal of Occupational Therapy, 41*(9), 595-600. https://doi.org/10.5014/ajot.41.9.595

Keptner, K. M., & Klein, S. M. (2019). Collaborative learning in a faculty-led occupational therapy Level I fieldwork: A case study. *Journal of Occupational Therapy Education, 3*(3). https://doi.org/10.26681/jote.2019.030308

Koski, K. J., Simon, R. L., & Dooley, N. R. (2013). Valuable occupational therapy fieldwork educator behaviors. *Work, 44*(3), 307-315. https://doi.org/10.3233/WOR-121507

Leonardelli, C. A., & Caruso, L. A. (1986). Level I fieldwork: Issues and needs. *American Journal of Occupational Therapy, 40*(4), 258–264. https://doi.org/10.5014/ajot.40.4.258

Mattila, A., Martin, R. M., DeIuliis, E. D. (2020). Simulated fieldwork: A virtual approach to clinical education. *Education Sciences, 10*, 272. https://doi.org/10.3390/educsci10100272

National Board for Certification in Occupational Therapy. (2004). A practice analysis study of entry-level occupational therapist registered and certified occupational therapist assistant practice. *OTJR: Occupation, Participation and Health, 24*(1).

National Board for Certification in Occupational Therapy. (2020). *NBCOT Certification renewal activities chart.* https://www.nbcot.org/-/media/NBCOT/PDFs/Renewal_Activity_Chart.ashx?la=en

Nielsen, S., Jedlicka, J. S., Hanson, D., Fox, L., & Graves, C. (2017). Student perceptions of non-traditional Level I fieldwork. *Journal of Occupational Therapy Education, 1*(2). https://doi.org/10.26681/jote.2017.010206

Platt, N. P., Martell, D. L., & Clements P. A. (1977). Level I placement at a federal correctional institution. *American Journal of Occupational Therapy, 31*, 385-387.

Presseller, S. (1983). Fieldwork education: The proving ground of the profession. *American Journal of Occupational Therapy, 37*, 163-165.

Rydeen, K., Kautzmann, L. & Cowan, M. K., & Benzing, P. (1995). Three faculty-facilitated, community-based Level I fieldwork programs. *American Journal of Occupational Therapy, 49*(2), 112–118. https://doi.org/10.5014/ajot.49.2.112

Roberts, M. E, & Simon, R. L. (2012). Fieldwork challenge 2012. *Occupational Therapy Practice, 17*(6), 20.

Rodger, S., Fitzgerald, C., Davila, W., Millar, F., & Allison, H. (2011). What makes a quality occupational therapy practice placement? Students' and practice educators' perspectives. *Australian Occupational Therapy Journal, 58*(3), 195–202. https://doi.org/10.1111/j.1440–1630.2010.00903.x

Shalik, L. D. (1990). The Level I fieldwork process. *American Journal of Occupational Therapy, 44*(8), 700-707. https://doi.org/10.5014/ajot.44.8.700

Snow, T., & Mitchell, M. M. (1982). Administrative patterns in curriculum clinic interactions. *American Journal of Occupational Therapy, 36*, 251-256.

Swinth, Y. (2016). Why should you take a fieldwork student? *Journal of Occupational Therapy, Schools, & Early Intervention, 9*(3), 223-225. http://dx.doi.org/10.1080/19411243.2016.1212536

Teske, Y. R., & Spelbring, L. M. (1983). Future impact on occupational therapy from current changes in higher education. *American Journal of Occupational Therapy, 37*, 667-672.

Thomas, Y., Dickson, D., Broadbridge, J., Hopper, L., Hawkins, R., Edwards, A., & McBryde, C. (2007). Benefits and challenges of supervising occupational therapy fieldwork students: Supervisors' perspectives. *Australian Occupational Therapy Journal, 54*, S2-S12.

Varland, J., Cardell, E., Koski, J., & McFadden, M. (2017). Factors influencing occupational therapists' decision to supervise fieldwork students. *Occupational Therapy in Health Care, 31*(3), 238-254. https://doi.org/10.1080/07380577.2017.1328631

Yanoshek, M. C., Fuguet, L., & Rose, A. (1997). *Group models: A creative approach to fieldwork education.* In *The reference guide to fieldwork education and program development* (pp. 68-76). Philadelphia Region Fieldwork Consortium.

Thinking Like an Educator
Theoretical Frameworks for Level I Fieldwork

Nancy R. Dooley, MA, PhD, OTR/L

As an occupational therapist or occupational therapy assistant, you can probably recall some of your Level I fieldwork experiences. Most of us also have a mixture of emotions that go along with these memories ranging from fear and confusion to excitement and interest. You may have a client story or interaction that stays with you years or decades later. As students, we may not have used the term "experiential learning," but we knew we were about to see real people with the problems or difficulties we had been reading and learning about in the classroom. We would also get an opportunity to try things out that we had seen in books, videos, online, or modeled in the occupational therapy classroom setting.

Level I fieldwork represents the first real actions we take toward becoming occupational therapists, so it requires thoughtful planning. As students, we are often not acutely aware of the purpose behind every learning activity placed before us. Educators, including occupational therapy practitioners serving as Level I fieldwork educators (FWeds), must be purposeful in choosing the learning activities that best suit their learners and contexts. This chapter will introduce experiential learning theory and describe the learning frameworks that are commonly used in occupational therapy curricula. It will provide the FWed with examples of how to apply the learning frameworks to different types of Level I fieldwork and provide the reader insight as to the value of theoretical frameworks in learning to think like an educator.

Hanson, D., & DeIuliis, E. D. (Eds.).
Fieldwork Educator's Guide to Level I Fieldwork (pp. 27-42).
© 2023 Taylor and Francis Group.

LEARNING OBJECTIVES

By the end of reading this chapter and completing the learning activities, the reader should be able to:

1. Differentiate between four frameworks for learning that are commonly used in occupational therapy programs.

2. Apply each element of the frameworks for learning to different types of Level I fieldwork education.

3. Appreciate the value of theoretical learning frameworks to the design of student learning experiences during Level I fieldwork.

The faculty of each occupational therapy and occupational therapy assistant education program are required to create a curriculum design and philosophy that meets the standards of the Accreditation Council for Occupational Therapy Education (ACOTE). Educational programs identify a philosophy including underlying beliefs about how people learn (ACOTE, 2018). This generally includes a *framework for learning*, the most common of which will be described here.

While academic programs have freedom to structure Level I fieldwork in unique ways in their curriculum, accreditation standards ensure that the fieldwork program, including Level I, clearly reflects the curriculum design of the program. Occupational therapy education programs are free to determine how many Level I fieldwork experiences students have, their format or structure, when they occur in the program, how long they are, and their educational focus. Occupational therapy education programs now have a variety of methods for incorporating Level I fieldwork into their curriculum designs. For example, Level I fieldwork may be a stand-alone course or embedded in a course focused on a variety of topics, such as occupational therapy practice with a specific population or certain grouping on the lifespan. Students may make the connection of Level I fieldwork to their other coursework through learning activities, such as assignments related to Level I fieldwork, journaling or other online discussions, seminars, and discussion within a related course.

In summary, the ACOTE (2018) standards and interpretive guidelines provide latitude for educational programs to organize information and pass it on to students in many different ways. Variability in curriculum designs, including theoretical frameworks for learning, produce differences in the layout and details of Level I fieldwork from one occupational therapy program to another.

THEORETICAL FRAMEWORKS FOR LEARNING

Since fieldwork education is by nature experiential, this chapter will begin with the educational framework of *experiential learning theory* as described by Kolb (2015). We will then explore Vygotsky's *social constructivism*, which is the basis for collaborative learning (Cohn et al., 2001; Vygotsky, 1978). Lastly, this chapter will describe two frameworks or *taxonomies of learning*: Bloom's Revised Taxonomy (Anderson et al., 2001) and Fink's (2003, 2013) Significant Learning Taxonomy. Each approach to learning will be applied to the different instructional methods to deliver Level I fieldwork—simulation, faculty practice, faculty-led site visits, and traditional one-on-one supervision by a FWed. As noted previously, educational activities require planning, and this chapter is meant to help FWeds approach their work with students systematically and assist them in organizing student learning activities that promote learning and skill acquisition.

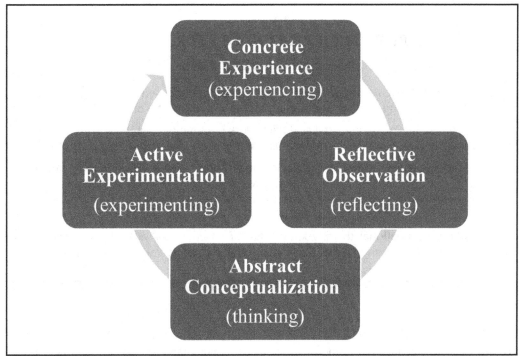

Figure 2-1. Kolb's Learning Cycle. (Adapted from Kolb, A. Y., & Kolb, D. A. [2017]. Experiential learning theory as a guide for experiential educators in higher education. *Experiential Learning and Teaching in Higher Education, 1*[1], 7-44 and Kolb, D. A. [2015]. *Experiential learning: Experience as the source of learning and development.* [2nd ed.]. Pearson Education.)

Experiential Learning Theory

David A. Kolb first described experiential learning and applied it to educating graduate students in business management in the early 1970s (Kolb, 2015). Kolb brought together the work of many theorists, who you might remember from a psychology course, including William James, John Dewey, Carl Rogers, and Lev Vygotsky. Kolb sees experiential learning theory as a holistic approach that can be applied to all aspects of life. Experiential learning is a dynamic theory that includes the central concepts of learning cycle, learning style, and learning space (Kolb & Kolb, 2017).

The first element of Kolb's Learning Cycle, *concrete experience*, or simply experiencing, is what it sounds like: having an experience or doing something. For example, a student in a faculty-led community Level I placement tries to extend the elbow of a person with high muscle tone due to a stroke. *Reflective observation*, or reflection, is the second step and is defined as reviewing the experience and connecting it with past learning. This will be different for each person because people's lives and learning styles are different. The student might recall a lecture or lab activity about muscle tone and the application of continuous tendinous pressure, while another might remember how it felt to help bathe her grandmother who had a similar problem. Next in the process is *abstract conceptualization*, or thinking. This is the point at which people make conclusions or theorize about their experience. Here, a student who has just co-led a group at a mental health day program might consider their client interactions to decide on the approach to take the next day. Continuing that example, the final step is *active experimentation*. The student takes action to apply what they learned when they co-lead the group again in what Kolb calls active experimentation or acting. The student has now had a new experience and the learning cycle continues (Kolb, 2015; Kolb & Kolb, 2017). See Figure 2-1 for a depiction of Kolb's Learning Cycle. Although Kolb uses the term cycle, it is important to note that learning can begin at any of his four points. Kolb

---

BOX 2-1

FIELDWORK EDUCATOR TIPS FOR USING KOLB'S EXPERIENTIAL LEARNING THEORY

- Use all parts of the learning cycle: just doing is not enough. Experiencing *must be combined with* reflecting, thinking, and acting for maximum effect (Kolb & Kolb, 2017).

- Know you are having an impact. Level I fieldwork is a time of growth for students, and the nature of direct experience makes this learning especially memorable (Kolb, 2015).

- Help students connect what they have learned in class to your unique Level I circumstances. Ask questions to prompt alternative explanations of what students see and experience. Do not forget to follow-up with *so what?* questions to help them make conclusions or theorize about what to do next.

- Apply your occupational therapy knowledge of interpersonal and physical environments to create learning spaces that initially foster comfort and later encourage students to try new actions.

---

suggested that people prefer different ways to start the learning process, and he called these preferences *learning styles* (Kolb, 2015). Kolb and Kolb (2017) recently expanded their learning style inventory to categorize people in nine different styles. Occupational therapy practitioners who have educated a few fieldwork students will have noticed that some students like to jump right in and try something (*Kolb's initiating style*). Others make a lot of meaning from a situation in their minds before acting (*Kolb's analyzing style*). More detail on the learning styles can be found online at: https://experientiallearninginstitute.org/resources/what-is-experiential-learning/ (Institute of Experiential Learning, 2020), and tips for applying Kolb's Learning Cycle are provided in Box 2-1. Kolb emphasizes that there is no need to match the learning styles of teachers to learners as is sometimes recommended when learning style is considered a personal trait. Kolb and Kolb think of the nine learning styles as "dynamic states" (2017, p. 9) and suggest that people should seek to maximize their flexible use of multiple styles in order to benefit most easily from new experiences. The last component of experiential learning theory is *learning space*, a term Kolb uses in the same way that occupational therapy practitioners use context and environment (American Occupational Therapy Association, 2020; Kolb & Kolb, 2017).

A great resource for helping Level I fieldwork coordinators and FWeds to apply Kolb's Learning Cycle is provided in Box 2-2. The Kolb Educator Role Profile (KERP) helps educators identify their preferred teaching approach for each of the elements of Kolb's Learning Cycle.

Social Constructivism

Social constructivism, part of the theoretical base for experiential learning (Kolb, 2015), has broad implications for human development and occupational therapy practice. Social constructivism was developed by Lev Vygotsky, a Russian psychologist who worked in the early 20th century. Vygotsky felt that people collaborate and converse with others to build knowledge in response to external stimuli (Berkley Graduate Division, 2021). Students' experiences during Level I fieldwork are a form of external stimuli and FWeds, other professionals, and Level II fieldwork students are what Vygotsky (1978) called more knowledgeable others. Students build knowledge together when they participate in collaborative or group supervision. An example is when supervision for a Level I FWed is being provided by an adjunct faculty member for three students at a university-affiliated

---

BOX 2-2

FIELDWORK COORDINATOR AND
EDUCATOR PROFESSIONAL DEVELOPMENT

KERP helps educators identify their preferred teaching approach according to the elements of Kolb's Learning Cycle: experiencing, reflecting, thinking, and acting. This **free, online self-assessment** categorizes educators as Facilitator, Subject Expert, Standard-Setter/Evaluator, or Coach. The results assist occupational therapy practitioners in teaching roles to see how they currently prefer to structure learning experiences, and how they could use other learning modes to meet the needs of more students (Kolb & Kolb, 2017).

Access it here: https://learningfromexperience.com/themes/kolb-educator-role-profile-erp/

---

child development center with preschool-aged children. The students work together to plan group activities and pass their ideas to the FWed for final approval. The group is completed with about six 4-year-olds and the Level I fieldwork students carry out different leadership roles. After the group, the students discuss their observations about the children's participation with the FWed's input and questions as needed to push the students' learning to greater sophistication.

Occupational therapy practitioners use the *zone of proximal development* (Vygotsky, 1978), another key principle of social constructivism, every day with clients, so it should be easy to apply to educating fieldwork students. The zone of proximal development is the difference between what someone can learn or do independently and what they can do with help from a mentor or peer (McLeod, 2020; Vygotsky, 1978). Occupational therapy practitioners are constantly observing and monitoring this area for potential growth when we upgrade client intervention activities or provide the just-right challenge. New FWeds will notice that they must also gauge students' readiness to respond to additional challenges when they begin supervising Level I fieldwork students.

Occupational therapy practitioners must be comfortable stepping out of the educator spotlight when they use Vygotsky's social constructivist approach in collaborative fieldwork education. When you are in the FWed role, students will ask you questions and expect you to respond with an answer. You are the clinician and probably project a sense of ease in interpersonal interactions and professional reasoning that students notice. Yes, even if you are a newer practitioner and do not feel it yet, you know more than the Level I fieldwork student! So, when asked a question, the Level I FWed using a collaborative approach requires students to discuss possible answers amongst themselves. Only then does the educating therapist weigh in with opinions. Remember that the idea is for students to build knowledge amongst themselves. Hanson et al. (2019) provided more details about key points and the pragmatics of collaborative fieldwork education. See Box 2-3 for an example.

Bloom's Revised Taxonomy

Benjamin Bloom and his colleagues developed a classification of educational outcomes rather than a new theory of learning (Bloom, 1956). Bloom originally described learning outcomes at the college level, but his taxonomy, widely known as *Bloom's Taxonomy*, has now been applied at all levels of education. The continuum of cognitive skills or processes is well known in education, but Bloom and colleagues also described learning in *affective* and *psychomotor* domains (Dettmer, 2006; Hoque, 2016; Kirk, 2021). The *affective* domain described attitudinal learning,

---

Box 2-3

Social Construction of Knowledge in a Collaborative Level I Fieldwork Experience: How Does the Conversation Go?

Using the situation described earlier, the FWed meets with the three occupational therapy students who have just led a group with preschool children, most of whom are developing typically. In this simulated conversation, Joe is the FWed. Eileen, Maria, and Samia are the students.

Joe: "How do you think it went?"

Maria: "Pretty good. It looked like they had fun, and all the kids were engaged. What did you think, Joe?"

Joe: "I would like to hear what you all think before I chime in. Samia, what is your impression of the group and your choice of activities?"

Samia: "I had a great time with the puppets, and it looked like the kids did too. We got a bit more interaction today from the boy who has more needs than the others. What about you, Eileen?"

Eileen: "Better than last week. I think this activity was a better fit for the developmental level of these kiddos."

Joe: "Great. What makes you say this was a better fit for the group? What did you see today?"

---

and the *psychomotor* domain detailed the development of skills or hands-on techniques, both of which are relevant to the purpose of Level I fieldwork: "to apply knowledge to practice and develop understanding of the needs of clients" (ACOTE, 2018, p. 41). It is common to see Bloom's Revised Taxonomy referenced in occupational therapy curriculum documents. A few different hierarchies of psychomotor learning have been described (Hoque, 2016), and some that seemed most suited to occupational therapy are presented in Table 2-1.

It is important that all three domains (cognitive, affective, and psychomotor) are considered when engaging students in Level I fieldwork experiential learning. It is common that a student might be more skilled in one domain than another. For example, a Level I fieldwork student might have the ability to create group intervention plans that are a great fit for an acute care mental health setting. Although the student might know what to do and say, they may have difficulty with psychomotor skills, such as word choice and using accurate pacing and voice tone when speaking to the group, as evidenced by blushing and having difficulty with their choice of words. Some Level I fieldwork experiences have psychomotor learning objectives that require students to carry out techniques they have learned in class and lab, such as manual muscle testing or a standardized cognitive outcome measure (Box 2-4).

Level I fieldwork in simulated environments provides opportunities to combine all three of Bloom's domains in a safe and controlled space with the added benefit of decreasing student anxiety and improving performance (DeFelippo et al., 2020). Simulation allows students to learn from situations they will not encounter in every Level I experience. Examples of simulation are provided in Box 2-5.

TABLE 2-1
BLOOM'S REVISED TAXONOMY APPLIED TO LEVEL I FIELDWORK

DOMAIN	DEFINITION	APPLICATION
Cognitive Domain		
Remember	Simple recall of facts, memory of concepts from a lecture or lab. Remember is the lowest cognitive skill in Bloom's Taxonomy.	FWed asks a pair of students in a collaborative supervision model to **list the contraindications** related to ultrasound as they prepare to treat a client with carpal tunnel syndrome.
Understand	Articulate or work with concepts, may involve classifying, locating, or translating.	Student completing fieldwork in a university occupational therapy clinic **explains the steps** in the occupational therapy process to a client or family member using terms they can understand.
Apply	Use previously acquired information in novel circumstances.	Student **completes** manual muscle testing with a client at an adult day program who has trouble understanding directions.
Analyze	Make connections or differentiate between ideas, compare, or distinguish one case from another.	A group of students working with a FWed at a skilled nursing and rehabilitation center **discuss the differences** between two residents who have had a cerebrovascular accident.
Evaluate	Appraise or critique process or ideas, argue a position or defend a stand.	FWed asks a pair of students to **appraise** if the client they have seen for 4 days is ready for discharge.
Create	Design or develop new plans or activities. Create is considered the highest level skill in the cognitive taxonomy.	Students **develop** a group to meet the needs of members of a mental health drop-in center during a faculty-led fieldwork.
Affective Domain		
Receiving	Being sensitive and open to new ideas, concepts, client stories, and situations. Able to tolerate differences encountered.	Listening without judgment to someone whose substance use disorder led to losing custody of their child.
Responding	Beginning to show commitment to new ideas, situations, and ways of living by actively responding with words or actions.	Student practices completing an occupational profile in a telehealth Level I fieldwork experience, incorporating appropriate verbal and nonverbal feedback to client's answers.

(continued)

TABLE 2-1 (CONTINUED)

BLOOM'S REVISED TAXONOMY APPLIED TO LEVEL I FIELDWORK

DOMAIN	DEFINITION	APPLICATION
Valuing	Openly demonstrating stronger commitment to different ideas or ways of living. Communicating new values verbally, in actions, online, etc.	After completing Level I fieldwork with people experiencing mental health and housing challenges, student speaks up to someone who makes a disparaging comment about a person on the street.
Organizing	Prioritizing some values over others to create one's own value system.	Level I FWed hears a student tell a paraprofessional that the process of a client's art project is more important than how it looks.
Characterizing	Internalizing values, integrate value system into daily life. Would not necessarily be seen by Level I FWeds.	After a Level I placement in a school system, students choose to volunteer in a summer program with the same children.
Psychomotor Domain		
Imitation	Doing a skill someone else does— the most basic element of the psychomotor domain.	Student holds a spoon the same way the therapist holds it while helping children during a feeding group.
Manipulation	Becoming more practiced at using skills so they are more habitual.	Student becomes capable of raising and removing wheelchair leg rests from different chairs and with various clients.
Precision	Becoming more accurate and at ease with a skill.	During their third Level I fieldwork experience, a student completes an occupational profile comfortably with a conversational tone.
Articulation	Demonstrating ability to alter skill application to new circumstances. This level of psychomotor learning would not be a common outcome of Level I fieldwork.	Student watches an experienced therapist modify their therapeutic approach during a session in response to client needs.
Naturalization	Skills come naturally and without thinking. This level of skill or psychomotor learning is not an expected outcome of Level I fieldwork.	A hand therapist creates custom orthoses quickly, efficiently, and without errors or wasted materials.

Adapted from Hoque, M. E. (2016). Three domains of learning: Cognitive, affective and psychomotor. *The Journal of EFL Education and Research, 2*(2), 45-52 and Kirk, K. (2021). What is the affective domain anyway? Science Education Resource Center at Carlton College. https://serc.carleton.edu/NAGTWorkshops/affective/intro.html

---

Box 2-4

ACADEMIC FIELDWORK COORDINATOR TIP

AFWCs are often called upon to write specific learning objectives for use in Level I fieldwork experiences. If your curriculum uses Bloom's Revised Taxonomy, you should use terms consistent with this framework when writing your learning objectives. Be sure to include objectives in the affective and psychomotor domains since learning in Level I fieldwork goes far beyond the cognitive domain. There are many lists of verbs categorized for use in writing learning objectives with Bloom's Taxonomy in mind.

Box 2-5

EXAMPLE OF FIELDWORK SIMULATION WITH BLOOM'S REVISED TAXONOMY

At Johnson & Wales University, students in the entry-level occupational therapy doctorate program complete 15 hours of simulation and 30 hours of faculty-led or traditional Level I fieldwork with each of four occupational therapy practice courses. In the first course, which focuses on mental health, a simulation involves a man responding to psychotic symptoms, played by an experienced therapist. The student who is role playing the occupational therapist attempts to apply their knowledge to encourage him to engage in the group, when he suddenly picks up scissors and walks away, creating an immediate safety hazard. The fieldwork student must respond in a way that is therapeutic to the client and keeps all players in the simulation safe. A thorough debriefing discussion follows in which questions include how the student playing the therapist and those observing felt, as well as whether the student therapist's actions, words, and body language were effective. In this simulation scenario, students must maintain their composure (Bloom's affective domain) in order to apply their knowledge (cognitive domain) with appropriate tone and volume of voice, nonverbal communication, etc. (psychomotor domain).

Fink's Taxonomy of Significant Learning

Fink (2003, 2013), an educator and leader in faculty development, created another framework for learning that is actively applied in many occupational therapy programs. In his 2007 Eleanor Clarke Slagle Lecture, Jim Hinojosa, one of occupational therapy's leading educators and writers, proposed that it was vital to equip students to cope with change rather than only having them demonstrate the profession's current skills. Hinojosa (2007) believed that occupational therapy education programs must ensure that graduates have learned *how* to learn. Learning how to learn is one of six interacting types of learning in Fink's Significant Learning Taxonomy.

Fink uses the term *significant learning* for the knowledge, skills, and attitudes that students actually use in the working world after graduation. The significant learning framework includes foundational knowledge, application, integration, human dimension, learning how to learn, and caring. Consistent with Level I fieldwork in occupational therapy, Fink (2003) views learning very holistically, understanding that learning in one area triggers additional types of learning. *Foundational knowledge* is basic information that is needed to support later learning. *Application* is the ability to use knowledge in practice. In Fink's Taxonomy, *integration* involves the ability to make connections between different people, perspectives, and situations or ideas. Educators hope this will be achieved during Level I fieldwork, but students' ability to integrate may be best seen in later Level I experiences and certainly in Level II fieldwork. Fink uses the term *human dimension* to describe learning about the self, others, and interpersonal interactions. Both *human dimension* and *application* learning fit very well with ACOTE's overall goals for Level I fieldwork (2018). *Learning how to learn* is when students analyze their learning styles and needs to become better at learning. They reflect on their own assets and areas for improvement. Finally, Fink's conception of caring emphasizes students' individual learning interests and values, rather than empathy toward others, similar to Bloom's affective learning (Fink, 2003, 2013). See Table 2-2 for application of Fink's Model of Significant Learning to Level I fieldwork.

As discussed early in this chapter, occupational therapy programs design curricula based upon a philosophy rooted in learning frameworks. See Box 2-6 for an example of how an occupational therapy program uses Fink's Model.

APPLYING THEORETICAL FRAMEWORKS TO LEVEL I FIELDWORK

As was previously discussed in this chapter, a great deal of planning and intention is given to the application of learning theories in the design of both academic and fieldwork coursework. Through application of the learning theories discussed in this chapter, the reader can "think like an educator" when designing learning experiences to facilitate best practices in the profession. This is the topic of Chapter 3. Because application of best practices involves a cycle of planning, doing, and reflection, Kolb's model is evident. Social constructivism influences students as they take ownership for their own learning and the development of professionalism to better fit within the community of practice at the fieldwork site. Taxonomies of learning, such as Bloom's and Fink's, are often applied by occupational therapy faculty (often the AFWC) when developing learning objectives for the Level I experience and considered by the Level I FWed when developing a Level I fieldwork learning plan. This involves tailoring learning objectives to experiences available onsite and determining learning experiences that are a good fit for the learning objectives. This is addressed in more detail in Chapter 8. Various components of learning theories shape how FWeds engage students in developing clinical reasoning skills, the topic of Chapter 5. For example, students benefit from a review of knowledge and opportunities to clarify understanding before applying skills directly to clients. The Level I FWed is best able to take advantage of emerging or "in-the-moment" learning activities onsite when actively applying learning theory. Recognition of the elements of learning suggested in the learning taxonomies allows the FWed to be highly strategic when choosing learning opportunities that are a best fit for the needs of the student; this is the topic of Chapter 9. Learning theory is also considered when the FWed is helping students to navigate psychosocial stressors on fieldwork as addressed in Chapter 11. Finally, experiential learning theory might also be applied at any point in the student's learning experience, from the time of the student's arrival through the conclusion of their final assessment, and, therefore, plays a powerful role in shaping many elements of the student's learning experience.

SUMMARY

This chapter has described four commonly used theoretical frameworks, as well as practical applications to Level I fieldwork. Kolb's Experiential Learning includes the concepts of learning cycle and learning styles. Vygotsky's Social Constructivism serves as the basis for collaborative learning and other times when students learn from each other. The frameworks described in this chapter, Bloom's Revised Taxonomy and Fink's Significant Learning Taxonomy, are often used to structure curricula, as well as Level I fieldwork objectives. Elements of all the learning frameworks provide ideas for FWeds in structuring learning for students throughout the Level I fieldwork experience.

TABLE 2-2

SIX TYPES OF SIGNIFICANT LEARNING APPLIED

TYPE	DEFINITION	APPLICATION
Foundational Knowledge	Understanding basic information and concepts. Students are often asked to apply foundational knowledge from the classroom or lab during a Level I fieldwork experience.	A student reviews muscles innervated at different spinal cord levels in preparation for next day's faculty-led trip to an adaptive sports program for people living with spinal cord injuries. A student on Level I fieldwork might learn to navigate an electronic medical record system to familiarize themselves with an assigned client.
Application	Skills to use knowledge in practice, to begin to think critically or implement professional reason. Although students may not be assessed on skill competency during Level I fieldwork, application is often key to the experience.	A student leading a group during a traditional Level I experience at a mental health partial hospital uses cognitive behavioral therapy techniques that they recently studied in class.
Integration	The ability to make connections between different people, perspectives, and situations or ideas.	A student recalls using sensory-based interventions during their simulation Level I experience in mental health and incorporates similar strategies during their faculty-led placement at an adult day program for people with dementia. A student employed as a nursing home activity assistant collaborates with classmates during a Level I experience. They share a technique that worked for them in the past.
Human Dimension	Learning about the self, others, and interpersonal interactions. Fits well with occupational therapy's therapeutic use of self, a frequent focus of Level I fieldwork.	A student evaluates a client at the university's faculty practice who has a tattoo that is offensive to them. Students discuss feelings this encounter generates, and how they handled the situation with their faculty mentor.
Caring	Students develop individual learning interests or become invested in an area of expertise. In Fink's Taxonomy, caring is not about empathy toward others.	A student who had been dreading a fieldwork experience in a skilled nursing facility discovers they love working with older adults and asks their AFWC for a Level II placement in a similar setting.

(continued)

TABLE 2-2 (CONTINUED)

SIX TYPES OF SIGNIFICANT LEARNING APPLIED

TYPE	DEFINITION	APPLICATION
Learning How to Learn	Using self-direction and inquiry to become a better student. Level I fieldwork experiences should help students determine how best to succeed during Level II fieldwork and beyond.	A quiet student receives feedback from a FWed, "I don't know if you understand everything or nothing." After conversation, the student learns that asking more questions will demonstrate their engagement in the fieldwork experience.

Adapted from Fink, L. D. (2003). *Creating significant learning experiences: An integrated approach to designing college courses.* John Wiley & Sons.

BOX 2-6

CASE APPLICATION OF FINK'S MODEL OF SIGNIFICANT LEARNING TO OCCUPATIONAL THERAPY CURRICULUM DESIGN

I was introduced to Fink's significant learning when I was developing an entry-level master's degree program designed to serve only certified occupational therapy assistants. Using our knowledge of occupational therapy practice and education, we chose Fink's significant learning as a learning framework for the Master of Science in Occupational Therapy program at New England Institute of Technology. Fink's model emphasizes change in the way the students think, which was appropriate as students transition from certified occupational therapy assistant to registered occupational therapist, which requires a significantly different mindset and role identification. We designed learning activities throughout the program to reinforce the reflection on this process and help students synthesize this change in their professional selves. Course objectives and student outcomes were structured using Fink's significant learning terminology to bring consistency to the curriculum. Structuring the curriculum around Fink's model allowed students to build a foundation upon which they could develop leadership and interpersonal skills, ethics, character, and the ability to adapt to change.

Reflection from Chapter Author—Nancy R. Dooley, PhD, OTR/L

LEARNING ACTIVITIES

1. Kolb's Experiential Learning and you as a learner and teacher.

   Think about how you prefer to enter the learning cycle as Kolb defines it. Are you more comfortable starting with experiencing, reflecting, thinking, or experimenting? Now complete KERP at https://learningfromexperience.com/themes/kolb-educator-role-profile-erp/ to determine your preferred teaching approach. After reading the assessment feedback, consider how you can structure learning opportunities from any point in the learning cycle, emphasizing one that is less comfortable.

2. Social constructivism in your fieldwork setting.

   Experienced FWeds:

   - Think about one of your recent Level I fieldwork student interactions when you thought the student could do more with your support than they could independently. What did you do to nudge the student to more skilled performance?

   - Do you naturally scaffold learn to assist students in reaching higher levels of performance during Level I experiences?

   - How could you add learning activities or structure to help students accomplish more skilled performance during their Level I fieldwork with you?

3. Bloom's Revised Taxonomy in your fieldwork setting.

   For FWeds, think about the ways in which Bloom's Revised Taxonomy can be applied to your fieldwork setting. This might be an interesting activity for a staff meeting in an occupational therapy setting to prompt a discussion of the ways in which different practitioners interact with Level I fieldwork students and create learning opportunities for them.

LEARNING OPPORTUNITIES RELATED TO BLOOM'S REVISED TAXONOMY

DOMAIN	DEFINITION	SITE-SPECIFIC LEARNING ACTIVITIES
Cognitive Domain		
Remember	Simple recall of facts, memory of concepts from a lecture or lab. Remember is the lowest cognitive skill in Bloom's Taxonomy.	
Understand	Articulate or work with concepts, may involve classifying, locating, or translating.	
Apply	Use previously acquired information in novel circumstances.	
Analyze	Make connections or differentiate between ideas, compare, or distinguish one case from another.	
Evaluate	Appraise or critique process or ideas, argue a position or defend a stand	
Create	Design or develop new plans or activities. Create is considered the highest level skill in the cognitive taxonomy.	

(continued)

DOMAIN	DEFINITION	SITE-SPECIFIC LEARNING ACTIVITIES
Affective Domain		
Receiving	Being sensitive and open to new ideas, concepts, client stories, and situations. Able to tolerate differences encountered.	
Responding	Beginning to show commitment to new ideas, situations, and ways of living by actively responding with words or actions.	
Valuing	Openly demonstrating stronger commitment to different ideas or ways of living. Communicating new values verbally, in actions, online, etc.	
Organizing	Prioritizing some values over others to create one's own value system.	
Characterizing	Internalizing values, integrate value system into daily life. Would not necessarily be seen by Level I FWeds.	
Psychomotor Domain		
Imitation	Doing a skill someone else does – the most basic element of the psychomotor domain.	
Manipulation	Becoming more practiced at using skills so they are more habitual.	
Precision	Becoming more accurate and at ease with a skill.	
Articulation	Demonstrating ability to alter skill application to new circumstances. This level of psychomotor learning would not be a common outcome of Level I fieldwork.	
Naturalization	Skills come naturally and without thinking. This level of skill or psychomotor learning is not an expected outcome of Level I fieldwork.	

4. Fink's Taxonomy of Significant Learning in your fieldwork setting.

For FWeds, think about the ways in which Fink's Taxonomy of Significant Learning can be applied to your fieldwork setting. With a colleague, discuss the ways in which different situations at your fieldwork site can foster learning opportunities for students in the different domains of learning.

LEARNING OPPORTUNITIES RELATED TO FINK'S TAXONOMY		
DOMAIN	**DEFINITION**	**SITE-SPECIFIC LEARNING ACTIVITIES**
Foundational Knowledge	Understanding basic information and concepts. Students are often asked to apply foundational knowledge from the classroom or lab during a Level I fieldwork experience.	
Application	Skills to use knowledge in practice, to begin to think critically or implement professional reason. Although students may not be assessed on skill competency during Level I fieldwork, application is often key to the experience.	
Integration	The ability to make connections between different people, perspectives, and situations or ideas.	
Human Dimension	Learning about the self, others, and interpersonal interactions. Fits well with occupational therapy's therapeutic use of self, a frequent focus of Level I fieldwork.	
Caring	Students develop individual learning interests or become invested in an area of expertise. In Fink's Taxonomy, caring is not about empathy toward others.	
Learning How to Learn	Using self-direction and inquiry to become a better student. Level I fieldwork experiences should help students determine how best to succeed during Level II fieldwork and beyond.	

ADDITIONAL RESOURCES

- **Access KERP here:** http://survey.learningfromexperience.com/survey/Login/Agreement
- **Free resources about Fink's Significant Learning** are widely available on the internet, particularly at Fink's site www.designlearning.org
- **Useful for AFWCs writing Level I fieldwork objectives:** Affective Domain of Bloom's Revised Taxonomy https://uwaterloo.ca/centre-for-teaching-excellence/sites/ca.centre-for-teaching-excellence/files/uploads/files/affective_domain_-_blooms_taxonomy.pdf

REFERENCES

Accreditation Council for Occupational Therapy Education. (2018). *2018 accreditation council for occupational therapy education standards and interpretative guide, 72*(Suppl. 2), 7212410005p1-721241005p83. https://doi.org/10.5014/ajot.2018.72S217

American Occupational Therapy Association. (2020). Occupational therapy practice framework: Domain and process (4th ed.). *American Journal of Occupational Therapy, 74*, 7412410010. https://doi.org/10.5014/ajot.2020.74S2001

Anderson, L. W., Krathwohl, D. R., Airasian, P. W., Cruikshank, K. A., Mayer, R. E., Pintrich, P. R., Raths, J., & Wittrock, M. C. (2001). *A taxonomy for learning, teaching, and assessing: A revision of Bloom's taxonomy of educational objectives.* Pearson Education.

Berkley Graduate Division. (2021). *Social constructivism.* Graduate Student Instructor Resource Center. https://gsi.berkeley.edu/gsi-guide-contents/learning-theory-research/social-constructivism/

Bloom, B. S. (1956). *Taxonomy of educational objectives: The classification of educational goals.* Longmans.

Cohn, E. S., Dooley, N. R., & Simmons, L. A. (2001). Collaborative learning applied to fieldwork education. In P. Crist & M. Scaffa (Eds.), *Education for Occupational Therapy in Health Care: Strategies for the New Millennium* (pp. 69-83). Haworth.

DeFelippo, A. M., Flowers, E., King, J. C., & Leger, R. (2020). Simulations offer transformational learning and anxiety reduction. *The Exchange, 33*, 19-22.

Dettmer, P. (2006). New Bloom's in established fields: Four domains of learning and doing. *Roeper Review, 28*(2), 70-78.

Fink, L. D. (2003). *Creating significant learning experiences: An integrated approach to designing college courses.* John Wiley & Sons.

Fink, L. D. (2013). *Creating significant learning experiences: An integrated approach to designing college courses (revised and updated).* [Ebook]. Jossey-Bass.

Hanson, D. J., Stutz-Tanenbaum, P., Rogers, O., Turner, T., Graves, C., & Klug, M. G. (2019). Collaborative fieldwork supervision: A process model for program effectiveness. *American Journal of Educational Research, 7*(11), 837-844. https://doi.org/10.12691/education-7-11-13

Hinojosa, J. (2007). Becoming innovators in an era of hyperchange. *American Journal of Occupational Therapy, 61*(6), 629-637. https://doi.org/10.5014/ajot.61.6.629

Hoque, M. E. (2016, September). Three domains of learning: Cognitive, affective and psychomotor. *The Journal of EFL Education and Research, 2*(2), 45-52.

Institute of Experiential Learning. (2020). *What is experiential learning?* https://experientiallearninginstitute.org/resources/what-is-experiential-learning/

Kirk, K. (2021). What is the affective domain anyway? Science Education Resource Center at Carlton College. https://serc.carleton.edu/NAGTWorkshops/affective/intro.html

Kolb, D. A. (2015). *Experiential learning: Experience as the source of learning and development.* (2nd ed.). Pearson Education.

Kolb, A. Y., & Kolb, D. A. (2017). Experiential learning theory as a guide for experiential educators in higher education. *Experiential Learning and Teaching in Higher Education, 1*(1), 7-44.

McLeod, S. (2020). Lev Vygotsky's sociocultural theory. *Simply psychology.* https://www.simplypsychology.org/vygotsky.html

Vygotsky, L. S. (1978). *Mind in society: The development of higher psychological processes.* Harvard University Press.

3

Mentoring in Professional Best Practices During the Level I Fieldwork Experience

*Hannah Oldenburg, EdD, OTR/L, BCPR
and Cherie Graves, PhD, OTR/L*

The previous chapter led you through the process of thinking like an educator as you are getting ready to host a Level I fieldwork student. This chapter will provide foundational knowledge as well as relevant strategies to support the integration of best practice principles for students during Level I fieldwork experiences across a variety of contexts (e.g., academic, community, educational, clinical settings). Regardless of the type of experience, the goal of Level I fieldwork continues to be consistent: "to introduce students to fieldwork, apply knowledge to practice, and develop understanding of the needs of clients" (Accreditation Council for Occupational Therapy Education [ACOTE], 2018, p. 41). Application opportunities for students during Level I fieldwork may address numerous competencies, such as professional reasoning, professional behaviors, therapeutic use of self, technical skills, the occupational therapy process, and the best practice principles.

The best practice principles presented in this chapter are derived from professional literature that identify key features of occupational therapy practice. *The Occupational Therapy Practice Framework, Fourth Edition* (OTPF-4; American Occupational Therapy Association [AOTA], 2020a) provides a structure and description of occupational therapy practice and service delivery. It presents components that are of utmost importance, the cornerstones, and contributors of occupational therapy practice. The "contributors" include (1) client-centered practice, (2) cultural humility, (3) ethics, (4) evidence-informed practice, and (5) occupation-based practice. These are foundational and directly influence the cornerstones of the profession, which describe the "distinct knowledge, skills, and qualities that contribute to the success of the occupational therapy process" and that are within each occupational therapy practitioner (AOTA, 2020a, p. 6).

Hanson, D., & DeIuliis, E. D. (Eds.).
Fieldwork Educator's Guide to Level I Fieldwork (pp. 43-73).
© 2023 Taylor and Francis Group.

In addition, Boyt Schell et al. (2019) identified client-centered practice, occupation-based practice, evidence-based practice (EBP), and culturally relevant practice as the key principles guiding contemporary occupational therapy practice. The best practice principles are complete by adding ethical practice. As a student, it is critical to observe and apply the best practice principles during Level I fieldwork to strengthen their professional identity development. As a practitioner, integrating the best practice principles not only strengthens practitioner professional identity, but also ensures our clients are receiving the best possible care.

Academic programs are required to demonstrate, through the accreditation process, how students are prepared to be competent in the implementation of the best practice principles (ACOTE, 2018). Teaching methods and assignments emphasize the importance of these principles and require students to incorporate them into their daily work. Following application of these principles in the classroom environment, students hope to identify and apply these best practice principles into practice during Level I fieldwork.

Unfortunately, students often report observing discrepancies between best practice principles emphasized in the classroom and the realities of practice experienced in fieldwork (Di Tommaso et al., 2016; Gupta & Taff, 2015; Ripat et al., 2013; Towns & Ashby, 2014). For example, they may see more emphasis on tasks to prepare clients for occupational performance rather than use of occupations and activities and therapy that is protocol driven rather than individualized to the client. Rather than using evidence to direct practice, students may see use of treatment approaches that are supported by tradition but not by recent evidence.

Every practitioner and fieldwork site experiences challenges in enacting best practice from time to time. Fieldwork educators (FWeds) who are intentional in their efforts to model best practices and engage students in discussion of best practice strategies, even during challenges, are highly regarded by students, clients, and their colleagues. Students report that this type of experience prepares them for the realities of their future practice.

As an educator and practitioner, it is important to reflect on your own strengths and challenges in understanding and implementing best practice principles to ensure success in bridging this knowledge to students in the field. Furthermore, it is important to identify and address the challenges at your site to aid in successful implementation of best practice principles during Level I fieldwork experiences. Have you developed strategies for engaging Level I students in the examination and implementation of best practice principles at your site?

LEARNING OBJECTIVES

By the end of reading this chapter and completing the learning activities, the reader should be able to:

1. Articulate the five best practice principles of the occupational therapy profession.

2. Describe the value of integrating best practice principles during Level I fieldwork experiences.

3. Identify your own facilitators and barriers to implementation of best practice principles across Level I fieldwork experiences.

4. Apply teaching and learning strategies to support implementation of best practice principles during Level I fieldwork experiences.

BEST PRACTICE PRINCIPLES ARE FOUNDATIONAL TO OCCUPATIONAL THERAPY PRACTICE

According to the most recent accreditation standards for occupational therapy education, Level I fieldwork experiences "may be met through one or more of the following instructional methods: simulated environments, standardized patients, faculty practice, faculty-led site visits, and supervision by a FWed in a practice environment" (ACOTE, 2018, p. 41). The multitude of variations in which Level I fieldwork can occur are new for the profession and allow academic programs to be flexible and creative.

Throughout academic coursework, students learn about each of the professional best practices, and this learning is strengthened with opportunities provided during Level I fieldwork. Exposure to occupation-based practice on Level I fieldwork helps to solidify the emerging professional identity of occupational therapy students. Observing client-centered and culturally relevant practice allows students to recognize the significant value of using these principles to mitigate bias. EBP observed during Level I fieldwork promotes the importance of lifelong learning, while the presence of ethical practice instills the core values and ethical principles students are learning about in the classroom.

Level I fieldwork experiences are often the first opportunity that students have in their academic program to apply their classroom knowledge to hands-on practice with clients, including standardized patients and simulated experiences, while under the supervision of a FWed. When students are unable to observe or participate in best practice during their Level I placement, the student's roots to the profession are compromised, and they may become disillusioned with the educational process. Furthermore, they will not have established a foundation for carrying out the best practice principles in their Level II fieldwork and into their beginning years of practice. Although there are many aspects of learning that occur during the Level I placement, understanding and implementation of best practice principles are foundational to everything else, and, therefore, merit individual review.

OVERVIEW OF THE BEST PRACTICE PRINCIPLES

This first section of the chapter will provide a brief literature review to help the FWed build a strong foundation of the five best practices principles.

Occupation-Based Practice

Occupation-based practice is the "bread and butter" of the profession. The fourth edition of the *OTPF-4* identifies four "cornerstones" of occupational therapy, distinguishing the profession from other professions (AOTA, 2020a). Occupation is embedded within two of these cornerstones, exemplifying the significance of occupation to the profession. First, the core values and beliefs of the profession are rooted in occupation. Second, occupational therapy practitioners have distinct knowledge and expertise in the therapeutic use of occupation (AOTA, 2020a). The presence of occupation in our work with clients is paramount to the identity of the profession and the value which occupational therapy contributes to a person's health and well-being. *Occupation-based practice* occurs when a practitioner uses evaluation and intervention to engage a client in occupation (Fisher & Marterella, 2019). A deep understanding of the meaning of occupation, particularly to clients served, is imperative to practice from an occupation-based perspective. This concept is demonstrated in the scenario described in Box 3-1.

> ### Box 3-1
> ## DEMONSTRATION OF OCCUPATION-BASED PRACTICE
>
> A 65-year-old client was admitted to the inpatient rehab facility following a severe stroke, impacting the client's ability to care for oneself. Prior to admission, the client was independent with all activities of daily living (ADLs). The occupational therapist completes the initial evaluation indicating maximum assist needed for all ADL tasks, including grooming, dressing, bathing, and toileting. Goals are created for the client to be independent with ADLs. After meeting with the client's family, they communicate that, in their culture, independence is not of primary value. The family expresses that they will provide any assistance needed upon discharge. The occupational goal shifts from independence with ADLs to caregiver education for safe discharge home with family.

Client-Centered Practice

Client-centered practice has been recognized from the early days of the profession as a key component to practice (Mroz et al., 2015). The *OTPF-4* identifies client-centered practice as one of the "contributors" that influences the "cornerstones" of the profession (AOTA, 2020a). One of these cornerstones being therapeutic use of self, a key concept and skill that distinguishes the occupational therapy profession from other professions, and which significantly impacts the relationship occupational therapy practitioners develop with clients.

While the profession has always focused on the client, it was not until the 1980s that the profession began to define *client-centered practice*. There have been a variety of definitions for client-centered practice in the literature; however, most share common tenets including establishing an effective partnership and collaboration with clients, encouraging shared decision making, respecting diversity, recognizing power, and identifying strategies to realign and equally distribute power in the therapeutic relationship (Law et al., 1995; Sumsion & Law, 2006). See Box 3-2 for examples of what client-centered practice might look like in practice.

Evidence-Based Practice

Decades after the founding of occupational therapy, the medical model gained strength increasing the emphasis on scientific evidence. By the 1980s, *evidence-based practice,* or EBP, had emerged in the medical field and slowly gained traction in occupational therapy in the late 1990s. EBP is described as the process in which practitioners develop a question, search the evidence, evaluate the evidence, and implement the evidence while considering the wishes of the client and their family (Law & MacDermid, 2014). There are several ways in which evidence can be incorporated into the daily practice of occupational therapy practitioners. See a list of EBP examples in Box 3-3. Additionally, see Appendix B for an example of an activity that can be used to have students actively review and appraise standardized tools that are applicable to a variety of practice settings and populations.

Ethical Practice

Professional behaviors and dispositions represent another cornerstone of occupational therapy practice, indicating the importance of ethical practice within the profession (AOTA, 2020a). The first document reflecting the ethical principles of the profession was introduced and passed by the Occupational Therapy Board of Management in 1926 (Doherty, 2019). It was not until 1975

BOX 3-2

EXAMPLES OF CLIENT-CENTERED PRACTICE

- **Early intervention:** Collaborate with parents to prioritize goals most important to family, one of which is using culturally accepted utensils for self-feeding.
- **Outpatient pediatric:** Collaborate with the client and family to arrange for therapy to occur at daycare to identify potential triggers for behavior client exhibits while at daycare.
- **School system:** Collaborate with the client to identify a plan for therapy that is mutually agreeable. If the client refuses the initial plan, adjust the plan to complete activities. For example, the client may be more agreeable to complete therapy outside on the playground rather than in the therapy room.
- **Acute care hospital:** Collaborate with the client to identify appropriate time for the therapy session. For example, the client scheduled for a morning dressing session following a back surgery. Client reports not having any clothes at the hospital yet. Alternative therapy time arranged.
- **Home health:** Respect client diversity. For example, the client is seen for initial evaluation and reports being unable to eat with family because of fear of getting down on the floor and not being able to get back up. Practitioner collaborates with client and family to safely complete floor transfer to allow client to participate in meaningful and culturally relevant occupation of eating as a family.
- **Skilled nursing facility:** Collaborate with the client to adjust evaluation procedures. For example, recognizing client fatigue and pain, the practitioner gathers occupational profile and then arranges with client to complete evaluation later in the day, allowing client time to rest and receive pain medication.
- **Community mental health:** Support an effective partnership by meeting client needs. For example, client calls at 8:30 a.m. describing an increase in anxiety symptoms and requesting a 10 a.m. appointment to be conducted via telehealth rather than in person. Therapy practitioner agrees to complete the appointment via telehealth.

BOX 3-3

USE OF EVIDENCE IN PRACTICE

- Evaluate effectiveness of an intervention approach prior to use.
- Identify outcome measures with best psychometric properties.
- Select outcome measures for use with specific client population.
- Critique best practice for a specific client population.

---

when the first AOTA Ethics Commission was established, and the first Principles of Occupational Therapy Ethics was published by AOTA in 1977. Since then, the Code of Ethics has been revised seven times, most recently in 2020 (AOTA, 2020b).

In the last decade, the increased complexity of health care and education sectors have challenged practitioners and educators in their decision making and use of ethical knowledge, skills, and behaviors in practice. Adhering to the Code of Ethics, applying ethical frameworks for decision making, and responding appropriately to ethical issues in practice ensures that occupational therapy practitioners continue to uphold the ethical standards of the profession and provide *ethical practice* to all clients. See a list of strategies to ensure ethical practice in Box 3-4.

Box 3-4

STRATEGIES FOR ETHICAL PRACTICE

- Display a copy of the most recent Code of Ethics in your practice setting.
- Be an active member in professional organizations, such as AOTA, to help inform you of resources to support ethical practice.
- Participate in continuing education and professional development opportunities that support professional values and principles of occupational therapy.
- Review, discuss, and reflect on case scenarios from practice, apply ethical principles, and strategize solutions to optimize ethical practice.

Box 3-5

STRATEGIES FOR CULTURALLY RELEVANT PRACTICE

- Reflect and identify your own bias or cultural unknowns.
- Actively educate yourself on cultural unknowns of your client, cultural environment, and resources.
- Develop partnerships with people or groups that advocate for others.
- Appreciate differences and highlight the unique strengths of a variety of groups and populations.
- Model respect for diversity.

Culturally Relevant Practice

Culture is a multidimensional concept that is crucial for occupational therapy practitioners to understand. Broadly speaking, culture encompasses the values, beliefs, behaviors, expressions, etc. that influence a group of people and is passed down through generations (Black & Wells, 2007). A person's culture shapes their roles, habits, and routines (Getty, 2016), in addition to the occupations that bring meaning and which they choose to participate in (Black, 2019). *Culturally relevant practice* involves recognizing and providing occupational therapy services that fit within the "complex social, political, and cultural milieu" of where the services are provided (World Federation of Occupational Therapists, 2010), while also recognizing because occupations are shaped by culture, practitioners must attend to the culture of their clients (Black, 2019). Having a detailed understanding of the client's roles, habits, and routines is the first step in understanding the client's perspective of occupational performance. As an occupational therapy practitioner, it is important to recognize and integrate cultural considerations into your evaluation and intervention process to ensure occupational therapy services are meaningful and specific to the client's culture. See a list of strategies to provide culturally relevant practice in Box 3-5.

Although best practice principles are lofty, they can best be accomplished by starting small. Pick one that you would like to improve upon in your role as a Level I FWed. Focus on that one until it becomes part of your routine, then aim to improve upon another. There is great value in providing therapy services that are consistent with best practice. Table 3-1 presents summary statements about how to pursue each of the best practice principles, and what value it brings to the client, the practitioner, and to the entire profession.

TABLE 3-1

BEST PRACTICE PRINCIPLES: HOW TO AND FOR WHAT VALUE?

	HOW DO I DO IT?	WHY SHOULD I DO IT?
Evidence-Based Practice	Develop a question, search, and evaluate the evidence, and implement the evidence while considering the wishes of the client and their family (Law & MacDermid, 2014).	Improves client outcomes at a quicker rate, ultimately saving health care dollars (Wilkinson et al., 2012).
Client-Centered Practice	Enhance skills in therapeutic use of self, using the Intentional Relationship Model (Taylor, 2020). Demonstrate professional behaviors and dispositions, such as collaboration, empathy, and humility (AOTA, 2020a, 2020b). Challenge the status quo or the institutional culture that does not enact client-centered practice.	Greater patient satisfaction; improved patient compliance; improved treatment outcomes (Korner & Modell, 2009; Plewnia et al., 2016; Zimmerman et al., 2014).
Occupation-Based Practice	Gather occupational history and occupations that are of concern (occupational profile). Identify resources that are available to you (either from yourself, workplace, or the client). Challenge the status quo or the institutional culture that does not value or enact occupation-based practice.	It is our distinct value and advances the understanding of occupational therapy. It separates us from other members of the interdisciplinary team. More enjoyable, rewarding, effective, and client and family centered (Estes & Pierce, 2012). Strengthens practitioner professional identity (Ashby et al., 2013; Estes & Pierce, 2012).
Ethical Practice	Identify and challenge the ethical scenarios with the principles and values of the occupational therapy profession. Apply AOTA Code of Ethics principles when managing ethical considerations with use of the principles and values in your decision making.	Upholds occupational therapy values and trust with delivering occupational therapy services with clients, groups, and populations. Supports clinical reasoning to ensure ethical decisions are rooted in principles and values of occupational therapy profession (AOTA, 2020b).

(continued)

	TABLE 3-1 (CONTINUED) BEST PRACTICE PRINCIPLES: HOW TO AND FOR WHAT VALUE?	
	HOW DO I DO IT?	**WHY SHOULD I DO IT?**
Culturally Relevant Practice	Identify cultural perspectives that support and inhibit occupational engagement across lifespan. Reflect on self and environment to be aware of bias that may inhibit occupational engagement. Demonstrate an attitude and intelligence that is receptive and knowledgeable on cultural aspects at a macro and micro level.	Strengthen therapeutic relationship with client and optimize client-centered approach. Ensures individualized care that is inclusive of norms, beliefs, attitudes, and behaviors of different cultural groups (AOTA, 2020b). Challenges practitioners to be lifelong learners of cultural relevance and knowledge to ensure safety and intelligence that is supportive of the unique needs of the client (AOTA, 2020b).

BACKGROUND OF THE PROBLEM

As previously mentioned, students often report observing discrepancies between best practice principles emphasized in the classroom and the realities of practice experienced on fieldwork (Di Tommaso et al., 2016; Gupta & Taff, 2015; Ripat et al., 2013; Towns & Ashby, 2014). See Box 3-6 for examples of discrepancies students may experience while on Level I fieldwork.

Many barriers to incorporating best practice principles are present in occupational therapy settings across the nation with no setting being immune. These barriers have also been identified in the literature and can be grouped into the categories of institutional barriers, organizational barriers, and personal barriers (Table 3-2).

Barriers to professional best practice will always be present, and it may be overwhelming to think about how to overcome these barriers. However, through collaboration with others, strategic analysis, and use of a cyclic process of reflection and action, incremental progress is possible. If you are feeling overcome by the barriers that you experience at your setting, consider partnership with your academic institution in offering fieldwork to students as an opportunity to learn about each of the best practice principles and to continue to grow in implementing them into practice.

PREPARATION FOR BEST PRACTICE

There are various steps that can be taken to help prepare for the implementation of best practice during Level I fieldwork. The next section will overview a few steps, such as identifying the roles and responsibilities of those involved, reflecting on facilitators and barriers of fieldwork context, and planning ways to scaffold student learning.

Box 3-6

REALITIES OF PRACTICE EXPERIENCED BY STUDENTS WHILE ON FIELDWORK

- Greater use of methods and tasks to prepare clients for occupational performance rather than use of occupations and activities.
- Difficulty in remaining client centered when practice setting defines the primary role of occupational therapy services.
- Difficulty incorporating culturally relevant care when others (manager, reimbursement) may dictate the amount of time a practitioner will have with a client.
- Difficulty implementing best practice with each client because the case load is too large, and time is limited.
- Difficulty incorporating use of evidence because there is not enough time in the workday.

Table 3-2

BARRIERS TO BEST PRACTICE PRINCIPLES

Institutional Barriers	Lack of time, space/storage, supplies, philosophical perspective
Organizational Barriers	Lack of support, power differentials, workplace culture
Personal Barriers	Lack of skills, lack of creativity, personal mindset

Roles and Responsibilities

During a Level I fieldwork experience, the student is beginning to identify their role and responsibility as an occupational therapy student and future practitioner. Students have the responsibility to keep an open mind, be curious about the use of best practice, and consider what their role is to strengthen the implementation of the best practice principles. Academic educators and FWeds have a role in introducing and fostering the start of best practice principles during Level I fieldwork. It is essential that academic educators and FWeds mentor students within the practice setting, classroom, or community setting to help them identify, understand, and begin to apply the best practice principles.

Reflecting on Fieldwork Context

From an academic and FWed perspective, it is important to analyze the facilitators and barriers that could arise when delivering a Level I fieldwork experience in different contexts (e.g., simulation vs. faculty-led clinic vs. practice environment). A SWOT (strength, weakness, opportunity, and threat) analysis can be used to assess the strengths, weaknesses, opportunities, and threats of a given context, to help academic and FWeds reflect and determine methods to best support implementation of the best practice principles during a Level I fieldwork experience. In review of each of the areas, it is important to consider internal and external factors that may influence the implementation of the best practice principles in the various Level I fieldwork opportunities (e.g., simulation, standardized patient, faculty-led clinic, faculty practice, fieldwork traditional site). Table 3-3 provides questions, using the SWOT approach, that may help academic and FWeds in identifying strengths and challenges when facilitating a Level I fieldwork experience. It may also be a tool to foster ongoing conversations with students about the practical realities that must be considered to provide care that is consistent with best practice.

Scaffolding Student Learning

Faculty and FWeds can foster student growth by supporting the understanding and application of best practice principles, starting in the classroom, and progressing to Level I and Level II fieldwork experiences. Scaffolding is a teaching strategy that encompasses social interaction between the educator and learner with the educator aiding the learner with external assistance and then progressing to less external assistance with a given knowledge or performance element (Sanders & Welk, 2005). This concept is part of Vygotsky's Sociocultural Learning Theory (introduced in Chapter 2), which provides a framework that considers sociocultural elements, as well as the use of teaching strategies, such as scaffolding, social modeling and culture, and reflection on a learner's progression toward autonomy in their knowledge processing and performance (Sanders & Welk, 2005).

Scaffolding the learning experiences within Level I fieldwork experiences can be facilitated through deliberate and progressive activities in the classroom, clinic, and community contexts. The goal of scaffolding is for the educator to provide support initially, with the goal of decreasing the support needed from the educator, with the learner internalizing the learning and performing independently. The example in Box 3-7 demonstrates scaffolding applied to ethical practice. This progression of scaffolding ethical considerations is demonstrated in Figure 3-1.

The learning process that occurs during scaffolding is active, and students are encouraged to take ownership in identifying their strengths and areas of growth, to ensure progression toward active use of the best practice principles. Faculty and FWeds need to provide guidance and perspective to students when applying the principles to ensure the application is accurate, feasible, and meaningful for the student, site, and client. Furthermore, educators should use discussion-based activities (e.g., live or asynchronous) to help students identify, analyze, and apply best practice principles.

The use of peer support through discussion within live or asynchronous format is a social learning activity that may help students be more explicit in their knowledge gains, as well as support each other in providing examples or considerations for background and application of best practice ideal implementation. This learning activity may provide a foundation for the student to use as they progress from Level I to Level II fieldwork experiences. Box 3-8 includes examples of discussion prompts that can be used to foster discussion and help identify areas of strength and areas of growth in the best practice principles.

STRATEGIES FOR INTEGRATION

A variety of strategies can be used while working with Level I fieldwork students to foster integration of best practice principles. Some FWeds may have a preferred strategy that comes naturally, while others may use a variety of strategies with students. There is no single best strategy to foster integration of best practice principles, rather the key is to do something and always try to progress. The following are a few common strategies that can be incorporated by FWeds while working with students: *modeling, active learning,* and *reflection.* The key to all strategies mentioned is the cyclic process of learning that was introduced earlier in Figure 3-1.

TABLE 3-3

SWOT ANALYSIS FOR LEVEL I FIELDWORK EXPERIENCE

	FIELDWORK FORMAT (e.g., simulated environment, standardized patient, faculty-led, faculy site visist, fieldwork site)	ACADEMIC/FACULTY STAKEHOLDER	FIELDWORK EDUCATOR STAKEHOLDER
STRENGTH (S)		What facilitators are present to support the FWed and student in bridging knowledge of best practice principles into practice?	What facilitators are present to foster best practice principles with a Level I fieldwork student at your practice site? *Consider the environment, practitioner skill set, clientele, administration, attitudes at site.*
WEAKNESS (W)		What are the potential barriers to consider when supporting the FWed and/or student in implementing best practice principles at a given site?	What are potential barriers to hosting and mentoring a Level I fieldwork student at your practice site? *Consider the environment, practitioner skill set, clientele, administration, attitudes at site.*
OPPORTUNITY (O)		What opportunities are available to you to support the educator and student in implementation of best practice principles during fieldwork? Are there opportunities that can come out of your strengths?	What opportunities are available to you to support a student in implementing best practice principles during fieldwork? Are there opportunities that can come out of your strengths at your facility?
THREAT (T)		What threats are present that may hinder your ability to assist the educator and/or student in implementing best practice principles during fieldwork?	What threats are present that may hinder your ability to assist the student in implementing best practice principles during fieldwork at your site?

> ### Box 3-7
> ## DEMONSTRATION OF SCAFFOLDING TO ETHICAL PRACTICE
>
> 1. Faculty provide support for knowledge and examples of identifying and articulating best practice principles with the AOTA Code of Ethics. *(Identify)*
>
> 2. Faculty provide examples to grow understanding of each ideal. *(Understanding)*
>
> 3. Faculty provide case scenarios for students to apply the knowledge and determine the ethical value challenged. *(Application)*
>
> 4. Faculty or FWeds progress the learning by providing students with specific scenarios or conditions and student needs to identify ethical considerations with a specific client and how to best serve the needs of that client. *(Application)*
>
> 5. Faculty or FWeds facilitate student reflection on scenario and identify strengths and areas of growth. *(Reflection)*

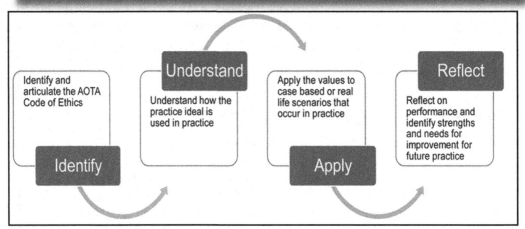

Figure 3-1. Example of scaffolding for Level I experience.

Modeling

Modeling is an instructional strategy that FWeds can use to teach or demonstrate application of a concept or skill. According to Ahn et al. (2020), modeling occurs when an observer attempts to imitate similar behaviors that are exhibited by a model. An effective role model demonstrates competence and success in the skills that are being modeled (Ahn et al., 2020) while the learner observes and interacts with the instructor during the modeling.

In all fieldwork learning opportunities, modeling is a strategy that can be incorporated. Before Level I fieldwork, students may have limited exposure to observing occupational therapy practice in action. They have gained knowledge related to the provision of services but have not yet themselves applied their knowledge with a client population. Modeling can be a valuable strategy for students to observe their FWed demonstrating a particular concept or skill, which can then be maximized by offering the student an opportunity to practice the concept or skill.

When using modeling, it is imperative that the FWed also verbally describe their actions and provide rationale to ensure the professional reasoning is explicit and accessible for the student to understand. For example, Box 3-9 shares a quick tip that is helpful when modeling during a Level I fieldwork experience. See Appendix A for several examples to assist academic fieldwork coordinators (AFWCs), FWeds, and faculty in incorporating modeling in the classroom, community, and practice settings.

Box 3-8

LEARNING ACTIVITY: DISCUSSION (LIVE OR VIRTUAL ENVIRONMENT)

During a Level I fieldwork experience, academic faculty and FWeds have a role in fostering growth in best practice. Discussion through live or virtual environments (e.g., discussion boards) may guide students to recognize, apply, and reflect on their understanding and implementation of best practice principles in a safe learning environment. The following questions can be posed to students to help them recognize their strengths and areas of growth.

Discussion prompts or questions to consider:

1. Describe a time you witnessed or experienced one of the best practice principles during your fieldwork experience.
2. How were best practice principles managed in this scenario?
3. Describe other considerations to ensure best practice is upheld.
4. What facilitators to best practice were experienced in this scenario?
5. What barriers to best practice were experienced in this scenario?
6. What more would you want to do to ensure best practice principles were upheld in future, similar scenarios?
7. How do you plan to implement those best practice principles in the future?

Box 3-9

MODEL DURING LEVEL I FIELDWORK

Quick Tip

Best practice principles are not always visible; therefore, students benefit from FWeds explicitly verbalizing their reasoning, and how they arrived at their decision. For example, a FWed selects intervention X to use with a client. The student wonders, "Why did they select intervention X over intervention Y?" The evidence-based decision-making process used to select intervention X was not visible to the student. The FWed verbalizing the reasoning to the student will allow the student to make a connection to EBP, and how it is implemented in practice (Stube & Jedlicka, 2007).

FWed to student: "Our next client is a 68-year-old woman who is on the unit following a right cerebrovascular accident. Her occupational challenges include dressing, bathing, toileting, meal prep and several other ADL and instrumental activities of daily living tasks. She is also an avid piano player and gardener."

Student to FWed: "What are we going to work on today?"

FWed to student: "I would like to do some neuromuscular reeducation to facilitate increased occupational performance in her left upper extremity. I prepared to complete a gardening activity during our session today. I try to incorporate as many occupation-based interventions as possible. There is stronger evidence in motor learning that supports the use of occupation-based interventions over biomechanical interventions, such as range of motion exercises. It is also more meaningful and enjoyable for the client."

> ## Box 3-10
> ## Active Learning During Level I Fieldwork
>
> Ask your student to …
> - Document their observations of a therapy session.
> - Verbally summarize their assessment of the therapy session.
> - Write a subjective, objective, assessment, and plan note on a therapy session.
> - Create three intervention ideas using the materials available onsite.
> - Locate evidence on a particular client population.
> - Prepare to complete an occupational profile on a new client.
> - Review a particular assessment tool and prepare to administer to a client.
> - Demonstrate application of an occupational therapy theory to a client.

Active Learning

Active learning is an instructional approach that requires the learner to be actively engaged in the learning process. This approach is aligned with constructivist philosophy, which surmises that knowledge is within the learner and the role of the educator is to facilitate the learner in constructing their own knowledge (Jonassen, 1999). This philosophy contrasts with the antiquated objectivist philosophy, which surmises that knowledge is within the educator (expert) and is transferred to the learner. The assumptions within objectivist philosophy contribute to instructional approaches in which educators (experts) lecture to learners as a means of transferring their knowledge to passive learners (Freeman et al., 2014).

Unfortunately, students are often passive learners during Level I fieldwork, which can be attributed to a variety of factors. One factor is due to occupational therapy practitioners fulfilling an additional role as FWed while their primary role is providing services to a client population, which requires a significant amount of their attention, naturally leading to a student being a passive learner. Another factor is the student's own hesitancy or lack of confidence in being an active learner during the experience.

It is important to invite and encourage students to be active learners in their application of best practice principles during Level I fieldwork experiences. See Box 3-10 for strategies to invite students to be active learners during Level I fieldwork. With active learning occurring during Level I experiences, students will transition to Level II fieldwork and into practice with more experience and confidence in their ability to implement best practice. Furthermore, Appendix B provides several examples to assist AFWCs, FWeds, and faculty in incorporating active learning strategies in the classroom, community, and practice settings. One specific example that is provided is to help facilitate student learning in identifying and understanding components of standardized tools that may be available on fieldwork or in the classroom.

Reflection

Reflection is an instructional approach that requires mindful awareness of one's thoughts, actions, or behaviors for a given situation, as well as for planning of future situations (Yazdani et al., 2020). Teaching and incorporating reflection in education encourages students to be self-directed and ensures the development of lifelong learning (Sandars, 2009; Winkel et al., 2017). The primary aim of reflection is to develop in-depth thinking about self and situations to enhance understanding and enable better performance in the future (Schei et al., 2019; Winkel et al., 2017).

Box 3-11
REFLECTION DURING LEVEL I FIELDWORK

Ask your student to ...

- Identify and evaluate client response to treatment before, during, or after session.
- Identify theoretical concepts in a particular occupational therapy theory and/or frame of reference.
- Analyze theoretical concepts in application of a particular client.
- Describe the context of the practice setting and impact on the best practice principles.
- Reflect on personal and professional presentation.
- Identify clinical competencies in evaluation, treatment planning, and implementation.
- Identify an ethical dilemma and use AOTA Code of Ethics to guide reasoning.

In this way, reflection can serve as a valuable strategy to scaffolded student learning to ensure appropriate level of challenge for student competency. See Appendix D for suggestions on ways to scaffold student reflection.

Reflection involves the student using elements of metacognition for awareness of the situation, analyzing the situation, interpreting one's own behaviors, and articulating the next step to the situation (Yazdani et al., 2020). Reflection can occur before, during, or after a situation and may involve one student and an educator or a group of students and an educator. Reflection occurring before a situation is often referred to as anticipatory reflection and can be applied as mental preparation and planning (Botelho & Bhuyan, 2020). This type of reflection can be particularly helpful for students who are in new or challenging situations. Reflection during the moment (in action) may involve pointed questions from an educator during a situation to facilitate deep thinking about the situation and to emphasize if a different course of action is needed by the student. Reflection that occurs after the event (on action) requires a student to look back on their action and learn if their action led to the desired outcome (Botelho & Bhuyan, 2020).

See Box 3-11 for examples of reflective activities that can be incorporated into Level I fieldwork learning experience. In addition, Appendix C provides several examples to assist AFWCs, FWeds, and faculty in incorporating reflection in the classroom, community, and practice settings.

APPLICATION EXAMPLES

Faculty and FWeds can support best practice during Level I fieldwork experiences through a variety of individual and peer activities. Similarities and differences will be present when considering how to integrate best practice principles across various types of Level I fieldwork. These activities can be tailored to the classroom or fieldwork site. It is important that students have the professional resources to help support best practice during these activities. For example, having the background knowledge of the AOTA Code of Ethics is essential to begin the application within the Level I fieldwork context.

The following section will provide examples of learning activities that are primarily directed toward FWeds and faculty to facilitate integration of the best practice principles. The section is organized by the format in which the Level I fieldwork experiences occur (e.g., simulation, standardized patient, traditional). Within each section you will find two to three suggested learning activities with an example of the type of integration strategy it is representing. See Table 3-4 for ideas to facilitate best practice during Level I fieldwork experiences occurring in a simulated environment, Table 3-5 for Level I fieldwork experiences occurring with standardized patients,

Table 3-6 for Level I fieldwork experiences occurring within a faculty practice, Table 3-7 for Level I fieldwork experiences occurring with faculty-led site visits, and Table 3-8 for Level I fieldwork experiences occurring at a fieldwork site. Within the tables, the activities and suggestions can be facilitated by a FWed, faculty, or student.

COLLABORATION BETWEEN ACADEMIA AND FIELDWORK EDUCATORS TO SUPPORT BEST PRACTICE

Occupational therapy academic programs, including AFWCs, faculty, and students, have a unique opportunity to positively impact the use of the best practice principles by collaborating and supporting FWeds in their efforts to provide best practice. Over time, the ongoing collaboration and support between academic programs and fieldwork partners can lead to improved implementation of best practice. Additionally, academic programs can foster the connection between fieldwork partners and the occupational therapy profession by sharing information and facilitating discussion about topics of concern that are occurring in the profession (e.g., topics such as level of degree required for entry-level practice, professional association initiatives, updates to accreditation standards, licensure compact initiatives).

SUMMARY

Level I fieldwork provides an opportunity to help occupational therapy students identify, understand, apply, and reflect on best practice principles that are essential for entry-level practice. Unfortunately, students often report lack of opportunity to observe or carry out these principles during their Level I experience. However, through review of this chapter, the FWed is provided strategies to foster best practice principles across all types of Level I fieldwork experiences. Fostering learning activities that support active learning, modeling, and reflection can help students to develop foundational skills in the implementation of best practice principles and strengthen their own professional identity as an occupational therapy practitioner. AFWCs, faculty, and FWeds all have a role in fostering opportunities for students to actively participate in best practice principles contributing to the implementation of best practice principles within the occupational therapy profession.

LEARNING ACTIVITY

1. Please review learning activities provided in Appendices A to E. Highlight those that would be a best fit for your practice setting. What new insights do you gain about incorporating best practices into Level I fieldwork experiences?

The size, method, commitment, and persons involved in providing collaboration and support to fieldwork partners can vary widely, allowing great freedom and flexibility to identify what is feasible. See Box 3-12 for a variety of methods that can be used and modified to provide collaboration and support to fieldwork partners.

TABLE 3-4
APPLYING BEST PRACTICE IN SIMULATED ENVIRONMENTS

Occupation-Based Practice	• Develop an occupational profile using the AOTA occupational profile template (AOTA, 2020c) from a case scenario provided. ***(Active Learning)*** • Identify a client's roles, routines, and rituals that influence occupational engagement from a case scenario or situation developed in a live or asynchronous simulation environment. ***(Active Learning)***
Client-Centered Practice	• Video an interaction with a simulated client, and reflect on body language, tone, and approach. ***(Reflection)*** • Watch a video on a client and practitioner interaction. Identify client-centered behaviors the practitioner utilizes or could improve upon. ***(Active Learning)***
Evidence-Based Practice	• Review nonstandardized and standardized tools that are used for a given site (pediatric vs. adult). ***(Active Learning)*** • Facilitate a "flipped classroom," assign students in small groups with each individual student assigned a common cognitive screen used in a pediatric, adult, or older adult fieldwork setting with having the students teach each other the background, administration steps, and scoring elements of the screen. ***(Active Learning)*** • Role play the implementation of one of the screens with one student being the therapist and one student being the client. ***(Active Learning and Modeling)***
Ethical Practice	• Identify potential billing codes for a case scenario, as well as the collaborating ethical considerations in the use of those codes. ***(Active Learning)*** • After participating in a live or asynchronous simulated case, students apply the ethical principles that were supported and/or challenged in the session, as well as possible solutions for addressing challenges that arose. ***(Active Learning and Modeling)***
Culturally Relevant Practice	• Reflect and identify cultural considerations that facilitate and inhibit occupational engagement. ***(Reflection)*** • After individual participation in a live or asynchronous simulation experience, have students complete a small discussion, sharing each of their experiences surrounding cultural considerations within their assigned client. ***(Reflection and Modeling)***

Table 3-5

Applying Best Practice With Standardized Patients

Occupation-Based Practice	• Develop an occupational profile using the AOTA occupational profile template (AOTA, 2020c). ***(Active Learning)***
	• Identify three occupations for a client, based on the occupational profile, that may be a focus for intervention. ***(Active Learning)***
	• Identify appropriate methods to analyze a client's occupational performance. ***(Active Learning)***
Client-Centered Practice	• Identify an inevitable interpersonal event that occurred and analyze using the intentional relationship model (Taylor, 2020). ***(Reflection)***
	• Reflect on client interactions and identify actions that demonstrate client-centered practice. ***(Reflection)***
Evidence-Based Practice	• Identify and administer a standardized functional-, cognitive-, or psychosocial-based screen or assessment that matches the presentation of the client. ***(Active Learning)***
	• Identify the reliability and validity considerations when using this tool. What are the strengths and weaknesses of the tool as well as appropriate application? ***(Active Learning)***
Ethical Practice	• Identify the ethical considerations that the client's health care team needs to consider with the given scenario provided in class or with community partners. ***(Reflection and Active Learning)***
	• Articulate elements of the AOTA Code of Ethics that you demonstrated in your session with the client and role play how you approached the situation. ***(Modeling)***
	• Describe how beneficence can be ensured during therapy sessions. How did you demonstrate this with your client? ***(Modeling)***
Culturally Relevant Practice	• While completing the occupational profile, highlight cultural considerations and how they will impact goal setting with the client. ***(Active Learning)***
	• Reflect on cultural knowns identified in your assessment and do a secondary analysis of those unknowns. ***(Active Learning)***

TABLE 3-6

APPLYING BEST PRACTICE WITHIN A FACULTY PRACTICE

Occupation-Based Practice	• Develop an occupational profile using the AOTA occupational profile template (AOTA, 2020c). *(Active Learning)* • Identify two to three occupational challenges for a client. *(Active Learning)* • Develop one long-term and one to two short-term goals for a client, being focused on meaningful occupations identified by the client. *(Active Learning)*
Client-Centered Practice	• Observe a FWed complete an evaluation. Then reflect on the session and record examples of how the FWed demonstrated client-centered practice. *(Reflection)* • Collaborate with a client to establish goals. *(Active Learning)*
Evidence-Based Practice	• Conduct literature search on best practice for a particular client population. *(Active Learning)* • Model or role play how you will approach and describe to the client implementation of an intervention that is supported in the evidence you found for a population or a client's given diagnoses. *(Modeling)*
Ethical Practice	• Conduct a literature search exploring an example of an ethical dilemma that may be experienced in the fieldwork setting. *(Active Learning)* • Facilitate a discussion board or in class discussion, having each student in small groups read an article on ethics and share ethical considerations they experienced or observed onsite. *(Modeling and Reflection)*
Culturally Relevant Practice	• Describe the cultural considerations of the clientele or population you are observing or assisting with your faculty mentor and/or community partner. *(Active Learning)* • Articulate the cultural considerations of the clientele, and how those considerations should be considered in the evaluation and plan of care. *(Active Learning and Modeling)*

TABLE 3-7

APPLYING BEST PRACTICE WITH FACULTY-LED SITE VISITS

Occupation-Based Practice	• Develop an occupational profile using the AOTA occupational profile template (AOTA, 2020c). *(Active Learning)* • Explore possible resources within the therapy space that can be used to provide occupation-based services. *(Active Learning)* • Identify and provide rationale for three occupation-based interventions for a client. Role play the discussion with a peer being the client and how you will facilitate the conversation regarding the plan of care development with the three interventions. *(Active Learning and Modeling)*
Client-Centered Practice	• Develop an occupational profile. *(Active Learning)* • Discuss a situation of working with a difficult client and strategies to maintain therapeutic rapport. *(Reflection)*
Evidence-Based Practice	• Identify and review the standardized tools, such as screens and assessments used at the site. Ask to observe your educator and/or role play with your educator one of the screens or assessment tools you reviewed. *(Active Learning and Modeling)* • Conduct literature search on commonly used interventions noted at the fieldwork site and share one finding with your FWed. *(Active Learning)*
Ethical Practice	• Identify and analyze an ethical dilemma experienced during fieldwork. *(Reflection)* • Process through the decision-making process using an ethical framework. *(Active Learning)* *see Appendix E for an example of an ethical framework*
Culturally Relevant Practice	• Identify the cultural considerations of the fieldwork site or community partner where you are completing your Level I placement. *(Active Learning)* • Articulate the cultural considerations of the clientele or populations you are observing or assisting during your Level I fieldwork placement. Consider how your educator fostered cultural considerations during the occupational therapy session. *(Active Learning and Reflection)*

TABLE 3-8

APPLYING BEST PRACTICE AT A FIELDWORK SITE

Occupation-Based Practice	• Develop an occupational profile for a given client you may encounter with your FWed. (AOTA, 2020c). *(Active Learning)*
	• Explore possible resources within the therapy space that can be used to provide occupation-based services. *(Active Learning)*
	• Reflect on frequently used interventions that are not occupation-based and consider alternative occupation-based interventions. *(Reflection)*
Client-Centered Practice	• Develop an occupational profile on a given client you may observe with a FWed. *(Active Learning)*
	• Journal on client-centered behaviors or routines the educator used when providing occupational therapy services to a client. *(Reflection)*
Evidence-Based Practice	• Select and review standardized screen or assessment frequently used at the fieldwork site. *(Active Learning)*
	• Identify an intervention observed in the clinic and search the literature for support of this intervention on the condition and goals of the client. *(Active Learning)*
Ethical Practice	• Reflect ethical considerations experienced during fieldwork and apply what AOTA Code of Ethics principles apply to the identified scenarios (e.g., discussion board, journaling). *(Active Learning)*
Culturally Relevant Practice	• Identify the client's social determinants of health and identify methods that may remove barriers to facilitate occupational engagement. *(Active Learning)*
	• Reflect on cultural routines at the site that support occupational therapy roles and responsibilities. *(Reflection)*
	• Identify a cultural aspect of a client that may be unfamiliar or unknown and research the background and application of your role to support the cultural aspects. *(Active Learning)*

Box 3-12

COLLABORATION AND SUPPORT FOR FIELDWORK PARTNERS

- Provide free live educational webinars on varying topics. Record them and post on a website for others to view asynchronously when convenient for them.
- Provide educational resources (in varying formats) on best practice principles.
- Create a Level I fieldwork assignment requiring students to share a new occupation-based assessment tool appropriate for the client population at the fieldwork site.
- Share a collection of stories in a newsletter (or other format) from across fieldwork sites, illustrating the best practice principles in action.
- Create awards that reflect best practice principles and encourage students (based on their experiences) to nominate fieldwork partners that demonstrate best practice principles during their Level I fieldwork. Several different types of awards can be created.
- Provide access to academic library resources for fieldwork partners to encourage EBP.
- Provide a webinar on how to use the academic library resources and incorporate evidence into practice.
- Create Level I fieldwork assignments requiring students to create an occupation-based kit for the fieldwork site.

REFERENCES

Accreditation Council for Occupational Therapy Education. (2018). *Accreditation council for occupational therapy education standards and interpretive guide.* https://www.aota.org/~/media/Corporate/Files/EducationCareers/Accredit/StandardsReview/2018-ACOTE-Standards-Interpretive-Guide.pdf

Ahn, J. N., Hu, D., & Vega, M. (2020). "Do as I do, not as I say": Using social learning theory to unpack the impact of role models on students' outcomes in education. *Social and Personality Psychology Compass, 14*(2), e12517. https://doi.org/10.1111/spc3.12517

American Occupational Therapy Association. (2020a). Occupational therapy practice framework: Domain and process–fourth edition. *American Journal of Occupational Therapy, 74*(Suppl. 2), 7412410010. https://doi.org/10.5014/ajot.2020.74S2001

American Occupational Therapy Association. (2020b). AOTA 2020 occupational therapy code of ethics. *American Journal of Occupational Therapy, 74*(Suppl. 3), 7413410005. https://doi.org/10.5014/ajot.2020.74S3006

American Occupational Therapy Association. (2020c). *Improve your documentation with AOTA's updated occupational profile template.* https://www.aota.org/Practice/Manage/Reimb/occupational-profile-document-value-ot.aspx

Ashby, S. E., Ryan, S., Gray, M., & James, C. (2013). Factors that influence the professional resilience of occupational therapists in mental health practice. *Australian Occupational Therapy Journal, 60*(2), 110-119. http://dx.doi.org/10.1111/1440-1630.12012

Black, R. M. (2019). Culture, diversity, and culturally effective care. In B. A. B. Schell & G. Gillen (Eds.), *Willard & Spackman's occupational therapy* (13th ed., pp. 223-239). Wolters Kluwer.

Black, R. M., & Wells, S. A. (2007). *Culture and occupation: A model of empowerment in occupational therapy.* AOTA Press.

Botelho, M., & Bhuyan, S. Y. (2020). Reflection before and after clinical practice–enhancing and broadening experience through self-, peer-, and teacher-guided learning. *European Journal of Dental Education, 25*(3), 480-487. https://doi.org/10.1111/eje.12623

Boyt Schell, B. A., Gillen, G., & Coppola, S. (2019). In Boyt Schell, B. A., & Gillen, G. (Eds.), *Willard and Spackman's Occupational Therapy* (13th ed., pp. 513-526).

Di Tommaso, A., Isbel, S., Scarvell, J., & Wicks, A. (2016). Occupational therapists' perceptions of occupation in practice: An exploratory study. *Australian Occupational Therapy Journal, 63*(3), 206-213, http://doi.org/10.1111/1440-1630.12289

Doherty, R. F. (2019). Ethical practice. In Boyt Schell, B. A., & Gillen, G. (Eds.), *Willard and Spackman's Occupational Therapy* (13th ed., pp. 513-526).

Estes, J. & Pierce, D. E. (2012). Pediatric therapists' perspectives on occupation-based practice. *Scandinavian Journal of Occupational Therapy, 19*(1), 17-25. http://doi.org/10.3109/11038128.2010.547598

Fisher, A. G., & Marterella, A. (2019). Powerful practice: A model for authentic occupational therapy. *Occupational Therapy in Health Care.*

Freeman, S., Leddy, S. L., McDonough, M., Smith, M. K., Okoroafor, N., Jordt, H., & Wenderoth, M. P. (2014). Active learning increases student performance in science, engineering, and mathematics. *Proceedings of the National Academy of Sciences in the United States of America, 111*(23), 8410-8415. https://doi.org/10.1073/pnas.1319030111

Getty, S. M. (2016). Assessing culture's impact on occupation. *SIS Quarterly Practice Connections, 1*(3), 15-17.

Gupta, J., & Taff, S. D. (2015). The illusion of client-centered practice. *Scandinavian Journal of Occupational Therapy, 22*(4), 244-251. http://doi.org/10.3109/11038128.2015.1020866

Jonassen, D. H. (1999). Designing constructivist learning environments. In C. M. Reigeluth (Ed.), *Instructional design theories and models: A new paradigm of instructional theory* (pp. 217-239). Lawrence Erlbaum.

Korner, M., & Modell, E. (2009). A model of shared decision-making in medical rehabilitation. *Rehabilitation, 48*(3), 160-165. https://doi.org/10.1055/s-0029-1220748

Law, M., Baptiste, S., & Mills, J. (1995). Client-centered practice: What does it mean, and does it make a difference? *Canadian Journal of Occupational Therapy, 62*(5), 250-257. https://doi.org/10.1177/000841749506200504

Law, M., & MacDermid, J. C. (2014). Introduction to evidence-based practice. In M. Law & J. C. MacDermid (Eds.), *Evidence-based rehabilitation: A guide to practice* (3rd ed.). SLACK Incorporated.

Mroz, T. M., Pitonyak, J. S., Fogelberg, D., & Leland, N. E. (2015). Client centeredness and health reform: Key issues for occupational therapy. *American Journal of Occupational Therapy, 69*(5), 6905090010. http://doi.org/10.5014/ajot.2015.695001

Plewnia, A., Bengel, J., & Korner, M. (2016). Patient-centeredness and its impact on patient satisfaction and treatment outcomes in medical rehabilitation. *Patient Education and Counseling, 99*(12), 2063-2070. http://doi.org/10.1016/j.pec.2016.07.018

Ripat, J., Wener, P., & Dobinson, K. (2013). The development of client-centeredness in student occupational therapists. *British Journal of Occupational Therapy, 76*(5), 217-224. https://doi.org/10.4276/030802213X13679275042681

Sandars, J. (2009). The use of reflection in medical education: AMEE Guide No. 44. *Medical Teacher, 31*, 685-695. https://doi.org/10.1080/01421590903050374

Sanders, D., & Welk, D. S. (2005). Strategies to scaffold student learning: Applying Vygotsky's zone of proximal development. *Nurse Educator, 30*(5), 203-207. https://doi.org/10.1097/00006223-200509000-00007

Schei, E., Fuks, A., & Bordreau, J. D. (2019). Reflection in medical education: Intellectual humility, discovery, and know-how. *Medicine, Health Care, and Philosophy, 22*(2), 167-178. https://doi.org/10.1007/s11019-018-9878-2

Stube, J. E., & Jedlicka, J. S. (2007). The acquisition and integration of evidence-based practice concepts by occupational therapy students. *American Journal of Occupational Therapy, 61*, 53-61.

Sumsion, T., & Law, M. (2006). A review of the evidence on the conceptual elements informing client-centered practice. *Canadian Journal of Occupational Therapy, 73*(3), 153-162. https://doi.org/10.1177/000841740607300303

Taylor, R. R. (2020). *The intentional relationship: Occupational therapy and use of self* (2nd ed.). F. A. Davis.

Towns, E., & Ashby, S. (2014). The influence of practice educators on occupational therapy students' understanding of the practical applications of theoretical knowledge: A phenomenological study into student experiences of practice education. *Australian Occupational Therapy Journal, 61*(5), 344-352. https://doi.org/10.1111/1440-1630.12134

Wilkinson, S. A., Hinchliffe, F., Hough, J., & Chang, A. (2012). Baseline evidence-based practice use, knowledge, and attitudes of allied health professionals: A survey to inform staff training and organisational change. *Journal of Allied Health, 41*(4), 177-184.

Winkel, A. F., Yingling, S., Jones, A. A., & Nicholson, J. (2017). Reflection as a learning tool in graduate medical education: A systematic review. *Journal of Graduate Medical Education, 9*(4), 430-439. https://doi.org/10.4300/JGME-D-16-00500.1

World Federation of Occupational Therapists. (2010). *Position statement: Diversity and culture.* https://www.wfot.org/resources/diversity-and-culture

Yazdani, F., Stringer, A., Nobakht, L., Bonsaksen, T., & Tune, K. (2020). Qualitative analysis of occupational therapists' reflective notes on practicing their skills in building and maintaining therapeutic relationships. *Journal of Occupational Therapy Education, 4*(4). https://doi.org/10.26681/jote.2020.040414

Zimmerman, L., Michaelis, M., Quaschning, K., Muller, C., & Korner, M. (2014). The significance of internal and external participation for patient satisfaction. *Rehabilitation, 53*, 219-224. https://doi.org/10.1055/s-0033-1357116

Appendix A: Application of Modeling the Practice Principles

BEST PRACTICE PRINCIPLE	APPLICATION
Occupation Based	Incorporate use of occupation into client evaluation and/or intervention. For example, instead of using TheraBand (TheraBand) exercises for upper extremity strengthening, engage a client in a more meaningful occupation, such as laundry, working in the kitchen, or gardening.
Client Centered	Initiate discussion with client and/or family about their goals for occupational therapy and what goals are of greatest priority.
Evidence Based	Role play a conversation with a peer or AFWC prior to discussing with the FWed on the use of evidence and/or resources in practice.
Ethical	Present an ethical case scenario or current situation that challenges the AOTA Code of Ethics principles and values and articulate active solutions that provide perspective from the client, practitioner, and environment standpoint.
Culturally Relevant	Demonstrate how practitioners facilitate asking culturally relevant questions and respectful responses during the evaluation process in a respectful and safe manner. Show the student how you incorporated cultural considerations in your session.

Appendix B: Application of Active Learning to Practice Principles

BEST PRACTICE PRINCIPLE	APPLICATION
Occupation Based	Instruct students to create three occupation-based intervention ideas for a specific client and gather all resources needed to implement the interventions. Allow students to complete the intervention session with supervision.
Client Centered	Ask students to prepare to complete an occupational profile on a new client. To prepare for the session, instruct students to create a list of questions needed to ensure the plan of care created is client centered. Allow students to complete the occupational profile interview with supervision.
Evidence Based	Ask students to prepare to complete an intervention session for a client that is on the schedule for the next day. Instruct the student to find current literature to support the selected intervention. Allow students to complete the intervention session with supervision.
Ethical	Display the AOTA Code of Ethics in the practice environment and have the student identify and apply the principles that support the intervention the student chose for a given session. Provide examples from your own caseload to actively show students how the principles are used.
Culturally Relevant	During preparation for a new evaluation, have the student articulate the cultural considerations of the assigned client specific to cultural considerations, cultural unknowns, and next steps to understanding the cultural considerations of the client.

Evidence-Based Practice Active Learning: Review of Standardized Screen or Assessment

Directions: Review and analyze a standardized screen or assessment that is used in your Level I practice setting. Complete the following questions to guide you on the application to practice.

Practice setting	
Name of screen or assessment	
Date of publication	
Intended population	
• Diagnoses/conditions	
• Ages	
• Gender	
• Ethnicity/race	

Reliability • Test-retest • Inter-rater	
Validity • Construct • Content • Face	
Administration • Time to complete • Intended environment • Supply/equipment setup	
Scoring considerations • Sub-task score • Total score	
Interpretation considerations • Meaning of the score (ranges, rankings, etc.)	
Additional considerations/notes	

Other considerations:

  1. **Strengths of the screen or tool:**

  2. **Limitations of the screen or tool:**

  3. **What are cultural considerations when using this tool in practice?**

  4. **What are ethical considerations when using this tool in practice?**

  5. **How is this tool used in the practice setting?**

Appendix C: Application of Reflection to Practice Principles

BEST PRACTICE PRINCIPLE	APPLICATION
Occupation Based	Following a day of fieldwork, instruct the student to reflect on three clients that were seen that day. Reflection prompts could include (1) identify the client's reason for therapy, (2) problem areas observed, (3) interventions that were completed during the session, (4) strengths/challenges with the interventions that were used, and (5) identify three occupation-based interventions that would be appropriate for each of the clients identified.
Client Centered	Instruct students to journal about strategies that were utilized to ensure client-centered practice was provided. Identify both supports and barriers to client-centered practice, as well as strategies to overcome the identified barriers.
Evidence Based	Instruct students to reflect on and write down the approximate schedule and daily activities occurring during the Level I fieldwork experience. After writing down the daily activities, students will highlight specific areas in which EBP was evident or opportunities in which EBP could have been implemented. Identify barriers to EBP and strategies to overcome identified barriers.
Ethical	Facilitate a discussion board regarding ethical considerations for practice specific to considerations in practice that support beneficence, nonmaleficence, and veracity. Have the students articulate how they will uphold these values and their plan to continue to ensure ethical practice while in the field.
Culturally Relevant	Foster reflective journaling on current or potential cultural scenarios that occurred (or may occur) in practice, as well as the actions and behaviors to support growth with cultural considerations.

Appendix D: Scaffolding Student Reflection

LEVEL OF LEARNER	SITUATION	STRATEGY
Student at beginning of coursework	Student peer group meeting with fieldwork participant for the first time focusing on establishing rapport.	Prior to session, student peer group meets to plan therapy session targeting methods to establish rapport with fieldwork participant. Student peer group presents plan to FWed. *(Anticipatory Reflection)* After session, FWed debriefs with student peer group and asks questions such as "What went well?", "What did not go well?", and "What will you do differently next time?" *(Reflection on Action)*
Student halfway through coursework	FWed asks student peer group to plan and implement a client therapy session for the next day.	Prior to session, student peer group meets to plan therapy session including goal that is targeted, three intervention ideas, rationale for ideas, and strategies to grade intervention ideas. Student peer group reviews plan with FWed. *(Anticipatory Reflection)* During session, FWed poses questions to facilitate student critical thinking. *(Reflection in Action)* After session, FWed debriefs with student peer group and asks questions such as "What went well?", "What did not go well?", and "What will you do differently next time?" *(Reflection on Action)*
Student in last semester of coursework	Student independently facilitates occupational therapy group.	Prior to session, student plans the therapy group session. *(Anticipatory Reflection)* While clients are working on group activity, student writes down quick reflections on how group session has gone so far. *(Reflection in Action)* After session, FWed debriefs with student and asks questions such as "What went well?", "What did not go well?", and "What will you do differently next time?" *(Reflection on Action)*

Appendix E: Ethical Decision-Making Map

ETHICAL DECISION-MAKING MAP		
1. ISSUE	**2. PERSPECTIVES OF THOSE INVOLVED**	**3. LOCUS OF DECISION**
What is the situation or dilemma? (Outline briefly) □ Basic medical problem □ Medical indications for treatment □ What decision needs to be made? □ What are the patient/family preferences? □ What are the preferences of healthcare providers?	***Patient's/family's concerns*** □ Adequate disclosure □ Capacity to choose □ Ability to refuse therapy □ Coercion, duress or abandonment □ Advanced directives □ Surrogate decision makers □ Patient health vs family finances □ Religion, values & culture	***Who has authority to act?*** □ Does physician have authority to force care on the patient? □ Does patient have authority to refuse or demand care? □ Does family have authority to refuse or demand care? □ Does authority lie with other agent?
Who does what to whom and under what circumstances? □ Who is involved in the situation? □ What actions are planned? □ What information is being given & withheld? □ Who will experience consequences? □ How will the decision be achieved?	***The Healthcare Providers= concerns*** □ Professional codes □ Standard of care □ Awareness of community norms □ Trust and professional reputation □ Diagnosis & prognosis □ Goals of therapy □ Efficacy/inefficacy □ Futility/utility □ Loyalty issues □ Communication with family/pt □ Institutional concerns & financial constraints	***How was the decision actually made in terms of power?*** (who makes decisions?) □ Doctor □ Family □ Patient □ Nurse □ Administration □ Other
Is there a conflict of values? □ Between healthcare provider and patient/family □ Among healthcare providers □ Between healthcare provider(s) and organization □ Between the family and patient □ Between patient and 3rd party payer	***Contextual/systemic, & quality of life issues*** □ Relevance of benefits, harms and rights of others □ Interests of others □ Protection of others □ Cost of care □ Allocation of resources □ Legal obligations □ Effects on community and the medical practice relations? □ Life expectancy □ Potential for disability & suffering	***What ethical principles inform the situation?*** (Examples) *Autonomy:* □ Does the patient have the right to refuse care? □ Is the patient informed enough to accept/refuse care? *Competency:* □ Does the patient/family understand the diagnosis and treatment? *Truth-telling* □ How much information should the healthcare providers provide? □ Does the family have a right to know? *Harm:* □ Will not telling cause harm? □ Will telling cause harm? □ Will forcing care cause harm? □ Will not forcing care cause harm?

ETHICAL DECISION-MAKING MAP		
1. ISSUE	2. PERSPECTIVES OF THOSE INVOLVED	3. LOCUS OF DECISION
What is the situation or dilemma? (ethical principles) (Outline briefly)	*Patient's/family's concerns*	*Who has authority to act?*
Who does what to whom and under what circumstances?	*The Healthcare Providers= concerns*	*How was the decision actually made in terms of power?* (who makes decisions?)
Is there a conflict of values?	*Contextual/systemic, & quality of life issues*	*What ethical principles inform the situation?*

1. What are my ethical concerns (see the ethical decision making map)?

2. Identify the core values(s) and attitude(s):

3. What organizational policies and professional guidelines should I consider?

4. How can I include other people, with different perspectives and diverse ideas, in the decision-making process?

5. Am I treating this person differently than I would treat anyone else in this circumstance and is this a difference of values/beliefs or a valid concern (illegal, unsafe etc..)?

6. What if the roles were reversed? How would I feel if I were in the shoes of one of the clients/colleagues?

7. What are the possible consequences of my actions? Short term? Long term?

8. Can I clearly and fully justify my thinking and my decision? To my colleagues? To the stakeholders? To the public?

Reproduced with permission from Cook, Ann F & Hoas, Helenda. (2000). National Rural Bioethics Project. Available at: https://www.umt.edu/bioethics/. Accessed 9/22/2021.

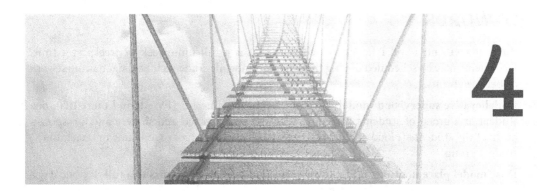

Context Matters
Application of Learning Frameworks in Context

Jaynee Taguchi Meyer, OTD, OTR/L; Becki Cohill, OTD, OTR/L;
and Lacey Spark, OTD, MOT, OTR

In the first three chapters, you have learned broadly about Level I fieldwork, frameworks for experiential learning, and best practices for Level I fieldwork. This chapter focuses on *contextual considerations* when designing Level I fieldwork learning experiences. The Accreditation Council for Occupational Therapy Education (ACOTE) standard C.1.9 enables academic programs to expand Level I fieldwork beyond established practice environments with and without occupational therapists to include faculty-led and faculty practice experiences, simulated environments, and standardized patients (ACOTE, 2018). This sets the stage for consideration of the many contextual elements that influence the student's learning experience on Level I fieldwork. The supervision structure, nature of the clientele, and contextual elements of the service delivery, as well as the curriculum model of the academic program, are expected to influence the Level I learning structure. Differences and similarities will be explored between the role emerging and established practice fieldwork structure. Temporal, environmental, and telehealth contexts will be considered. Student participation and supervisory models will also be discussed.

Hanson, D., & DeIuliis, E. D. (Eds.).
Fieldwork Educator's Guide to Level I Fieldwork (pp. 75-106).
© 2023 Taylor and Francis Group.

KEY WORDS

- **Block placement:** Level I fieldwork schedule that is a full-time week or weeks at a time. Placements may be scheduled during the school term while students take didactic coursework or between terms.

- **Collaborative supervision model:** Uses one fieldwork educator (FWed) and more than one student or a group of students. Learning is active, self-initiated and shared, and a responsibility of the students (Flood et al., 2010) with the FWed serving as facilitator or coach to the student group.

- **Dose model placement:** Level I fieldwork schedule that is a few hours to a full day one day a week or more but less than a full-time week, over several weeks or over the course of a semester/term.

- **Established practice fieldwork:** Practices in which occupational therapy service provision already exists. Some think of this as "traditional" Level I fieldwork.

- **Faculty-led site visits:** "Faculty-facilitated experiences in which students will be able to participate in, observe, and/or study clinical practice first-hand" (ACOTE, 2018, p. S75).

- **Role-emerging fieldwork:** Fieldwork in settings where no occupational therapy services exist. There is potential for occupational therapy services and for student learning experiences. Some think of this as "nontraditional" Level I fieldwork.

- **Same-site model:** Students complete Level I and Level II fieldwork at the same fieldwork site (Evenson et al., 2002).

- **Simulated environment:** "A setting that provides an experience similar to a real world setting in order to allow clients to practice specific occupations (e.g., driving simulation center, bathroom, or kitchen centers in a rehabilitation unit, work hardening units, or centers)" (ACOTE, 2018, p. S53).

- **Standardized patient simulation:** A simulation is where "an individual has been trained to portray, in a consistent, standardized manner, a patient/client with occupational needs" (ACOTE, 2018, p. S54).

- **Telehealth:** "The application of evaluative, consultative, preventative, and therapeutic services delivered through information and communication technology" (AOTA, 2018b, p. S81).

LEARNING OBJECTIVES

By the end of reading this chapter and completing the learning activities, the reader should be able to:

1. Describe the types of Level I fieldwork that meet the ACOTE standards.
2. Consider the types of contexts/settings where Level I fieldwork might occur.
3. Compare and contrast the contextual variables evident across types of Level I fieldwork.
4. Appreciate the impact of the chosen supervision model on student learning across Level I fieldwork types.
5. Understand the impact of curriculum design on Level I fieldwork format.
6. Identify special considerations for Level I fieldwork that occur in simulated or virtual contexts.

7. (Academic fieldwork coordinator [AFWC] and FWed) Apply knowledge of contextual variables in Level I fieldwork to determine a fieldwork type that is a best fit for your practice or academic setting and steps you would take to prepare for this type of placement.

8. (Student) Identify strategies for preparation for Level I fieldwork that are particularly suited to each Level I fieldwork type.

LEVEL I FIELDWORK TYPES AND SETTINGS

Although still regulated by ACOTE, the requirements and inherent structure of Level I fieldwork differs from Level II fieldwork. An overview of the types and settings commonly used for Level I fieldwork will be provided to give the reader a foundation for further Level I fieldwork development.

Level I Fieldwork in Established Practice

"The goal of Level I fieldwork is to introduce students to fieldwork, apply knowledge to practice, and develop understanding of the needs of clients" (ACOTE, 2018, p. S63). This goal is broad and allows for Level I fieldwork to occur in facilities with and without occupational therapy practitioners supervising them. The majority of Level I fieldwork experiences occur in established occupational therapy practices with an occupational therapist supervising the students. Johnson et al. (2006) found that 82% of Level I fieldwork experiences were supervised by an occupational therapist, and 2.5% were supervised by an occupational therapy assistant. Level I fieldwork experiences historically occurred in acute medical and psychiatric hospitals and schools (Shalik, 1990). Today, Level I fieldwork settings have expanded to include not only acute medical and psychiatric hospitals and schools but also inpatient and outpatient physical rehabilitation, home health, skilled nursing facilities, hand therapy practices, community-based mental health, and pediatric clinics and hospitals.

Accreditation standards allow other credentialed and/or licensed professionals to supervise Level I students, including physical therapists, nurses, teachers, psychologists, social workers, physician assistants, and others. FWeds, who are not occupational therapists, are required to have a good understanding about the profession and the learning objectives for the Level I fieldwork experience (ACOTE, 2018). Level I fieldwork experiences without occupational therapy practitioner supervision may occur in a very broad range of settings including, but not limited to, sheltered workshops, homeless shelters, child care centers, adult day care centers, etc. Though supervision by an occupational therapist is not required, students prefer and value Level I fieldwork experiences supervised by an occupational therapist more highly than those without an occupational therapist (Johnson et al., 2006; Box 4-1).

Faculty-Led Site Visits and Faculty Practice

ACOTE defines faculty led site visits as "Faculty-facilitated experiences in which students will be able to participate in, observe, and/or study clinical practice first-hand" (ACOTE, 2018, p. S75). Faculty practice is defined as "Service provision by a faculty member(s) to persons, groups, and/or populations" (AOTA, 2018a, p. S75). These broad definitions and newly included types of Level I fieldwork encourage academic programs to utilize occupational therapy faculty including AFWCs to supervise Level I fieldwork students in practice settings as part of their faculty roles. Experiences may be attached to practice-based didactic coursework in occupational therapy or occupational therapy assistant programs and could include campus-based probono onsite clinics

---

Box 4-1

AN AFWC'S PERSPECTIVE: SENDING STUDENTS TO LEVEL I FIELDWORK SETTINGS WITHOUT OCCUPATIONAL THERAPY PRACTITIONERS ONSITE

An AFWC from an occupational therapy assistant program shared her experience sending students to sites without occupational therapy practitioners onsite. "It's not really about watching an occupational therapist do occupational therapy. It's about getting to know clients and being able to identify deficits, [and] applying concepts learned in class." She continued, "A lot of times, even if you're with an occupational therapist, they don't have a lot of time … sometimes not having an occupational therapy or occupational therapy assistant there helps students get a wider range of experience." She said that in sites where occupational therapy was not already established, students were able to think very creatively and develop groups and individual interventions that are perhaps free of constraints of established practice. "When they first get there, they're really forced to put themselves out there more" (J. Padilla, personal communication, August 17, 2021).

(Erdman et al., 2020), student-run probono clinics (Kent et al., 2014; Lie et al., 2016; Seif et al., 2014, and role-emerging practice settings in the community (Brown & Mohler, 2020; Keptner & Klein, 2019; Mattila et al., 2018). Faculty may always be onsite with Level I students or part of the time, and supervision may be shared with professional staff at the facility (Box 4-2). Some academic programs hire occupational therapy practitioners as adjunct faculty exclusively to provide supervision for Level I students.

Oftentimes these experiences occur in emerging practice settings where faculty are occupational therapy consultants or direct service providers. Clark et al. (2019) posited that faculty-led fieldwork experience "closes a gap between academia and clinical practice by providing early carryover of classroom lectures and labs to real clients" (p. 26; Box 4-3).

Faculty knows students well and may be able to better individualize and tailor learning experiences for students. Johnson et al. (2006) found 19% of Level I fieldwork was provided in emerging practice contexts including senior centers, assisted living, sheltered workshops, services for homeless individuals, after school programs, and international settings.

Simulated Environments

As defined by ACOTE (2018), simulated environments are "a setting that provides an experience similar to a real world setting in order to allow clients to practice specific occupations (e.g., driving simulation center, bathroom, or kitchen centers in a rehabilitation unit, work hardening units or centers)" (p. S53). Simply put, simulated environment fieldwork experiences take place in an environment that is not a clinic setting but is meant to mimic a clinic or real world setting. In the same way that inpatient rehabilitation occupational therapists may train a patient in the simulated environment of the therapy kitchen in preparation for going home to prepare a meal, simulated environments in fieldwork are meant to allow students to practice in an environment that will be similar to environments they will encounter in Level II fieldwork and in clinical practice. Further identified in the literature, simulated environments can either be physical or virtual in context (DeIuliis et al., 2021; Mattila et al., 2020). Examples of physical contexts could include work hardening units, simulation centers that are built and set up to look like an inpatient ward of a hospital, or a classroom that has been transformed to look like an outpatient pediatric clinic with equipment and environmental setup. The virtual simulated environment could include the

---

BOX 4-2

AN ACADEMIC PROGRAM'S STRUCTURE OF FACULTY-LED COMMUNITY-BASED LEVEL I FIELDWORK

The academic program prepares students for these emerging practice fieldwork assignments by prebriefing to prepare them. Faculty facilitation during Level I fieldwork was onsite part of the time. Virtual facilitation in groups helped students process what they were seeing and how they felt about it. Students discussed what they would do at the site if they were occupational therapists. Faculty brainstormed with the students about how they could turn an interview "into a mini-evaluation," for example. Structured assignments supported student participation, reflection, and achievement of learning objectives (A. McNeil, MA, OTR/L, personal communication, August 20, 2021).

BOX 4-3

FACULTY FWED'S PERSPECTIVE: FACILITATING FACULTY-LED LEVEL I FIELDWORK

Jerilyn Callen, OTD, OTR, is a faculty educator who has experience facilitating faculty-led fieldwork in both community mental health and older adult living communities. When speaking on faculty-led fieldwork, Jerilyn states that it gives faculty an "ability to match the client, experience, and debriefing conversations to the specific learning objective that you are trying to meet." Additionally, she goes on to explain that she "really enjoys being able to support students who might be struggling before they have an opportunity to fail. You can build in supports for students as faculty that you can't when they are out with a practitioner" (J. Callen, OTD, OTR, personal communication, August 28, 2021).

---

use of a driving simulator, virtual reality, or computer-based programs and software that virtually place the student in different clinical environments and situations in which they must problem solve their way through.

Standardized Patients

Using standardized patients to fulfill Level I fieldwork requirements involves training people to act out a clinical case in a standardized way (ACOTE, 2018). In this type of simulated fieldwork experience, the developers of the simulation would design the scenario, case information, learning objectives, and possible actor responses within the scenario, as well as guides for the debriefing with the students afterward. A standardized patient simulation can occur in a simulated environment, over telehealth, or in a clinical setting as long as the actor is trained to act in a standardized manner within the simulated scenario. Students would go into the session with the patient actor as if they were going into a real clinical setting and perform as outlined by the simulation design. The FWed, along with other students, observes the participating student in the scenario. Students and the FWed can observe from another room via a video stream, through one-way glass, or in the same room. After the scenario is complete, the FWed guides all the students through debriefing to discuss and expand on observations, critiques, praises, and topics to address and explore the simulation learning objectives (Bajaj et al., 2018).

LEVEL I FIELDWORK CONTEXTUAL VARIABLES ACROSS LEVEL I FIELDWORK TYPES

When determining what type of Level I fieldwork would work best for the students, community, and academic program, there are multiple contextual variables to consider. It is the AFWC's responsibility to oversee the fieldwork program, including the various contexts. AFWCs work collaboratively with fieldwork sites, faculty, and students to ensure that all fieldwork experiences enhance students' didactic education, include learning experiences that fulfill Level I fieldwork objectives, and meet accreditation standards. Table 4-1 outlines each Level I fieldwork experience type and what considerations would need to be explored for each type.

SUPERVISION MODELS IN LEVEL I FIELDWORK

Many different supervisory models are used in Level I fieldwork. The apprenticeship model, collaborative model, and same site models are briefly presented here. The reader is encouraged to seek additional information about other supervisory models, including multiple mentoring model (Copley & Nelson, 2012; Graves & Hanson, 2014), intraprofessional occupational therapy–occupational therapy assistant model (AOTA, 2018a; Costa et al., 2012; Jung et al., 2008), and international fieldwork placements (Cameron et al., 2013).

Evenson et al. (2015) surveyed more than 800 occupational therapy practitioners who were FWeds. Approximately 78% used a one-to-one apprenticeship supervisory model for occupational therapy students. For occupational therapy assistant students, a one occupational therapy assistant fieldwork educator on one occupational therapy assistant student model was used 33% of the time, while one occupational therapist fieldwork educator on one occupational therapy assistant student was used more often at 54% of the time (Evenson et al., 2015). This is a familiar model for many occupational therapy practitioners, as it was the model in which they were educated and trained in established practice sites. Students observe their supervising practitioner who is usually an occupational therapist or less frequently an occupational therapy assistant. Most Level I students are afforded some amount of hands-on participation during Level I fieldwork. In fact, ACOTE (2018) standards require that Level I fieldwork include "directed observation and participation in selected area aspects of the occupational therapy process" (p. S64). Keeping this standard in mind when planning Level I fieldwork experiences is critical to ensure the experience includes active participatory learning and does not rely solely on observation. Evenson et al. (2015) found that the two-to-one supervisory model (two students to one FWed) was used much less frequently than the one-to-one model (15% of occupational therapy students and 2% of occupational therapy assistant students). Other models were used with approximately 17% of occupational therapy students to 28% of occupational therapy assistant students (Evenson et al., 2015).

The growing number of emerging practice fieldwork placements use multiple student supervision models. Students assigned to Level I fieldwork in emerging practice settings are often assigned in pairs or groups (Brown & Mohler, 2020; Flood et al., 2010; Grenier, 2015; Hagen et al., 2019; Hanson & DeIuliis, 2015; Keptner & Klein, 2019) and learn from facility staff who are not occupational therapy practitioners, from other students, and from a faculty FWed, if involved. Grenier (2015) identified facilitators and barriers to learning in occupational therapy fieldwork education through a survey of students. Students expressed a preference for collaborative education models and interprofessional education models. Of the students surveyed, 12 of the 29 students experienced nontraditional fieldwork placements with multiple FWeds. Of these 12 students, 10 reported multiple students at the same site created an opportunity for collaborative learning, which allowed students to work as a team. Keptner and Klein (2019) described a collaborative learning model using peer-to-peer and faculty-led supervision with groups of students. Their study described a

TABLE 4-1

LEVEL I FIELDWORK CONTEXTUAL VARIABLES ACROSS LEVEL I FIELDWORK TYPES

	ESTABLISHED PRACTICE	FACULTY-LED SITE VISITS	FACULTY PRACTICE	SIMULATED ENVIRONMENTS	STANDARDIZED PATIENTS
General Definition	Students go to an established site with occupational therapy services established and a practitioner as the supervisor. Supervision takes place with an occupational therapy assistant, occupational therapist, or other licensed professional with an understanding of the occupational therapy profession	Faculty lead visits to a community site and act as a consultant and FWed in that setting. Supervision may be shared by professionals at the facility	Faculty-led campus affiliated or community clinic where community members/clients come to the clinic for groups, individual appointments, and/or educational programs	Fieldwork occurs in a simulated environment, either virtual or physical environments, with faculty as the FWed	Actors are trained to play a client in a scenario in which students engage and/or observe the interaction and are supervised by faculty
Supervision Considerations	Availability of practitioners willing and able to take Level I fieldwork students Less direct oversight by the academic program on the fieldwork experience	Time availability of faculty Direct oversight and facilitation of experience by academic program Ability to hire affiliated faculty to supervise fieldwork students in community site	Time availability of faculty Direct oversight and facilitation of experience by academic program in collaboration with community facility staff	Time availability of faculty Direct oversight and facilitation of experience by program Ability to hire affiliated or adjunct faculty to supervise fieldwork	Time availability of faculty Direct oversight and facilitation of experience by program Ability to hire affiliated or adjunct faculty to facilitate fieldwork

(continued)

TABLE 4-1 (CONTINUED)

LEVEL I FIELDWORK CONTEXTUAL VARIABLES ACROSS LEVEL I FIELDWORK TYPES

	ESTABLISHED PRACTICE	FACULTY-LED SITE VISITS	FACULTY PRACTICE	SIMULATED ENVIRONMENTS	STANDARDIZED PATIENTS
	Students have varied experiences, share, and learn from each other and reflect on different supervision styles	Training of faculty to supervise in this setting and meet Level I fieldwork objectives	Ability to hire affiliated or adjunct faculty to supervise fieldwork at community site Training of faculty to supervise in this setting and meet Level I fieldwork objectives	Training of faculty to supervise and debrief in this setting and meet Level I fieldwork objectives	Training of faculty to supervise and debrief in this setting and meet Level I fieldwork objectives
Supervision Model Used	One-to-one, two-to-one, one-to-two, same-site model, group supervision model	Two-to-one or group supervision model	Two-to-one or collaborative group supervision model, same-site model	Collaborative group supervision model	Collaborative group supervision model
Financial Considerations	Inherently no added costs to occupational therapy/occupational therapy assistant programs	Possible workload overages of faculty may lead to increased costs Extra staffing costs if additional faculty is hired	Possible workload overages of faculty may lead to increased costs Extra staffing costs if additional faculty is hired Marketing to recruit clients to receive services at the clinic Cost of materials and resources to run clinic	Possible workload overages of faculty may lead to increased costs Extra staffing costs if additional faculty is hired Both virtually or physically simulated environments require purchase and can be costly	Workload overages of faculty may lead to increased costs Extra staffing costs if additional faculty is hired Extra staffing costs if simulation technicians are needed and hired to help run program

(continued)

Table 4-1 (continued)

Level I Fieldwork Contextual Variables Across Level I Fieldwork Types

	ESTABLISHED PRACTICE	FACULTY-LED SITE VISITS	FACULTY PRACTICE	SIMULATED ENVIRONMENTS	STANDARDIZED PATIENTS
			Grants can help finance on campus or community clinics Working with community clinic (when applicable) on scheduling and staffing	Grants can help programs build or purchase simulated environments	Actors may need to be paid or use contracts Grants can help programs build standardized patient programs
Environmental/Site Considerations	Students travel to sites— could be a considerable distance Need staff buy-in to have students Workspace, if possible, for students Capacity to take one or more students at scheduled times Ability to accommodate block, dose, or both models of scheduling Sites may become overwhelmed with taking students	Students travel to sites— could be a considerable distance Site must be willing and able to take groups of students with the faculty supervisor or a student who is supervised by a licensed professional at the site with oversight by faculty Students exposed to real world environments and practice settings	No added driving requirements for students (if on campus or telehealth) Students travel to sites— could be a considerable distance (to community clinic) Physical space needed to run clinic if not run via telehealth or at the community clinic	No added driving requirements for students Physical space needed if a physically simulated environment Computers, internet, and software needed for virtually simulated environment Additional headsets needed if using virtual reality technology	No added driving requirements for students Can take place in classroom, lab, simulation space, someone's home, or via telehealth If students are in groups and observing interactions, important to have setup where all students can see

(continued)

TABLE 4-1 (CONTINUED)

LEVEL I FIELDWORK CONTEXTUAL VARIABLES ACROSS LEVEL I FIELDWORK TYPES

	ESTABLISHED PRACTICE	FACULTY-LED SITE VISITS	FACULTY PRACTICE	SIMULATED ENVIRONMENTS	STANDARDIZED PATIENTS
	Students exposed to real world environments and situations as they are happening in practice	Opportunities to provide occupational therapy services in underserved and emerging practice settings	Parking and transportation needed for community members coming to clinic (if not telehealth) Physical clinic accessibility: Does building follow the Americans with Disabilities Act guidelines? Can community members get to clinic easily and safely? Telehealth accessibility: Access to stable internet for clients and students Schedule must accommodate faculty, groups of students, and community schedules and availability		

(continued)

TABLE 4-1 (CONTINUED)

LEVEL I FIELDWORK CONTEXTUAL VARIABLES ACROSS LEVEL I FIELDWORK TYPES

	ESTABLISHED PRACTICE	FACULTY-LED SITE VISITS	FACULTY PRACTICE	SIMULATED ENVIRONMENTS	STANDARDIZED PATIENTS
Legal Considerations	Contracts between university or college and established practice organization needed to send students to a site AFWC to ensure that site is appropriate for student learning	Contracts between university or college and community organization needed to send students to a site AFWC to ensure that site is appropriate for student learning Safety plan in place for instances where the faculty member is not always onsite with the students	Consider state practice act and billing guidelines as it relates to students providing services Client consents demonstrating their understanding that students are not licensed occupational therapists/occupational therapy assistants Academic programs work with legal department to develop clinic guidelines	Consider state practice act and billing guidelines as it relates to students providing services Contracts with clients to demonstrate understanding that students are not licensed occupational therapists/occupational therapy assistants Programs work with legal department to develop guidelines for simulated environments	Contracts in place for standardized patients regarding payment vs. volunteer status, conduct and behavior expectations, and training requirements
Preparation Considerations: AFWC Role	Placement of all students at a site with communication and confirmation of dates, supervisor, location, and times Confirmation of contracts for site	Contracts in place with the sites Confirmation of dates, location, times	Work with faculty to ensure all students are meeting requirements for engagement		Work with faculty to ensure all students are meeting requirements for engagement

(continued)

TABLE 4-1 (CONTINUED)

LEVEL I FIELDWORK CONTEXTUAL VARIABLES ACROSS LEVEL I FIELDWORK TYPES

	ESTABLISHED PRACTICE	FACULTY-LED SITE VISITS	FACULTY PRACTICE	SIMULATED ENVIRONMENTS	STANDARDIZED PATIENTS
	Training of FWeds when needed Ensure all FWeds are appropriately qualified (according to accreditation standards)	Train faculty as needed, but faculty will be more familiar with program requirements than practitioners in community Collaborate with faculty to plan and ensure learning activities will meet Level I fieldwork objectives and accreditation standards	May work with faculty on scheduling and marketing Work through legal considerations Collaborate with faculty and community facility staff to plan and ensure learning activities will meet Level I fieldwork objectives and accreditation standards	Depends on the simulated environment, but likely to collaborate with faculty to ensure learning activities will meet Level I fieldwork objectives Assist with scheduling and possibly fieldwork activity development	May work with faculty on scheduling and marketing to recruit actors Work through legal considerations May work with faculty on development of simulation scenario and training of standardized patient actors
Preparation Considerations: FWed and/or Faculty Roles	**FWed:** Become familiar with Level I fieldwork objectives Plan schedule to ensure there is time for student questions and feedback Determine Level I fieldwork schedule that works for clients, staff, and facility operations	**Faculty and site supervisor(s):** Collaborate with AFWC to develop Level I fieldwork objectives and learning activities Work with AFWC to determine Level I fieldwork schedule that works for clients, staff, and facility operations	**Faculty and site supervisor(s):** Collaborate with AFWC to develop Level I fieldwork objectives and learning activities May collaborate with AFWC on scheduling and marketing	**Faculty:** Plan Level I fieldwork objectives and learning activities with AFWC consultation May work with AFWC on scheduling and marketing	**Faculty:** Plan Level I fieldwork objectives and learning activities with AFWC consultation May work with AFWC on scheduling and marketing

(continued)

TABLE 4-1 (CONTINUED)

LEVEL I FIELDWORK CONTEXTUAL VARIABLES ACROSS LEVEL I FIELDWORK TYPES

	ESTABLISHED PRACTICE	FACULTY-LED SITE VISITS	FACULTY PRACTICE	SIMULATED ENVIRONMENTS	STANDARDIZED PATIENTS
	Collaborate with AFWC for guidance and training, especially if new to taking students. Help prepare student ahead of time by giving recommended readings, dress code, schedule, and other logistics of the site/population	Prepare students in advance by recommending readings, dress code, schedule, and other logistics. Work with and, get feedback from, site throughout fieldwork experience (and sometimes in conjunction with AFWC)	Prepare students in advance by recommending readings, dress code, schedule, and other logistics. Work with, and get feedback from, site throughout fieldwork experience (and sometimes in conjunction with AFWC). Prepare for debriefing and giving feedback to the students	Prepare students in advance by recommending readings, dress code, schedule, and other logistics. Prepare for debriefing and giving feedback to the students	Prepare students in advance by recommending readings, dress code, schedule, and other logistics. May work with AFWC on development of simulation scenario and training of standardized patient actors
Preparation Considerations: Student Role	Study site services/population. Communicate with FWed on dress code, schedule, and other logistics of the site. Study Level I fieldwork objectives ahead of time to ensure clear understanding of expectations	Study site services/population. Communicate with FWed on dress code, schedule, and other logistics of the site. Study Level I fieldwork objectives ahead of time to ensure clear understanding of expectations	Study site services/population. Communicate with supervisor on dress code, schedule, and other logistics of the site. Study Level I fieldwork objectives ahead of time to ensure clear understanding of expectations	Study site services/population. Communicate with supervisor on dress code, schedule, and other logistics of the site. Study Level I fieldwork objectives ahead of time to ensure clear understanding of expectations	Study site services/population. Communicate with supervisor on dress code, schedule, and other logistics of the site. Study Level I fieldwork objectives ahead of time to ensure clear understanding of expectations

---

Box 4-4

FWED's Perspective: Facilitating Collaborative Model Level I Experiences in Emerging Practices

Erin McIntyre, MOT, OTD, OTR/L, a faculty FWed in a community-based mental health setting described her experience as a group facilitator in emerging practice Level I fieldwork, stating that, "These kinds of experiences lend [themselves] to the social construction of knowledge, where students are partners in their own development."

She tells her students that, "We [FWeds] are here and available if you need us, but we are setting you up for going out and trying things. We also want to debrief and hear about your experiences, and to help you design interventions for your clients' needs." She adds, "Don't look at us as the experts. We are your collaborators." (E. McIntyre, MOT, OTD, OTR/L, personal communication, August 16, 2021).

---

three-phase process in the use of a collaborative learning model. The first phase included preparation for the experience including use of a peer-to-peer collaborative learning model, understanding the population to be served at the community facility, and activity plan brainstorming. The second phase (onsite) included observations, activity implementation, and group reflection at the end of each day facilitated by a faculty FWed to process the day's events and plan for the following day. Students also kept a journal during their experience. The third phase (reflection/follow-up) included writing subjective, objective, assessment and plan notes (often abbreviated as SOAP note); completing self and peer evaluations and reviewing them with the faculty FWed; and a final group meeting to debrief and summarize the experience. Students showed increased clinical reasoning ability and confidence in themselves resulting from these emerging practices, community-based Level I fieldwork experiences facilitated by an occupational therapy faculty member (Box 4-4).

A same site model for fieldwork supervision was used by Evenson et al. (2002). In this study, students had the option to go to the same fieldwork site for their first Level II fieldwork experience as they experienced in Level I fieldwork. Perceived benefits identified by both FWeds and students included reduced stress going into the Level II fieldwork placement. Familiarity with the site, and for FWeds, familiarity with the students were noted. Better student preparedness for Level II fieldwork was a perceived benefit of the same site model for FWeds (Barlow et al., 2020). Barlow et al. (2020) further asserted that using a trauma-informed approach to education supported the same site model with its main benefit to students of reducing anxiety and stress going into Level II fieldwork. Perceived limitations of this model by FWeds and students included a reduced range of fieldwork settings experienced, and concerns that the same site model should not be considered best practice for fieldwork placement (Barlow et al., 2020). One faculty FWed used the same site model for an emerging practice Level I experience in pediatric mental health fieldwork, stating "[the students] liked it so much they wanted to come back" (J. DeBrun, MOT, OTD, OTR/L, personal communication, August 16, 2021).

LEVEL I FIELDWORK BY CURRICULUM DESIGN

Academic programs have flexibility to design and responsibility to ensure that Level I fieldwork is in alignment with their curricular design, mission, and values to support didactic coursework in accordance with ACOTE (2018) standards. The type and number of Level I experiences, sequence, situatedness in the curriculum, and focus of learning are determined by the academic program. An academic program may require all students to have a Level I fieldwork experience

---

Box 4-5

An Academic Program's Perspective: Using Curriculum Design and Student Feedback to Create and Improve Level I Fieldwork Design

One academic occupational therapy program highly valued the psychosocial aspects of care as part of their curriculum design. The students' first Level I fieldwork experiences were in psychosocial settings and, to ensure that all students were placed, community-based settings without occupational therapists were used. Students were challenged to identify what occupational therapy could bring and how it could exist in these environments at this early stage in their academic program. Design of the learning experience evolved into students going to sites in pairs or groups. Doing so added peer support to the students' learning and helped the academic program ensure placement of all its students in psychosocial settings. Faculty-led facilitation was added in response to student feedback asking for help to connect concepts learned in coursework to what they were experiencing in their community Level I fieldwork. Clinical reasoning and professional development were also fostered using faculty facilitation.

---

with older adults, for example. Students may be assigned to a hospital, skilled nursing or assisted living or memory care facility, continuing care and retirement community, or senior center in the community. Another academic program valuing service to the community may require that all students complete a Level I fieldwork in a community-based setting that does not provide occupational therapy services. Examples may include homeless shelters, adult day care centers, facilities providing services for young adults with intellectual disabilities, and drop-in centers for individuals with mental illness (Box 4-5).

Academic programs have flexibility in the number of Level I fieldwork experiences they require. ACOTE standards (2018) do not specify the number of hours, weeks, or number of Level I fieldwork experiences, allowing academic programs to determine them in accordance with the curricular designs. One academic program might sequence Level I fieldwork experiences developmentally following the lifespan of the individual starting with pediatrics, followed by adolescents, adult, and older adult Level I fieldwork experiences.

Situatedness of a Level I fieldwork experience within a program's curriculum is important to know. A first-term Level I student will have very different learning needs and occupational therapy knowledge than a last-term Level I student who completed most of the didactic portion of the academic program and is ready for Level II fieldwork a few weeks after completion. Consider the occupational therapy program that sends students out to community-based psychosocial settings without occupational therapy practitioners onsite in their first term. In subsequent terms, students then go to pediatric and physical dysfunction settings. As students progress through their academic programs, they experience more practice settings and populations and acquire more knowledge.

One academic program sent students out early in the curriculum to community-based psychosocial settings without an occupational therapy practitioner onsite for their first Level I fieldwork. The AFWC's observations and experience were that students seemed most open when experiencing their first Level I fieldwork, relative to what occupational therapy could offer these settings, precisely because occupational therapy is not set up or structured there already (A. McNeil, MA, OTR/L, personal communication, August 20, 2021). Knowing where the students are in their curriculum can help FWeds adjust expectations of the students' knowledge and professional development accordingly.

Box 4-6

Block Versus Dose Model Level I Fieldwork Scheduling

An occupational therapy academic program sends Level I fieldwork students out for a full-time (40 hour) week. The AFWC shared "almost all sites preferred 1 week block and won't take them unless they come for a chunk of time. [It seems] a lot easier for the site to schedule it" (L. Kleine, personal communication, August 12, 2021).

Finally, the focus of learning in Level I fieldwork experiences will be determined by the academic program. Professionalism and exposure to different populations of people in a variety of practice settings may be the focus. In settings where no occupational therapy exists, the focus may be on developing rapport and interviewing skills or determining the occupational needs of the setting and clients. In other academic programs, Level I fieldwork is paired with practice-based courses. Thus, the focus of Level I fieldwork may be on observing and performing parts of the evaluation, goal setting, documentation, and intervention planning. One former faculty FWed was teaching a mental health practice course and facilitating a corresponding community-based Level I fieldwork in an emerging practice. She taught course content on group dynamics, and in "Level I fieldwork, [students were] enacting what they were learning [in class]" (B. Doherty, personal communication, August 16, 2021). Students ran groups and then wrote subjective, objective, assessment, and plan (SOAP) notes on one client each afterward. Academic programs are required to communicate the academic program's learning objectives for the fieldwork experience to fieldwork sites and educators.

Finally, it is the academic program's responsibility to ensure that Level I fieldwork experiences across its curriculum have comparable rigor (AOTA, 2018a). This complex task may be accomplished using one Level I fieldwork evaluation tool, such as AOTA's *Level I Fieldwork Competency Evaluation for OT and OTA Students* (2017) across all settings, or a tool generated by the academic program that demonstrates consistency across Level I fieldwork settings. The AOTA Fieldwork Resource webpage (n.d.) has examples of other programs' evaluation tools.

TEMPORAL CONTEXT CONSIDERATIONS

Academic programs will determine the schedule of Level I fieldwork, and schedules for Level I fieldwork will vary from program to program. Blocked Level I fieldwork schedules are immersive, short-term (e.g., 1 or 2 weeks) experiences, whereas a *dose model* Level I fieldwork experience may include 1 half or 1 full day per week over several weeks (Box 4-6).

A survey of more than 800 FWeds nationwide showed a preference for week-long (53%) over weekly (41%) schedules (Evenson et al., 2015). Additional study results showed either a preference for mid-semester Level I fieldwork (41%) or no preference (37%).

Imagine a blocked model, 1-week experience in an inpatient mental health setting, and how that experience would differ from a dose model experience in the same setting. Consider an outpatient pediatric clinic or private hand therapy clinic in a blocked or dose model experience. In what ways would an inpatient acute hospital experience be a different learning experience from an outpatient rehabilitation experience? How would a blocked or dose model Level I fieldwork work in your setting? In what ways would you be able to infuse active participation into each model?

ENVIRONMENTAL FACTORS AND STUDENT PARTICIPATION

Designing quality Level I fieldwork experiences requires consideration of the environment in which the learning experience occurs. Consider your setting, daily practices, and client population served. Do you see clients every 30 minutes or on the hour? Are clients seen individually one-to-one, in groups, or both? Do both occupational therapists and occupational therapy assistants work with clients in your setting? What other professionals work in the setting? How are inter-professional relationships cultivated and communication handled? What is the expectation and turnaround time to complete documentation, and how is it handled? Does your practice include virtual contexts, such as telehealth or phone consultations with clients, in addition to in-person face-to-face contact?

How much will students participate in the daily activities of your practice? ACOTE (2018) standard C.1.9 requires that academic programs "ensure that Level I fieldwork enriches didactic coursework through directed observation and participation in selected aspects of the occupational therapy process …" (p. 64). Johnson et al. (2006) reported that students valued Level I fieldwork experience independent of variables that included type of setting and type of FWed (occupational therapist or nonoccupational therapist personnel). Students primarily valued experiences when they were provided opportunities to practice clinical skills, observe theory in practice, and partici-pate in occupation-based practice. Consider your clients, their level of complexity, and opportuni-ties for student participation in addition to observation. You may need to consult your institution's policies around student participation in service delivery, as these policies may influence how stu-dents engage in the occupational therapy process at your facility or organization.

EMERGING PRACTICE: COMMUNITY AGENCIES PARTNERING WITH ACADEMIC OCCUPATIONAL THERAPY/OCCUPATIONAL THERAPY ASSISTANT PROGRAMS

Level I fieldwork experiences in emerging practices have existed since the 1970s (Shalik, 1990). Not surprisingly, practice contexts changed over the years as new practices emerged. Johnson et al. (2006) conducted a study of Level I fieldwork contexts and student perceptions of their experi-ences. Emerging practice was included in this study, in addition to role-established practices in physical disabilities, mental health, and pediatrics. They defined emerging practices in their study as sites that met the following criteria:

a. No occupational therapist onsite

b. No Level II fieldwork students onsite providing supervision

c. Potential existed for clients to benefit from occupational therapy services

d. Potential existed for students to engage in program development or service learning (Johnson, 2006, p. 280)

Gat and Ratzon (2014) found that students expressed higher levels of self-identified profes-sional and personal growth in areas of cultural competence and personal responsibility when par-ticipating in a nontraditional community-based fieldwork, more than their peers who participated in a traditional fieldwork setting. Nontraditional community-based experiences were defined as those without occupational therapy services provided onsite, and traditional experiences as those who were supervised by an occupational therapy FWed in an established occupational therapy practice.

An effective way to create new fieldwork experiences for students is to establish collaborative relationships between community-based organizations who provide services to individuals with or without disabilities that do not include occupational therapy services and academic occupational therapy programs. Some examples of community-based organizations include those providing social services to homeless individuals; community mental health services for at-risk youth, transition age youth, and adults; older adult service agencies; senior centers; centers for children, adolescents, and young adults with developmental disabilities; intimate partner violence shelters; recuperative care centers, etc. For many organizations, having occupational therapy students can be a welcome addition to their services.

Consider the contextual factors discussed earlier including the population served, professionals and other staff involved in service provision, potential for occupational therapy services, and potential for students to be engaged in service learning and/or program development. Informative discussion between both parties includes, but is not limited to:

- Education about the occupational therapy profession
- Ways in which Level I students could benefit and align both the organization and academic program
- Learning objectives for the Level I fieldwork experience
- Expectations of FWeds who are not occupational therapists
- Temporal structure including hours, scheduling, and duration of the experience

If a faculty-led or faculty practice experience is being developed, the role of the occupational therapy faculty needs to be clearly developed and agreed upon. Having a shared understanding of the mission and values of both academic program and community agency is important. You are creating a shared purpose and clear understanding about the Level I fieldwork experience, including who will supervise the students, and how student participation and performance will be evaluated. See Box 4-7 for an excerpt of a fieldwork preparation checklist.

Understanding the roles and responsibilities of each party involved is critical to success of emerging practice Level I fieldwork experiences. Table 4-2 outlines roles and responsibilities of the academic institution and faculty, the potential Level I fieldwork site/community organization, and the AFWC in community-based Level I fieldwork in emerging practice.

SPECIAL CONSIDERATIONS FOR LEVEL I FIELDWORK

Virtual Context-Telehealth

Telehealth is the broad term that is used to describe occupational therapy services to include consultative, preventative, and therapeutic services using communication technology (Cason, 2012). Telehealth is defined by the AOTA (2018b) as "the application of evaluative, consultative, preventative, and therapeutic services delivered through information and communication technology" (p. 1). Additionally, the World Federation of Occupational Therapists published a telehealth position statement providing a global perspective of the use of telehealth (2014). Telehealth is recognized as an effective and viable service delivery model for occupational therapy practitioners. Telehealth technology can be used to assist clients with developing skills, incorporating adaptive techniques and assistive technology, environmental modifications, creating satisfying routines,

> **BOX 4-7**
>
> # FIELDWORK PREPARATION CHECKLIST FOR AFWCS AND FWEDS
>
> ☐ Contact an occupational therapy or occupational therapy assistant program to speak with an AFWC about your interest in hosting a fieldwork student (an AFWC can help you navigate the following steps).
>
> ☐ Speak with your site (and parent company) administrators to request approval to host students and advocate on the benefits of hosting fieldwork students (ask your AFWC for email templates or ways to ask and communicate with your team).
>
> ☐ Ask the AFWC for a copy of the following so you can prepare for future students:
>
> - Fieldwork Performance Evaluation (Level I and II)
> - Sample syllabi that include fieldwork objectives
>
> ☐ Work with your AFWC to create sample objectives as needed and confirm that your site meets fieldwork course and supervision requirements.
>
> - AOTA's website has many resources and samples to view
>
> (A. McNeil, MA, OTR/L, personal communication, August 20, 2021).

and coordinating care (Cason, 2012). Occupational therapy practitioners can utilize telehealth technology to provide evaluation (tele-evaluation), intervention (teleintervention), consultation (teleconsultation), monitoring (telemonitoring), and supervision of students and practitioners (AOTA, 2018b).

Telehealth can be used by occupational therapy practitioners in a variety of settings, including early intervention, schools, hospitals, rehabilitation centers, and outpatient settings. The use of telehealth as a service delivery model promotes engagement and participation of clients in the natural context. This may be the client's home environment, work, school, or community center and can be anywhere that the client participates in meaningful life activities. The opportunity to support participation in the authentic environment can be especially beneficial for a Level I fieldwork experience. Figure 4-1 explains the considerations that need to be considered prior to initiating a telehealth session for a Level I fieldwork experience.

It is important to understand that telehealth is a *service delivery model* and occupational therapy practitioners should adhere to the same regulations as in-person experiences. This includes adherence to federal, state, documentation, and ethical guidelines for occupational therapy practitioners. FWeds need to hold a license in both the state that they are physically located in and the state in which the client is located. AOTA has initiated adoption of license portability, which will allow for occupational therapy practitioners to provide occupational therapy in states participating in the compact (Willmarth & Conway, 2019).

Technology is another important consideration in providing telehealth as a Level I fieldwork experience (Table 4-3). A Health Insurance Portability and Accountability Act, also known as HIPAA, complaint platform (Zoom, WebEx) and encrypted emails should be used to connect the client with the session. The occupational therapist will need to consider their environment when connecting with a client via telehealth. The occupational therapist environment should be private, with a door that can be closed, with no identifiable information visible. There are additional considerations for both the occupational therapist and the client. In addition to a HIPAA-compliant platform, the occupational therapist should ensure that the client has access to an internet-ready device, such as a smartphone, tablet, or laptop. It is often beneficial to do a test session or in-person session to assist the client to access the occupational therapy session.

TABLE 4-2

ROLES AND RESPONSIBILITIES IN COMMUNITY-BASED LEVEL I FIELDWORK IN EMERGING PRACTICE

ROLES/ RESPONSIBILITIES	OCCUPATIONAL THERAPY/ OCCUPATIONAL THERAPY ASSISTANT (FACULTY, ADMINISTRATION)*	LEVEL I FIELDWORK SITE/ COMMUNITY ORGANIZATION	AFWC
Identify academic course content areas to be enhanced by Level I fieldwork experiences	X*		X
Develop learning objectives reflecting purpose and performance expectations to be achieved	X*		X
Sequence objectives from concrete to conceptual (simple to complex)	X*		
Identify organizations/ settings that may be able to provide necessary learning experiences	X	X	X
Determine occupational needs of clients served by identified organization (needs assessment)		X	X
Assess whether learning objectives can be met at the site		X	X
Coordinate administrative issues (memorandum of understanding/contract, scheduling, deadlines, evaluation of students, number of students to be assigned at a time)		X	X
Discuss academic curriculum, skill level of students, and expectations of observation and active participation		X	X

(continued)

TABLE 4-2 (CONTINUED)
ROLES AND RESPONSIBILITIES IN COMMUNITY-BASED LEVEL I FIELDWORK IN EMERGING PRACTICE

ROLES/ RESPONSIBILITIES	OCCUPATIONAL THERAPY/ OCCUPATIONAL THERAPY ASSISTANT (FACULTY, ADMINISTRATION)*	LEVEL I FIELDWORK SITE/ COMMUNITY ORGANIZATION	AFWC
Determine fieldwork experience type (with or without occupational therapy FWed, faculty led/ faculty practice, etc.)	X		X
Determine if administrative aspects of Level I fieldwork will impact effectiveness and quality of experiential learning		X	X
Identify learning activities at the Level I fieldwork site that will meet objectives	X	X	X
Assess Level I fieldwork experience on ongoing basis to determine if needs of both parties continue to be met		X	X
*Applies to Level I fieldwork associated with practice courses in the academic curriculum.			

Telehealth engages clients and caregivers to be active participants in the occupational therapy process. Engaging the caregiver is an important consideration for occupational therapy FWeds who want to utilize telehealth as a service delivery model for Level I fieldwork experiences. Telehealth allows occupational therapy students to use technology to understand the unique roles of caregivers in the everyday context of clients. Educational opportunities may include learning to coach a family to promote routines-based intervention in early intervention, home safety evaluation for a client who is leaving an inpatient rehabilitation setting, or promoting carryover for an adult with dementia from the day program routine to the home setting (Proffitt et al., 2021). Students and FWeds should understand that there are additional considerations when preparing and conducting a telehealth session (Figure 4-2).

"We are living in a time of rapid and unpredictable change. Advances in knowledge and technology have made our lives more interconnected and complex" (Hinojosa, 2007, p. 6). The use of telehealth in Level I fieldwork can provide opportunities for AFWCs, FWeds, and students to

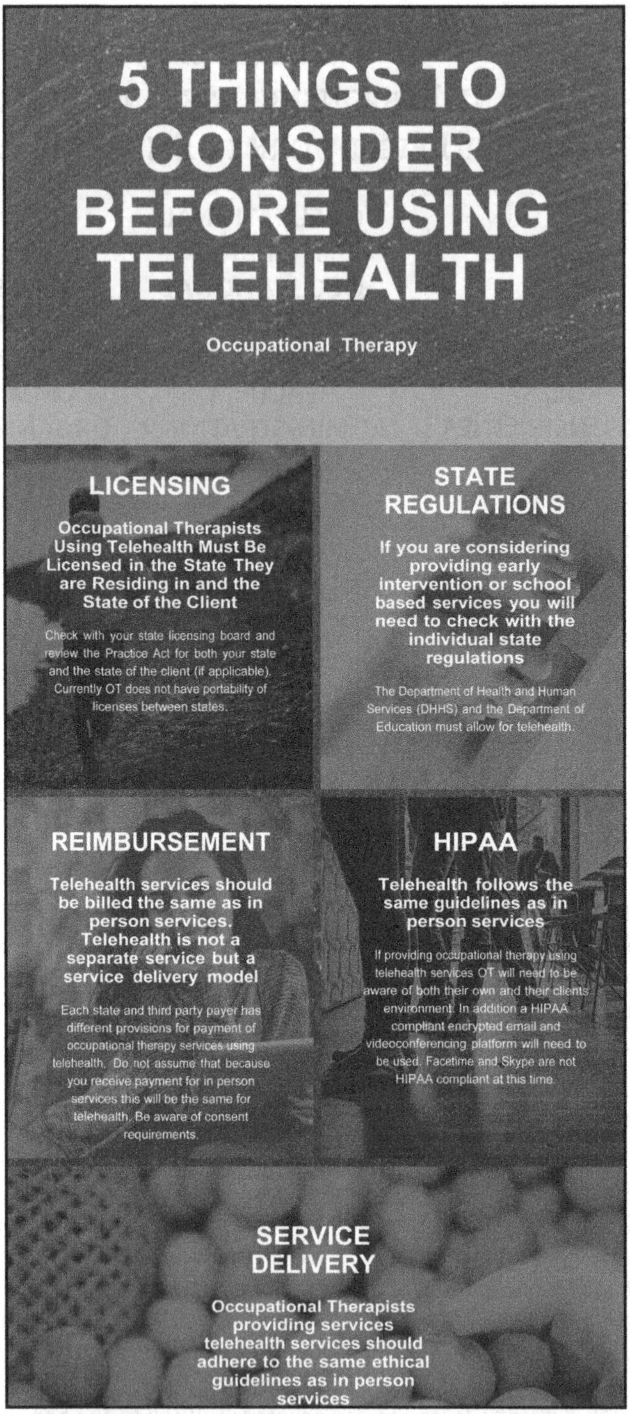

5 THINGS TO CONSIDER BEFORE USING TELEHEALTH

Occupational Therapy

LICENSING

Occupational Therapists Using Telehealth Must Be Licensed in the State They are Residing in and the State of the Client

Check with your state licensing board and review the Practice Act for both your state and the state of the client (if applicable). Currently OT does not have portability of licenses between states.

STATE REGULATIONS

If you are considering providing early intervention or school based services you will need to check with the individual state regulations

The Department of Health and Human Services (DHHS) and the Department of Education must allow for telehealth.

REIMBURSEMENT

Telehealth services should be billed the same as in person services. Telehealth is not a separate service but a service delivery model

Each state and third party payer has different provisions for payment of occupational therapy services using telehealth. Do not assume that because you receive payment for in person services this will be the same for telehealth. Be aware of consent requirements.

HIPAA

Telehealth follows the same guidelines as in person services

If providing occupational therapy using telehealth services OT will need to be aware of both their own and their clients environment. In addition a HIPAA compliant encrypted email and videoconferencing platform will need to be used. Facetime and Skype are not HIPAA compliant at this time.

SERVICE DELIVERY

Occupational Therapists providing services telehealth services should adhere to the same ethical guidelines as in person services

Figure 4-1. Five things to consider before using telehealth occupational therapy. (Reproduced with permission from Becki Cohill, 2020.)

TABLE 4-3

TECHNOLOGY CONSIDERATIONS

- Confidentiality (security, privacy)
- Integrity (HIPAA)
- Availability (information, services)
- Cost/benefit
- Socioeconomic considerations
- Cultural considerations
- Existing infrastructure
- Connection requirements (bandwidth)
- Sound and image quality
- Accessibility of equipment
- Provider and user expertise with technology

---

participate in valuable experiences that allow for equitable access to occupational therapy services. See Box 4-8 for an example of the use of telehealth used as a service delivery model in pediatric practice.

The roles and responsibilities of the AFWC, FWed, and student are presented in Table 4-4 using the pediatric telehealth scenario in Box 4-8.

Simulated Environment

When discussing the topic of simulations, it is important to understand that there is a continuum of fidelity with simulations. There are low-fidelity simulations, which are not generally interactive and can include case studies, clinical vignettes, skills practice with realistic tools, or guided discussions on clinical situations with a faculty member (Munshi et al., 2015). High-fidelity simulations are more immersive, complex, and authentic to the real world experience than low-fidelity simulations (Munshi et al., 2015). While there are many types of simulations along the fidelity continuum, ACOTE allows for occupational therapy programs to utilize the higher-fidelity simulations of simulated environments and standardized patient to fulfill Level I fieldwork requirements (ACOTE, 2018).

ACOTE (2018) defines simulated environments as "a setting that provides an experience similar to a real world setting in order to allow clients to practice specific occupations (e.g., driving simulation center, bathroom or kitchen centers in a rehabilitation unit, work hardening units or centers)" (p. 54). While ACOTE has outlined some specific and built environment examples in the standard, a simulated environment can be fulfilled using virtual platforms, such as Simucase (DeIuliis et al., 2021; Matilla et al., 2020).

Simucase and other health care–based simulation software aims to take students through clinical scenarios where they will interact and respond in real time as a scenario unfolds and is just one example of a simulated environment. While some simulation programs may integrate avatars that mimic client reactions, other programs, such as Simucase, use authentic audio and video recordings of real client scenarios. A patient in Simucase can have adverse reactions,

AN OVERVIEW OF A TELE-INTERVENTION SESSION

PREPARING FOR AND CONDUCTING A TI SESSION

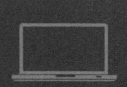

PREPARING

Planning therapy sessions may require more time and logistics due to a pure coaching model.

For quality you may consider, high-quality microphones at both sites, headphones to cancel echo effect, or the use of a document camera to show smaller toys, books

Planning activities and communicating them in advance with the family.

Gathering of toys/materials

Identifying toys/materials that the family needs prior to the session.

Doing a bandwidth and platform check prior to first session.

Prepared for educational purposes by Leah Foreman, OTD and Becki Cohill, OTD

CONDUCTING

The actual TI session can be divided into 3 main phases:

Reviewing goals and activities
- Discussion of strategies from last session
- Update on new milestones or progress
- Review of goals for current session

Conducting the lesson/activity
- Demonstration of strategies and activities using modeling, demonstrating or coaching
- Coaching Model to create success
- Discussion integrating goals/activities into the daily routines
- of the home

Debriefing
- Questions and problem solving about potential barriers
- Discussion of goals
- Summarizing of the session and goals for the coming week

Figure 4-2. Overview of a teleintervention session. (Reproduced with permission from Leah Foreman & Becki Cohill, 2020.)

Box 4-8

PEDIATRIC TELEHEALTH CASE EXAMPLE

MMC is a privately owned occupational therapy clinic that provides early intervention services in rural communities and internationally. The occupational therapist has offered to collaborate with a local Master of Occupational Therapy/Occupational Therapy Doctorate academic program for a Level 1 fieldwork experience. Level I occupational therapy students will participate in the mutlidisciplinary evaluation process including Individualized Family Services Plan (IFSP) development for infants who are 0 to 3 years old at MMC. The Master of Occupational Therapy/Occupational Therapy Doctorate academic program has integrated Level I fieldwork experiences into a Pediatric Clinical Intervention course. For instance, the students can engage with the MMC remotely when learning about the early intervention arena of practice, family-centered care, routines based interventions, and human development within the Pediatric Applications course.

---

complications, respond negatively or positively, and ask questions based on how a student chooses to interact with the simulation. Students report that they enjoy and feel that they professionally and educationally benefit from these types of simulated learning experiences (Mattila et al., 2020).

When a student is using a program like Simucase and interacting through a computer screen, it is more specifically called a *computerized software simulation* (DeIuliis et al., 2021). When the scenario is being conducted through virtual reality where the physical movement of the student becomes the movement within the simulation, it is called a *virtual-immersive reality simulation*. Lastly, another simulated environment is called a *human patient simulation* where students interact in a simulated environment with a mannequin in the place of a real-life person. Health care mannequins also have a continuum of fidelity from mannequins that look like people but do not interact to mannequins that can verbally respond, mimic physiological responses, and react in real time to student intervention (Lee et al., 2008).

When considering using simulated environments for Level I fieldwork, there are several steps that an AFWC, FWed, and student can take to make the most out of the learning experience. As the lead organizer of fieldwork experiences, the AFWC can take inventory of the simulated environment resources available to their occupational therapy program, both within the program and community. There may be opportunities to partner with community organizations or other programs to borrow or share resources, avenues for funding and obtaining mannequins or computer software, or businesses who would welcome occupational therapy students using their real world clinic environments for this type of fieldwork. Additionally, the AFWC would want to ensure that the FWed and students have access to the simulated environments at the designated times. In the case of a computer-based simulated environment, the AFWC would want to ensure that all students had a functional login assigned, that the FWed had instructor privileges on the software where applicable, and that equipment would be ready for the simulations.

The FWed can best prepare for simulated environments by becoming familiar with the equipment and physical space. The FWed can run through the simulation beforehand, set up the space, and become familiar with the objectives of the simulation. Further, the FWed would want to ensure that they are prepared for debriefing after the simulation experience and that the focus of the debriefing is related to addressing the learning objectives of the simulation.

A Level I fieldwork student would want to be sure that they have any and all logistical setup completed before the day of the simulation. That would include the logins and passwords set up for any computer-based simulation, as well as any computer program training or education to ensure that the simulation runs smoothly. For simulated environments with or without a computer component, it would be helpful for a student to review course materials related to the case,

TABLE 4-4

ROLES AND RESPONSIBILITIES IN TELEHEALTH OCCUPATIONAL THERAPY

AFWC/FACULTY	FIELDWORK EDUCATOR	FIELDWORK STUDENT
• Ensure that proper contracts and documentation are in place between university/college and facility. • Propose opportunity to faculty teaching the pediatric course. • Collaborate with university faculty to determine scoffolding of the students' learning experience and scheduling of Level I fieldwork experience. • Educate students on telehealth etiquete and HIPAA requirements in collaboration with faculty. • Ensure that supervision of Level I fieldwork meets the needs of the students. • Prepare students for telehealth sessions prior to the experience using role playing a telehealth session.	• Ensure that all consents are signed for virtual sessions. • Complete test session with students and FWed. • Determine learning objectives for Level I fieldwork experience in collaboration with university/college AFWC or faculty. • Introduce students to multidisciplinary team and caregiver and family prior to eligibility assessment. • Provide necessary resources to students and AFWC/faculty to prepare for experience. • Perform eligibility assessment with multidisciplinary team. • Participate in debriefing/reflection with occupational therapy students following multidisciplinary evaluation. • Facilitate debriefing sessions following evaluation and IFSP with students.	• Prepare for telehealth session by ensuring environment is free of distractions, is private, and has adequate internet connection. • Observe multidisciplinary eligibility assessment for early intervention. • Complete screening tool for telehealth eligibility evaluation for early intervention and determine percent delay and adjusted age of child during observation. • Complete occupational profile of child. • Observe routine-based interview and IFSP process (session 2). • Keep camera off during sessions and camera on for debriefing. • Develop family-centered/routines based goal for child for review with FWed following session. • Complete clinical observations worksheet that includes observations of the child, parent, environment, and other team members.

environment, or situation of the simulation ahead of time and be prepared to discuss and explore ideas after the simulation concludes.

Simulated environments can be a great tool for occupational therapy programs to use for Level I fieldwork. This fieldwork approach for Level I can help ease the burden on community sites that take students for fieldwork rotations since simulated environment simulations would typically take place at the school. It also allows occupational therapy programs to ensure students are connecting the information from didactic coursework to clinical scenarios and settings because the program has control and direct oversight in running these simulations. Further, because simulated environments rely on mannequins, computer programs, or built environments, they can be easily replicated and do not require recruitment of actors or real patients like some of the other Level I fieldwork methodologies do.

However, the technologies that simulated environments rely on tend to cost a lot of money. Simucase, mannequins, virtual reality headsets, driving simulators, and building out the space to have a functional kitchen environment all require funding to obtain. This can be prohibitive for programs without a lot of resources. These systems can sometimes also require maintenance, updates, trouble shooting, and technical skills that may be an extra challenge for some AFWCs, FWeds, or students.

Standardized Patients

Standardized patient simulations include training an actor to mimic the symptoms, history, mannerisms, and behaviors of someone with specific conditions that a student may encounter when practicing clinically (Gardner et al., 2018; Riopel et al., 2018). These simulations bring to life real world scenarios for the student clinician to be able to practice clinical reasoning, patient interaction, and other clinical skills as outlined by the objectives set forth in the scenario (Gardner et al., 2018). Gaba (2004) argued that the use of simulations and standardized patients assist with improving the safety of the general public because students could make critical mistakes and learn from them in the simulated cases instead of making mistakes with real patients. Giles et al. (2014) were one of the first to explore the use of standardized patient simulations within occupational therapy education in their study that explored a method of using these simulations to assess student preparedness for Level II fieldwork. They found that simulations were an effective tool for assessing student readiness for clinical internship and assisted students with improving their confidence going into their fieldwork experiences (Giles et al., 2014).

One example of a standardized patient case could involve an occupational therapy student seeing a patient in their home, in home health services, following a total hip replacement. The simulation could take place in a classroom that has been set up to look like someone's home or use a home environment lab space. It could be set up to have one actor portray a person who is recovering from a total hip replacement and another actor portray that person's spouse. Before the simulation takes place, the actors would be trained on the condition, how to portray the condition, their back story, and what to say in response to students' questions. The student would be given brief information on the case, as well as objectives of what is to be completed in the simulation. Other students can observe the simulation unfold either from the room, from a viewing space, or virtually using cameras streaming to another room. Afterward, the students and FWed would debrief the experience and talk through the learning objectives of the simulation. As mentioned previously, these types of educational experiences are beneficial in preparing students for Level II fieldwork.

Some other benefits of standardized patient simulations are that it mimics the real world of occupational therapy practice because the students are interacting with humans directly as they would in practice. Many of the benefits of a simulated environment are also applicable to standardized patient simulations, such as the occupational therapy program being able to ensure connection from didactic learning to fieldwork experiences and easing the burden on community fieldwork placement sites.

Also similar to simulated environments, standardized patient simulations require a lot of resources and time to conduct. There is a lot of scenario building, simulation writing, recruiting and training of actors, and overall planning in the beginning of building a standardized patient simulation program. Additionally, there is the cost of the environments that are set up for these simulations, hiring and training actors, and equipment to record and stream for viewing by other students. Some programs that rely on standardized patient simulations heavily for Level I fieldwork may also decide to hire simulation technicians to help take some of the planning and organizing burden off the AFWC, which would be an additional cost.

The AFWC, FWed, and student would have similar steps to take to prepare for standardized patient simulations as they would for simulated environments with some alterations. For the AFWC, there would be more time focused on training the actors and organizing those schedules instead of managing login information. For the FWed, they would want to familiarize themselves with the case from both the standardized patient and student side, as well as prepare for the debriefing by being focused on the simulation objectives. The student would prepare very similarly but would not have to worry about the logistics of computer logins. Regardless of how each stakeholder prepares for simulated environments or standardized patient simulations, it is important that efficacy of implementation is a focus.

Educational institutions should be certain the techniques of simulation are effectively implemented. This is where, as discussed earlier, effective debriefing of the experience comes in and where you start to see a differentiation of a simulated experience being utilized in lab experiences vs. Level I fieldwork experiences.

LAB VERSUS LEVEL I FIELDWORK

It is not a question of whether simulations are effective learning tools but how occupational therapy programs can ensure they are effective for their students, and how they are differentiated from lab experiences. Additionally, there are other important factors that must be implemented to have a successful fieldwork simulation program for Level I fieldwork.

Regardless of the setting used for student Level I fieldwork, it is important to keep in mind fidelity to ensure that these experiences are preparing the student for practice in a variety of contexts. It is not enough to have students practice on a driving simulator or answer questions on a virtual case. A faculty member, FWed, or AFWC must help guide the student through debriefing of that experience to ensure the students are meeting Level I fieldwork objectives. It is vital that students are truly learning and processing this valuable information from the experiences to carry forward into their education and practice. Adequate debriefing is not only essential to an effective simulation but students report learning the most from their simulation experience during the debriefing process (INACSL Standards of Best Practice: Simulation-Simulation Design, 2016; Mattila et al., 2020). This is true for both simulated environments and standardized patient simulations.

Further, it is also important for a program to differentiate between lab and Level I fieldwork activities. A professor may choose to use a scenario in Simucase as a lab activity, and Simucase can also be used to meet a Level I fieldwork objective. There is not a consensus or guidance from ACOTE yet on how to distinguish between these two items, so it is up to individual programs to decide how they are best going to navigate that within their curriculum (Box 4-9). We suggest that it may be helpful for programs to make their lab and fieldwork objectives specific and differentiated and build their Level I program according to those overarching principles.

> ### Box 4-9
> ### Differentiating Lab Versus Level I Fieldwork (Faculty Led)
>
> One former faculty member recalled how she differentiated lab vs. Level I fieldwork to her students. Level I fieldwork day was Fridays. When questions about fieldwork arose earlier in the week in class, she would say "we'll talk about that on Friday." In fieldwork, she made it clear that she and other FWeds who were adjunct instructors, "shared [our] experiences as FWeds and didn't talk about class assignments." Grading in class assignments vs. fieldwork performance was different too, as the academic institution's fieldwork evaluation tool was used (B. Doherty, personal communication, August 16, 2021).

SUMMARY

Attending to context matters are critical for successful Level I fieldwork experiences. It is important and essential to have a clear understanding of accreditation requirements that are minimal standards for Level I fieldwork experiences. Knowledge of the various types of Level I fieldwork that ACOTE (2018) allows affords academic programs and community service organizations unique expansion opportunities to design and implement creative learning experiences for students and meet client and population needs. Academic programs and community service organizations can partner to expand services and develop meaningful learning experiences for occupational therapy and occupational therapy assistant students to create outcomes that benefit all. Level I fieldwork settings may assess their own capacities to benefit from occupational therapy and occupational therapy assistant student involvement, including the contextual variables discussed in this chapter. Contacting local academic occupational therapy and occupational therapy assistant programs can support needs assessments and lead to provision of evidence-based services. New and established academic programs are encouraged to assess and reassess their Level I fieldwork experiences within the context of their curricula, considering new accreditation standards, and in line with their institution and program's mission and values. Students need to be aware that Level I fieldwork can occur in a variety of contexts and within a range of different types, in addition to clinical practice in established settings. Special contexts including simulated and virtual contexts, including standardized patients and telehealth, can now be utilized to meet Level I fieldwork standards. Lastly, ensuring rigor and adequate debriefing and processing of special context experiences is critical to supporting students to meet learning objectives. These are exciting and ever-evolving times, with creative opportunities to utilize a variety of Level I fieldwork contexts and supervisory models to optimize learning, with the overall goal of educating and training entry-level occupational therapists and occupational therapy assistants through didactic education and practice experiences.

LEARNING ACTIVITIES

1. You are an **AFWC** in a growing occupational therapy program. The faculty teaching the pediatric coursework has received feedback from students that, while on their Level II fieldwork experiences, they felt unprepared with developmental milestones of children under 2 years old. There are 45 students in each cohort in the pediatric course, and one day a week for Level I pediatric fieldwork. What steps would you take to collaborate with faculty and potential sites? How might you use a virtual context to solve this problem?

2. You are a **Level I FWed** at a community-based program for individuals who are experiencing homelessness. The program has multiple programs including a wellness program, substance abuse program, transitional youth program, and senior food programs. You are currently supervising one occupational therapy assistant student in the wellness program. The director of the program sees the potential benefit of expanding the role of occupational therapy in all the programs they offer by increasing the number of Level I fieldwork students. What should you consider before you agree to taking on more students? What collaborations with occupational therapy and occupational therapy assistant programs might you consider?

3. You are a **student** on your first Level I fieldwork experience at an acute care hospital. This will be your first experience, and you have multiple supervisors, including a physical therapist and a speech-language pathologist. Your fieldwork educators are very busy but allow time at the end of the day for you to reflect on the day. During one of your debriefing sessions with your supervisors, they expressed concerns that you are not participating in the evaluation process and would like you to perform a 30-minute session independently the following day. How would you handle this situation? Is this an appropriate request for Level I fieldwork?

4. You are an **occupational therapist** whose child attends a center providing activities for adolescents and young adults with developmental disabilities. You volunteer at the center two mornings a week and wonder if it could be a Level I fieldwork site, even though the center does not provide occupational therapy services. You wonder if you could be the **FWed**. How do you pursue this idea? What are the first steps you can take to develop your idea?

5. You are a new **AFWC** for an occupational therapy assistant program at a local community college. Securing sufficient fieldwork placements for your students is challenging, and you want to expand fieldwork opportunities by utilizing emerging practice community-based experiences. Some of your students volunteered at a nearby nonprofit agency providing a range of social services, including temporary housing and mental health and vocational training services to veterans, homeless individuals and families, and at-risk youth. The students give the center high praise and tell you "It's too bad they don't have occupational therapists there." Write out a plan for developing this potential new Level I fieldwork site.

6. You are a new **student** in the first school term of your academic program. Your program provides Level I fieldwork using Simucase and telehealth, in addition to practice experience in an established occupational therapy practice. How can you prepare yourself for fieldwork in these different contexts? What resources will you use to ensure you are successful in these varied environments?

ADDITIONAL RESOURCES

American Occupational Therapy Association. (2020). *OT/OTA Fieldwork Councils/Consortia in the United States.* https://www.aota.org/-/media/Corporate/Files/EducationCareers/Educators/Fieldwork/Supervisor/Fieldwork-Consortiums.pdf

American Occupational Therapy Association & Rebuilding Together. (2015). *Student learning opportunities: Service learning and Level I fieldwork with rebuilding together.* https://www.aota.org/-/media/Corporate/Files/Practice/Aging/rebuilding-together/Student-Learning-Opportunities-Rebuilding-Together.pdf

Hanson, D., & Nielsen, S. K. (2015). Introduction into role-emerging fieldwork. In D. M. Costa (Ed.), *The essential guide to occupational therapy fieldwork education: Resources for educators and practitioners* (2nd ed., pp. 341-368). American Occupational Therapy Association.

International Clinical Educators. (n.d.). *ICE Learning Center.* https://www.icelearningcenter.com/

International Nursing Association for Clinical Simulation and Learning. (2019). *Health care simulation standards of best practice.* https://www.inacsl.org/inacsl-standards-of-best-practice-simulation/

Theatre in Tandem. (n.d.). *Theatre, allied health, and educational organization providing simulated skill development for students in higher education.* https://www.theatreintandem.com/

REFERENCES

Accreditation Council for Occupational Therapy Education. (2018). 2018 accreditation council for occupational therapy education standards and interpretive guide. *American Journal of Occupational Therapy, 72*(Suppl. 2), 7212410005p1-72121410005p83. https://doi.org/10.5014/ajot.2018.72s217

American Occupational Therapy Association. (n.d.). *Resources for fieldwork education*. https://www.aota.org/Education-Careers/Fieldwork/Supervisor.aspx

American Occupational Therapy Association. (2017). *Level I fieldwork competency evaluation for OT and OTA students*. https://www.aota.org/-/media/Corporate/Files/EducationCareers/Educators/Fieldwork/LevelI/Level-I-Fieldwork-Competency-Evaluation-for-ot-and-ota-students.pdf

American Occupational Therapy Association. (2018a). Importance of collaborative occupational therapist–occupational therapy assistant intraprofessional education in occupational therapy curricula. *American Journal of Occupational Therapy, 72*(Suppl. 2), 7212410030p1-7212410030p18. https://doi.org/10.5014/ajot.2018.72S207

American Occupational Therapy Association. (2018b). Telehealth in occupational therapy. *American Journal of Occupational Therapy, 72*(Suppl. 2), 7212410059p.1. https://doi.org/10.5014/ajot.2018.72s219

Bajaj, K., Meguerdichian, M., Thoma, B., Huang, S., Eppich, W., & Cheng, A. (2018). The PEARLS health care debriefing tool. *Academic Medicine, 93*(2), 336. https://doi.org/10.1097/ACM.00000000002035

Barlow, K. G., Salemi, M., & Taylor, C. (2020). Implementing the same site model in occupational therapy fieldwork: Student and fieldwork educator perspectives. *Journal of Occupational Therapy Education, 4*(3). https://doi.org/10.26681/jote.2020.040307

Brown, A. B., & Mohler, A. J. (2020). SELTEC: Service and experiential learning through engagement in the community: A Level I fieldwork model: Part 1. *Journal of Occupational Therapy Education, 4*(3). https://doi.org/10.26681/jote.2020.040317

Cameron, D., Cockburn, L., Nixon, S., Parnes, P., Garcia, L., Leotaud, J., Mashaka, P.A., Mlay, R., Wango, J., Williams, T. (2013). Global partnerships for international fieldwork in occupational therapy: Reflection and innovation. *Occupational Therapy International, 20*(2), 85-93. https://doi.org/10.1002/oti.1352

Cason, J. (2012). Telehealth opportunities in occupational therapy through the affordable care act. *American Journal of Occupational Therapy, 66*(2), 131–136. https://doi.org/10.5014/ajot.2012.662001

Clark, S., Grieves, H., Hock, N., Suarez, M., & Young, T. (2019). Faculty-facilitated clinics with a group supervision model. *OT Practice, 24*(6), 26-29.

Copley J., & Nelson, A. (2012). Practice educator perspectives of multiple mentoring in diverse clinical settings. *British Journal of Occupational Therapy, 75*(10), 456-462. https://doi.org/10.4276/030802212X13496921049662

Costa, D., Molinsky, R., & Sauerwald, C. (2012). Collaborative intraprofessional education with occupational therapy and occupational therapy assistant students. *OT Practice, 17*(21), CE-1–CE-7.

DeIuliis, E. D., Mattilla, A., & Martin, R. M. (2021). Level I FW in a simulated environment: A blueprint on how to use Simucase™. *Journal of Occupational Therapy Education, 5*(2). https://doi.org/10.26681/jote.2021.050215

Erdman E., Black J. D., Campbell S., Golder T., Grazioli S., & Palombaro K. M. (2020). Investigating the influence that service in a probono clinic has on a first full-time clinical education experience from the perspective of students and their clinical instructors. *The Internet Journal of Allied Health Sciences and Practice, 18*(4).

Evenson, M. E, Barnes, M. A., & Cohn, E. S. (2002). Perceptions of Level I and Level II fieldwork in the same site. *American Journal of Occupational Therapy, 56*(1), 103-106. https://doi.org/10.5014/ajot.56.1.103

Evenson, M. E., Roberts, M., Kaldenberg, J., Barnes, M. A., & Ozelie, R. (2015). National survey of fieldwork educators: Implications for occupational therapy education. *American Journal of Occupational Therapy, 69*(Suppl. 2), 6912350020. https://doi.org/10.5014/ajot.2015.019265\

Flood, B., Haslam, L. & Hocking, C. (2010). Implementing a collaborative model of student supervision in New Zealand: Enhancing therapist and student experiences. *New Zealand Journal of Occupational Therapy, 57*(1), 22-26.

Gaba, D. M. (2004). The future vision of simulation in health care. *Quality & Safety in Health Care, 13*(Suppl. 1), i2-i10. http://doi.org/10.1136/qshc.2004.009878.

Gardner, D. D., Wettstein, R., Hart, M. K., Bhasin, P., Tran, K., Sanchez, J., & Restrepo, R. D. (2018). Using standardized patients as part of a preclinical simulation. *Respiratory Care Education Annual, 27*, 43-55.

Gat, S., & Ratzon, N. Z. (2014). Comparison of occupational therapy students' perceived skills after traditional and nontraditional fieldwork. *American Journal of Occupational Therapy, 68*(2), e47-e54. https://doi.org/10.5014/ajot.2014.007732

Giles, A. K., Carson, N. E., Breland, H. L., Coker-Bolt, P., & Bowman, P. J. (2014). Use of simulated patients and reflective video analysis to assess occupational therapy students' preparedness for fieldwork. *American Journal of Occupational Therapy, 68*(Suppl. 2), S57-S66.

Graves, C., & Hanson, D. (2014). The multiple mentoring model of student supervision. *OT Practice, 19*(8), 20-21.

Grenier, M. (2015). Facilitators and barriers to learning in occupational therapy fieldwork education: Student perspectives. *American Journal of Occupational Therapy, 69*(Suppl. 2), 6912185070p1. https://doi.org/10.5014/ajot.2015.015180

Hinojosa, J. (2007). Becoming innovators in an era of hyperchange. *American Journal of Occupational Therapy, 61*(6), 629-637. https://doi.org/10.5014/ajot.61.6.629

International Nursing Association for Clinical Simulation and Learning. (2016). INACSL Standards of Best Practice: Simulation-Simulation Design. *Clinical Simulation in Nursing, 12*, S5–S12.

Johnson, C. R., Koenig, K. P., Piersol, C. V., Santalucia, S. E., & Wachter-Schutz, W. (2006). Level I fieldwork today: A study of contexts and perceptions. *American Journal of Occupational Therapy, 60*(3), 275-287. https://doi.org/10.5014/ajot.60.3.275

Jung, B., Salvatori, P., & Martin, A. (2008). Intraprofessional fieldwork education: Occupational therapy and occupational therapist assistant students learning together. *Canadian Journal of Occupational Therapy, 75*(1), 42-50. https://doi.org/10.2182/cjot.06.05x

Kent F., Drysdale P., Martin N., & Keating, J. L. (2014). The mixed-discipline aged-care student clinic: An authentic interprofessional learning initiative. *Journal of Allied Health, 43*(1), 51-56.

Keptner, K. M., & Klein, S. M. (2019). Collaborative learning in a faculty-led occupational therapy Level I fieldwork: A case study. *Journal of Occupational Therapy Education, 3*(3). https://doi.org/10.26681/jote.2019.030308.

Lee, K. H., Grantham, H., & Boyd, R. (2008). Comparison of high- and low-fidelity mannequins for clinical performance assessment. *Emergency Medicine Australasia, 20*(6), 508-514. https://doi:10.1111/j.1742-6723.2008.01137.x

Lie, D. A., Forest, C. P., Walsh, A., Banzali, Y., & Lohenry, K. (2016) What and how do students learn in an interprofessional student-run clinic? An educational framework for team-based care. *Medical Education Online, 21*(1). https://doi.org/10.3402/meo.v21.31900

Mattila, A., DeIuliis, E. D., & Cook, A. B. (2018). Increasing self-efficacy through role emerging placements: Implications for occupational therapy experiential learning. *Journal of Occupational Therapy Education, 2*(3). https://doi.org/10.26681/jote.2018.020303

Mattila, A., Martin, R. M., & DeIuliis, E. D. (2020). Simulated fieldwork: A virtual approach to clinical education. *Education Sciences, 10*(10), 272. https://doi.org/10.3390/educsci10100272

Munshi, F., Lababidi, H., & Alyousef, S. (2015). Review article: Low- versus high-fidelity simulations in teaching and assessing clinical skills. *Journal of Taibah University Medical Sciences, 10*(1), 12-15. https://doi.org/10.1016/j.jtumed.2015.01.008

Proffitt, R., Cason, J., Little, L., & Pickett, K. A. (2021). Stimulating research to advance evidence-based applications of telehealth in occupational therapy. *OTJR: Occupation, Participation and Health, 41*(3), 153–162. https://doi.org/10.1177/15394492211011433

Riopel, M. A., Litwin, B., Silberman, N., & Fernandez-Fernandez, A. (2018). Utilizing standardized patient feedback to facilitate professional behavior in physical therapist students: A pilot study. *Internet Journal of Allied Health Sciences & Practice, 16*(3), 1-14.

Seif, G., Coker-Bolt, P., Kraft, S., Gonsalves, W., Simpson, K., & Johnson, E. (2014). The development of clinical reasoning and interprofessional behaviors: service-learning at a student-run free clinic. *Journal of Interprofessional Care, 28*(6), 559-564/ https://doi.org/10.3109/13561820.2014.921899

Shalik, L. D. (1990). The Level I fieldwork process. *American Journal of Occupational Therapy, 44*, 700-707. https://doi.org/10.5014/ajot.44.8.700

Willmarth, C., & Conway, S. (2019). AOTA/NBCOT occupational therapy licensure compact initiatives moves forward. *International Journal of Telerehabilitation, 11*(2), 29-30. https://doi.org/10.5195/ijt.2019.6296

World Federation of Occupational Therapists. (2014). World federation of occupational therapists' position statement on telehealth. *International Journal of Telerehabilitation, 6*(1), 37-40. https://doi.org/10.5195/ijt.2014.6153

Unit II

Supporting the Student During a Level I Fieldwork

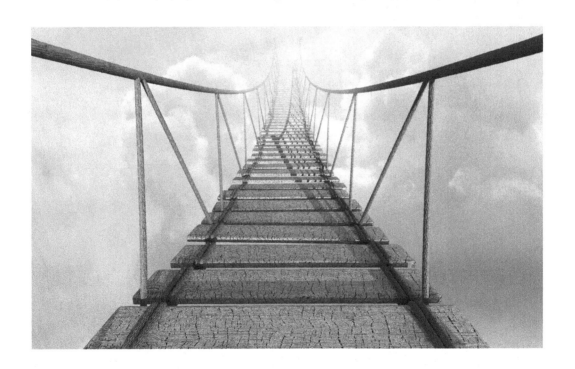

5

Fostering Clinical Reasoning During Level I Fieldwork

Debra Hanson, PhD, OTR/L, FAOTA
and Amy Mattila, PhD, OTR/L

Each unique learning format now available for Level I fieldwork offers rich opportunity for students to develop and refine clinical reasoning skills in preparation for Level II fieldwork and practice. According to the Accreditation Council for Occupational Therapy Education (ACOTE) accreditation standards, "The goal of Level I fieldwork is introduce students to fieldwork, apply knowledge to practice, and develop understanding of the needs of clients" (2018, p. 41). In other words, Level I fieldwork provides students the opportunity to take what they are learning in the classroom and apply it to practice. Through knowledge of clinical reasoning types, a continuum of clinical reasoning development, and application of educational theory, fieldwork educators (FWeds) can be intentional in the kinds of hands-on learning opportunities that they offer students. In addition to a better understanding of the occupational therapy process, opportunities to work directly with clients helps students gain an understanding of their therapeutic effectiveness, appreciate the affective aspect of practice, discover professional interests, and begin to internalize the values of the profession.

There are many challenges to clinical reasoning development, both from the FWed and the student's perspective. An understanding of the challenges will help the FWed address them in a mindful manner. Knowledge of specific strategies for clinical reasoning development gives the FWed tools to fit for the learning style of the student and the nature of the learning experiences available.

Hanson, D., & DeIuliis, E. D. (Eds.).
Fieldwork Educator's Guide to Level I Fieldwork (pp. 109-142).
© 2023 Taylor and Francis Group.

LEARNING OBJECTIVES

By the end of reading this chapter and completing the learning activities, the reader should be able to:

1. Understand types of clinical reasoning used in occupational therapy practice.

2. Recognize the continuum of clinical reasoning development and identify reasoning levels appropriate for Level I fieldwork learning.

3. Apply a theoretical learning framework (addressed in Chapter 2) to facilitate clinical reasoning development.

4. Become familiar with strategies used to promote clinical reasoning development.

CLINICAL REASONING SKILLS

While clinical reasoning has been explored extensively in the literature over the past 30 years, occupational therapy practitioners often still struggle to articulate what it is, and how it looks in practice. Rogers (1983) may have been one of the first to discuss the concept in her Eleanor Clarke Slagle Lecture, where she stated clinical reasoning is defined as, "the thinking that guides practice…[and that] cognitive activity constitutes the heart of the clinical enterprise" (p. 601). Even then, when Rogers asked therapists to comment on how they reached treatment decisions, many answered, "I have never really thought about it" or "I don't know how I reached that conclusion, I just know" (1983, p. 601). Similarly, when students are in the fieldwork setting, there can be a disconnect between the classroom knowledge around discussions around clinical reasoning with FWeds. Cohn (1989) describes that students are often looking for the "right way" to think in fieldwork experiences and that they tend to get easily frustrated with ambiguity. On the other hand, that same ambiguity can lead to the development of critical and creative thinking (Liu et al., 2000). This becomes the great challenge of fieldwork education: the balance between technical skills and competencies and the development of clinical reasoning.

To attempt to bridge these two challenges, it is important to first understand the foundations of clinical reasoning and *types of reasoning used in occupational therapy*. Next, it is important to understand the *continuum of clinical reasoning development* in order to help students to focus on types of reasoning that are appropriate for the Level I learning experience. Level I FWeds need to consider both the type of clinical reasoning they are trying to teach, as well as where the student stands in the continuum of clinical reasoning skills. This will then provide the foundational knowledge to choose the teaching style that will best meet the needs of the student, a hallmark of FWed quality (Rodger et al., 2011).

TYPES OF REASONING USED
IN OCCUPATIONAL THERAPY

Terms such as clinical reasoning, clinical judgment, problem solving, decision making, and critical thinking are often used interchangeably. Regardless, the goal of these collective concepts is ultimately to articulate a process by which practitioners can collect, process, and reflect on a client's needs and wants, then create the most appropriate plan of care. There are several forms of clinical reasoning that will be discussed in this chapter:

> **BOX 5-1**
> ## NARRATIVE REASONING EXAMPLE
>
> A client shares that prior to their spinal cord injury, one of their favorite things to do was ski each winter. The therapist picks up cues that when the client discusses this experience, they go through a range of emotions, from excitement to sadness at the potential loss of this occupation. The therapist turns this knowledge of the client's story into opportunity, by incorporating interventions and, ultimately, resources around adaptive skiing for the client's future story.

> **BOX 5-2**
> ## PROCEDURAL REASONING EXAMPLE
>
> A therapist is referred to a client in an outpatient clinic status post flexor tendon repair. The therapist immediately recognizes rather than going through a more open-ended evaluation, they should ensure the proper flexor tendon protocol is completed by verifying with the hand surgeon. Once the therapist has the recommended protocol, they are able to continue with a prescribed set of processes and procedures that will align with the client's needs based on the diagnosis at hand.

> **BOX 5-3**
> ## INTERACTIVE REASONING EXAMPLE
>
> A therapist is working with an individual experiencing homelessness at a women's shelter. The client expresses desire to return to school to finish their nursing degree. To ensure the therapist supports this goal, they and the client were equally involved in the discussion and shared in the problem solving around how to take the first steps toward this goal. The therapist was empathetic to the client's situation and utilized active listening as a key skill during this session.

Narrative reasoning utilizes story making or storytelling as a means to understand the client experience (Schell & Schell, 2018). It is a process that can explore where the client is now and where they wish to be in the future (Box 5-1).

Procedural reasoning focuses around the process. How do we get things done to maximize client performance? What is to happen next? This reasoning addresses the physical diagnosis and treatment techniques (Schell & Schell, 2018; Box 5-2).

Interactive reasoning explores the relationship between the therapist and the client. Often connected to therapeutic use of self, the therapist can use this form of reasoning to engage with and motivate the client in the therapeutic process (Schell & Schell, 2018; Box 5-3).

Conditional reasoning heavily focuses on context and environment. This context can be where and how the interventions occur, where the client performs occupations, and how to translate the client's needs into adaptations that will facilitate occupational performance (Schell & Schell, 2018; Box 5-4).

Scientific reasoning is a systematic approach to making decisions. It allows therapists to follow a prescribed method to derive conclusions that are reliable and generalizable (Schell & Schell, 2018). It is closely aligned with the use of evidence-based practice (Box 5-5).

Box 5-4
CONDITIONAL REASONING EXAMPLE

A therapist is working in the home health context with a client who has late stage dementia. The client's son is typically present for the sessions and very engaged. The therapist utilizes the son as an invaluable member of the therapeutic process. The therapist typically asks questions and talks to the son while simultaneously working with the client. The therapist asks particular questions to construct what a day typically looks like for the client, then uses the answers to visualize what the treatment and possible goals might look like. Through this process, the therapist is able to formulate an understanding of the past, present, and future for the client given the multiple variables at hand.

Box 5-5
SCIENTIFIC REASONING EXAMPLE

A client post–cereborovascular accident (CVA) mentions casually that this morning, they stumbled a bit when getting out of bed. The therapist starts considering the hypotheses: *Was it dark, and they tripped over something? Were they experiencing deteriorating sitting balance? Was their medication making them dizzy?* Using deductive reasoning and observation, the therapist was able to ascertain that their client was getting out of bed on their weak side and, therefore, lost balance during the task.

Box 5-6
DIAGNOSTIC REASONING EXAMPLE

A therapist is evaluating a client in an acute care hospital. The admission note from the attending physician states, "Rule out Parkinson's disease," and the therapist also has the current documentation from the social worker and charge nurse on the unit. Following the evaluation, the therapist particularly notes several critical cues, such as a mild resting tremor, slowed movements, jaw stiffness, and occasional speech changes. After reviewing the cues and patterns from the evaluation, the therapist feels confident their evaluation supports the plausible hypothesis of a Parkinson's diagnosis and shares this with the physician.

Diagnostic reasoning is a way for therapists to investigate and analyze the cause or nature of the client's condition. It is often considered a component of scientific reasoning and utilized to justify the need for occupational therapy services (Schell & Schell, 2018; Box 5-6).

Pragmatic reasoning encourages therapists to attend to and reflect on practical decisions and realities of providing services (Schell & Schell, 2018). It focuses on the therapist's personal context and the practical context of therapy itself (Box 5-7).

Ethical reasoning is the ability of therapists to make decisions based on ethical principles and actions. It provides a framework for ethical decision making, rooted in ethical theories (Schell & Schell, 2018; Box 5-8).

While there is significant literature around each of these eight components of clinical reasoning (see Additional Resources at the end of this chapter), this foundational knowledge can be used to provide context to the highly complex discussion around clinical reasoning. Each of these areas provide a blueprint for how to promote the fieldwork student's ability to *think about the*

Box 5-7

Pragmatic Reasoning Example

A therapist is working with a 16-year-old client with intellectual disability and their family on integrating a sensory diet. The family states the main concern is finding the time to schedule treatment, as the client's new school schedule runs from 7 a.m. to about 5 p.m. with the long bus ride. Instead of trying to navigate each week, the family and therapist coordinated a 5-times-per-week treatment plan for the 1 week of holiday break. The therapist was able to see the client daily, in many contexts at various times of the day, ultimately getting an even richer perspective than a typical schedule would have provided.

Box 5-8

Ethical Reasoning Example

A therapist is working in an outpatient clinic. The therapist certified in lymphedema management resigned, and there is no plan to replace them. The therapy manager has requested that the therapist begin treating patients with lower extremity lymphedema. The treating therapist attended a continuing education course 5 years ago and has occasionally used the techniques since. The therapist is not certified and has never worked to directly treat lymphedema. The therapist is being pressured by the clinic manager to treat these patients. The therapist recognizes this decision may not be in the patients' best interest or even safety and decides to have a conversation with the clinic manager around a better transition plan for the patients.

---

way they think, or even to be more aware of the different kinds of critical thinking skills used in occupational therapy practice. With that, it is vital that educators utilize intentional reflection and dialogue to assist students in moving beyond novice thinkers.

The Novice to Expert Continuum

First and foremost, it is important for FWeds to have realistic expectations around the student's abilities to clinically reason. The ability to utilize clinical reasoning can be graded along a continuum. Neistadt (1996) first described the continuum in occupational therapy through the stages of novice, advanced beginner, competent, proficient, and expert. Neistadt (1996) contends that even postgraduation, new clinicians are entering practice at the novice or advanced beginner at best, emphasizing the need to take a developmental approach for students at the Level I or Level II fieldwork stages. Table 5-1 further elaborates on these stages and key characteristics of the practitioner.

To further understand the connection between clinical reasoning and the novice to expert continuum, Unsworth and Baker (2016) conducted a systematic review of professional reasoning literature in occupational therapy. When presented with the findings, some results were unsurprising, such as experts having a higher frequency of instances of reasoning or similar use of reasoning during assessment. An interesting differentiation occurred between the types of clinical reasoning utilized along the continuum. A greater percentage of experts utilized interactive and conditional reasoning than novices. For example, Strong et al. (1995) found that experts are able to seamlessly understand their clients through both the lens of their diagnosis or disability, as well as the clients' perceptions or personal story. On the other hand, students placed a higher value on their knowledge of the illness or disability alone. Similar to the findings of Cohn (1989), a greater number

TABLE 5-1
STAGES OF KEY CHARACTERISTICS OF
CLINICAL REASONING SKILLS

STAGE	YEARS IN PRACTICE	KEY CHARACTERISTICS
Novice	0	Have knowledge of theories, frameworks, and principles around practice; usually rigid in application (textbook knowledge); limited experience to rely on
Advanced Beginner	< 1	Begins to incorporate context and may practice modification of rules to adapt to specific situations; still less flexible in that application and limited ability to prioritize well
Competent	3	Able to adjust therapy to specific needs of client and context; sorts relevant data and prioritizes intervention accordingly; lacks the speed and flexibility of proficient therapist
Proficient	5	Are flexible and have the ability to alter both evaluation and treatment plans as needed; has a perception of the case based on experience rather than deliberation; skillful in understanding the narrative of client's needs
Expert	10	Reasoning is a quick and intuitive process; anticipates and recognizes clients strengths and weaknesses based on experience; does not rely on rules and guidelines for decision making, but more on intuition (experts often find it difficult to explain this intuition)

Adapted from Dreyfus, H. L., & Dreyfus, S. E. (1986). *Mind over machine: The power of human intuition and expertise in the era of the computer.* Free Press and Neistadt, M. E. (1996). Teaching strategies for the development of clinical reasoning. *American Journal of Occupational Therapy, 50*(8), 676-684.

of novices relied on procedural reasoning alone in their decision making. In their study of home health practitioners, Mitchell and Unsworth (2005) found an interesting discrepency between novice and expert clinicians. While they also found procedural reasoning to be the highest amongst novice clinicians, the response "not knowing" was very different between the new and expert practitioners. The authors found that overall, the experts demonstrated very little discomfort in the "unknown" and seemed to have a better grasp on what to do about the gaps they needed to fill. The novices in the study shared great feelings of frustration and discomfort when they ran into issues with procedural or other types of reasoning. The authors of this chapter refer to this challenge as the *iceberg effect*, or the comparison of the novice clinican to see things for what they are, at the surface. The expert clinician can start to peel back the layers of the situation and better understand the full picture of the client they are working with. The illustration in Figure 5-1 demonstrates a visual of the novice to expert understanding of a client and their needs, based on the literature (Mitchell & Unsworth, 2005; Strong et al., 1995; Unsworth, 2001).

As academic educators and FWeds, we need to have an understanding of both the foundations of clinical reasoning and the developmental continuum of the learner to be able to effectively implement strategies to support their growth. Since Level I fieldwork occurs early in the students'

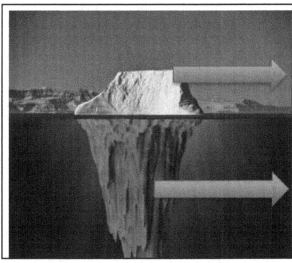

Novice: Diagnostic criteria, illness narrative, procedural understanding (task environment, problem space, etc.)

Expert: Relationship between diagnosis and personal narrative, communication skills, interactive skills, context, planning for future

Figure 5-1. Novice to expert understanding of client. (Unknown Author/CC-BY-SA.)

learning, students may be more oriented toward procedural and scientific reasoning and may have difficulty integrating this perspective with other reasoning types, such as narrative and interactional reasoning. In the next section, some challenges related to clinical reasoning development will be explored, as well as some of the frameworks used to apply clinical reasoning and practical ways to model the process. Be sure to complete Learning Activity 1 at the end of this chapter to consider your own understanding of the clinical reasoning continuum.

CHALLENGES OF CLINICAL REASONING DEVELOPMENT: THE FIELDWORK EDUCATOR PERSPECTIVE

FWeds have expressed concerns about the readiness of occupational therapy students for clinical reasoning in the practice setting (Hanson, 2011). They indicate that some students lack foundational communication, problem solving, and clinical skills, which then impacts their willingness to accept students for Level II placement. Generational differences may impact professional reasoning development. For example, Generation Y and Z students and FWeds desire feedback and preferably feedback that includes reference to their achievement or success, and they may not respond well to direct criticism of their efforts (Graen & Schiemann, 2013; Hills et al., 2015). Generation Y is more likely to value teamwork, whereas Generation X is more likely to pursue and value innovation (DeIuliis & Saylor, 2021); therefore, collaborative learning of clinical reasoning may be more difficult. Both generations, X and Z, favor a coaching model over a management model to enhance professional growth (DeIuliis & Saylor, 2021). A coaching model emphasizes the development of human relationships over a focus on task completion and skills mastery, which were hallmarks of the Baby Boomer generation (Bartz et al., 2017; Deloitte, 2016; DeIuliis & Saylor, 2021). High expectations for one's own and others' performance coupled with an efficient *skimming* approach to detailed information gathering may increase the anxiety and negatively impact the clinical reasoning development of Generations X to Z (DeIuliis & Saylor, 2021; Hills et al., 2015). Due to prevalence of technology use and expectations for instant gratification, these later generations may have less tolerance and experience with practicing skills over time to attain expertise. Fostering a growth mindset, which is believing intelligence is not fixed and can be developed (Claro et al., 2016), over a fixed mindset, defined as a "belief that one's talents are the result of inborn traits and are unchangeable" (Hochanadel & Finamore, 2015), is important for the development of persistence in addressing challenges. These generational attributes are highly likely to impact the readiness of students to make the most of their Level I learning experiences and to influence the types of active learning experiences and feedback offered to students by their FWeds. The readiness of students to engage in clinical reasoning during Level II fieldwork may be directly related to the opportunities they had for active participation during their Level I fieldwork experience.

EXPERIENTIAL LEARNING STIMULATES CLINICAL REASONING DEVELOPMENT

Do students get adequate opportunities to practice and develop their reasoning skills during Level I fieldwork? A common misunderstanding among FWeds is that Level I fieldwork should be primarily focused on observation. In a study examining 1,002 student reports on Level I fieldwork experience in occupational therapy, Johnson et al. (2006), found that student opportunities to practice skills other than communication were limited. For example, students reported opportunities to practice skills common to occupational therapy assessment of manual muscle testing, goniometry, transfers, feeding, and activities of daily living in 55% or less of their pediatric and physical disabilities Level I experiences. In a similar vein, occupational therapists employed in pediatric and adult rehabilitation settings expressed that they felt cautious about supervising students for their Level II fieldwork placement, citing potential concerns with foundational communication, problem solving, and clinical skills. Therapists felt that lack of opportunity for hands-on learning experience in the context of the curriculum, such as opportunity to complete an assessment process and write client notes using electronic documentation formats used in most facilities, would be particularly helpful for addressing these needs (Hanson, 2011).

Is fieldwork the setting in which these skills should be obtained? Chipcase et al. (2012) confirmed that knowledge and understanding needed for readiness to work in the clinical setting is definitely developed in the context of clinical learning. They advocate that students should be viewed as adult learners who take responsibility for their own learning, and that educators should promote clinical learning experiences with learners as a part of the clinical environment rather than a temporary adjunct experience.

Having opportunity for extensive hands-on time working with clients over time may be a critical element in student clinical reasoning development. Seif et al. (2014) found that students from medicine, pharmacy, occupational and physical therapy, and physician assistant programs who participated as volunteers in a student-run free clinic had a higher perception of clinical reasoning skills when compared to a control group of students who did not volunteer ($p = .002$). Coker (2010) examined the impact of participation in a 1-week experiential learning program on the critical reasoning skills of occupational therapy students. She found changes in both objective and subjective ratings of critical thinking and clinical reasoning ($p > .05$) in 25 participants, again supporting the value of hands-on learning in a practice context. Clearly, the opportunity for hands-on learning experiences over time contributes to clinical reasoning development. It appears that practicing specific skills needed for client interaction is foundational to preparation for learning. However, there must also be opportunity for genuine problem solving that involves face-to-face interaction with a recipient of services. In addition, the opportunity to connect various elements of the occupational therapy process in the context of client care is central to clinical reasoning development. For example, the opportunity to have input into the assessment tool chosen, to gather assessment data and then to interpret that data to write an overall treatment plan, and then to design the plan for a specific session serves to connect the clinical reasoning process.

TABLE 5-2

INFLUENCE OF THERAPY CONTEXT ON THERAPY PROCESS

Relationship between practitioner and client	**Interactive reasoning:** What is the nature of the relationships that develop between practitioners and clients at this site? What is considered acceptable or unacceptable?
Organization where therapy is provided	**Procedural reasoning:** What is the typical process or procedures that are used within this organization?
Influence of legislation and government policy	**Conditional reasoning:** How are intake and discharge procedures of this organization influenced by government policy or legislation? How does this impact the bigger picture of the options available to our clients?
Impact of social structures and culture	**Narrative reasoning:** What is the story behind the culture of the therapy department at this site, and how does that influence how therapists interact with clients to understand their stories within the therapy process?

These findings support the strong influence of context on reasoning development. Turpin and Hanson (2018) argue that it is during fieldwork that students develop a richly contextualized understanding of how to practice as an occupational therapy practitioner. Differing organizational contexts, such as a hospital, school, or the client's home, will influence what can be done in practice; what is appropriate in one context may not be relevant to another. In addition, the student must work hard to envision the many contexts that are relevant to the client's life and the role that each might play in the therapy process. Turpin and Iwama (2011) introduced the Model of Context-Specific Professional Reasoning (MCPR), identifying four layers of context that nest together and influence how occupational therapy practitioners engage in professional encounters. Their model includes attention to (1) the professional relationship between the therapy practitioner and client; (2) the organization where therapy is provided; (3) the influence of legislation and government policy; and (4) the impact of social structures and culture.

Although the first layer is the most obvious, the other layers also influence each professional encounter in some way. See Table 5-2 for an example of how each layer of context might impact the clinical reasoning process.

Because of the many layers that are brought together in an integrated reasoning process, it is essential that the student have multiple opportunities to "step back" from their practice to appreciate the situational nature of their knowledge and look actively for new knowledge that can add to their effectiveness. Efficiency of reasoning is supported by the use of frameworks, scripts, and exemplars to handle complex information (Carr & Shotwell, 2007; Schell, 2018). Based on the work of Roberts (1996), Schell (2018) described important parts of the process as (1) cue acquisition, (2) pattern recognition, (3) limiting the problem space, (4) problem formulation, and (5) problem solution (Table 5-3).

What are the implications of this information for Level I FWeds? It is important that FWeds help students to efficiently recognize cues and patterns in complex situations so that the student can focus on the most fruitful areas, formulate an explanation for observed problems, and identify a course of action based on problem formulation. During this process, FWeds will also need to help students appreciate the influence of the context on the entire reasoning process. This underscores the need for a planned orientation for any type of Level I experience. The student needs

TABLE 5-3
A PROCESS FOR CLINICAL REASONING

Scenario: Jane works in an acute care hospital and has orders to evaluate and treat Mrs. Landsom, who was recently admitted following a myocardial infarction. She also has a history of diabetes and heart and kidney failure. She is waiting for a pacemaker, pending stabilization of physical symptoms. The family would like her evaluated for inpatient rehabilitation, but, due to some confusion and physical weakness, she is also a candidate for transitional care in a skilled nursing facility. According to her chart, she has been a lifelong homemaker and takes pride in playing the piano for her rural church. She would like to return home and has two daughters who live locally who may assist with her caregiving. She is considered a fall risk due to balance issues and impulsivity. When she enters the room, Jane notes that the Mrs. Landsom is responsive to her name and asks to use the bathroom. Mrs. Landsom complains that she did not sleep well last night and needed a sleeping pill early this morning. Jane helps her to sit up and notes that she spontaneously swings her legs over the bed and reaches for her walker. Mrs. Landsom is able to walk using the walker with standby assistance but is unsteady when seating herself on the commode and needs cueing to use the bars to raise herself up rather than reaching for the walker to stand. Mrs. Landsom asks Jane if it is snowing outside and states that her daughter is coming to visit and bringing some comfortable clothes to wear if the roads are not too slippery. Jane asks if she would like to wash her face and brings her to the sink. She wets the washcloth but does not apply soap and leaves the water running while she washes her face. When asked if she would like to brush her teeth, Mrs. Landsom declines and states she has dentures so does not need to brush. She also states she is tired and would like to sit down.

Cue acquisition: The therapist searches and targets helpful information through observation and questioning.	Jane directs her attention to Mrs. Landsom's physical and cognitive abilities by watching how she responds to questions and what she initiates in conversation. She notes how she orients herself to her environment and her attention to safety issues.
Pattern recognition: Similarities and differences among situations are noted.	Jane notices Mrs. Landsom is responsive to her name as well as directions, but when not directed, does not spontaneously address safety (e.g., care of her dentures, using the bars when standing, shutting off the water). She is oriented to time and place as evident by comment about her daughter and the weather. She has some physical strength for walking and bed mobility but tires easily.
Limiting the problem space: Being mindful of cues and patterns to focus on most fruitful areas.	Since Mrs. Landsom is being considered for rehabilitation and possibly return home, Jane would like to evaluate her potential for rehabilitation with a focus on self-care skills and functional cognition to address safety concerns in her home.
Problem formulation: Explain what is going on and why and what might be a better situation or outcome.	Jane wonders if Mrs. Landsom's cognitive issues may be related to her physical condition with recent myocardial infraction, and medication taken for sleep aid. She is also questioning whether time of day impacts her physical or cognitive abilities.
Problem solution: Identify a course of action based on problem identified.	Jane plans to return to see Mrs. Landsom in the early afternoon to again assess physical endurance and cognitive ability while completing a dressing evaluation.

to understand the context of service delivery in order to understand the nature of the problems addressed. Table 5-4 provides an example of how the MCPR might be used as part of a successful orientation process for a Level I fieldwork taking place in the context of a state psychiatric hospital.

The Challenges of Professional Reasoning From the Student's Perspective

Understanding the challenges of professional reasoning from the student's perspective is helpful to thinking about strategies for teaching professional reasoning during fieldwork. Copley et al. (2010) used a phenomenological approach to describe students' experiences of learning to implement occupation-centered approaches when working with children. They found that students reported difficulty in keeping their focus on observing occupational performance as opposed to body structures and functions. When actually involved in therapy, they expressed how challenging it was to keep up with the spontaneous nature of therapy sessions, addressing unexpected issues while thinking on their feet. They particularly struggled with identifying performance breakdowns related to tasks that were difficult to observe or simulate in the clinical environment and establishing clear goals that tapped into the child's motivation. Learning how to use certain techniques and strategies was another area of difficulty, as students found it difficult to ask the right questions to facilitate realistic or helpful child-generated strategies and to use tools and models to address performance in tasks that were unfamiliar to them.

The authors of the study (Copley et al., 2011) suggested that students need consistent exposure to learning environments that provide authentic experiences in the implementation of occupation-centered approaches. They also suggested that challenges experienced by students in adapting their actions in response to unexpected outcomes reflected difficulty with *reflection-in-action*, as this is preliminary to the ability to experiment on the spot.

STRATEGIES TO ENHANCE LEARNING ON LEVEL I FIELDWORK

What can FWeds do to help students to develop clinical reasoning skills? When asked, students indicate that a quality student placement provides individualized opportunities to meet student learning needs. Students expressed that graded learning experiences across and between placements, as well as adequate opportunity for observation, therapist modeling, skills practice, and reflection, help them learn the skills that they need for practice (Rodger et al., 2011). In addition, they reported that feedback given routinely, generously, and without prompting was extremely useful to their development. Several specific techniques can be used to help the student to develop clinical reasoning more efficiently and effectively. Through engaging with reflection and dialogue, the supervising practitioner creates a safe place for students to share their thinking and questions. With intentional therapist modeling and reasoning out loud, students can come to appreciate the complex thinking behind the reasoning process, and how the therapist determines a focus for therapeutic interactions. Opportunities for active experimentation allows students to build on academic knowledge to practice skills in a clinical context. Students learn to identify specific cues and recognize patterns to limit the problem space of their reasoning when FWeds help them to "chunk" information through use of heuristics, domain-specific protocols, and observations sheet. Debriefing, feedback, and reflection help students to develop skills in evaluating their own performance to adjust their practice approach in future therapeutic encounters. Figure 5-2 provides an overview of helpful learning strategies that will be addressed in this section.

TABLE 5-4 INFLUENCE OF THERAPY CONTEXT ON THERAPY PROCESS	
Relationship between practitioner and client	At this facility, we emphasize a client-centered approach to therapy. Therefore, we use a treatment mall approach, where clients have the opportunity to choose the treatment groups they wish to attend. We collaborate with our clients to find topics and approaches to therapy that are a fit for their needs.
Organization where therapy is provided	As a state hospital, we take in clients from all over the state who desire services, from children through geriatric age group. We work with a variety of mental health issues including chemical dependency.
Influence of legislation and government policy	Because of government policy, clients can be committed for long-term treatment if they are deemed to be a danger to harm themselves and others.
Impact of social structures and culture	Occupational therapy services are provided in the context of the activities therapy department, which also includes recreation therapy and vocational services. The role of the occupational therapy is primarily directed toward activities of daily living, instrumental activities of daily living, education, and social participation. We collaborate with recreation therapy in working on leisure and social participation, and with vocational services when addressing work and education.

Engaging in Clinical Reasoning With Reflection and Dialogue

James Lang (2006), in his engaging text entitled *Small Teaching*, speaks of the power of internal motivation for learning. He suggests that internal motivation is evident when the learner cares more about what is being learned than a reward that will be achieved at the conclusion of the learning session. He provided an example of his daughter learning to play the violin, and the additional motivation she gained when he would join her on the piano. At those times, her practice became a shared social activity rather than a grueling practice session. When we as practitioners join with our students in reflection and dialogue, we can leverage the power of shared positive emotions as a motivational force for learning.

In doing so, we are likely using principles of social constructivism, which were discussed in Chapter 2 of this text. As you may recall, social constructivism highlights the collaborative relationships and conversation that might occur in a work context, where novices with less experience build their knowledge through interacting with individuals who are more knowledgeable or experienced (Berkley Graduate Division, 2021; Vygotsky, 1978).

As academics and FWeds, one of the most important ways to provide a positive learning experience and develop professional reasoning among novices is to promote reflection and consistent dialogue around what they see, what they do, and the thinking and emotions that make up their experience. This is woven into some strategies for adult learning. For example, Fink's Taxonomy of Significant Learning (Fink, 2003, 2013; discussed in Chapter 2) begins with foundational knowledge of the problem, but then branches out to knowledge of application, integration, exploring the human dimension, and caring elements of learning, as well as learning how to learn. As demonstrated in Table 5-5, all of these elements can be encouraged through reflection and dialogue with a student.

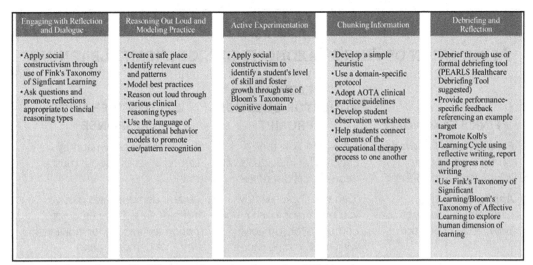

Engaging with Reflection and Dialogue	Reasoning Out Loud and Modeling Practice	Active Experimentation	Chunking Information	Debriefing and Reflection
• Apply social constructivism through use of Fink's Taxonomy of Signficant Learning • Ask questions and promote reflections appropriate to clincial reasoning types	• Create a safe place • Identify relevant cues and patterns • Model best practices • Reason out loud through various clinical reasoning types • Use the language of occupational behavior models to promote cue/pattern recognition	• Apply social constructivism to identify a student's level of skill and foster growth through use of Bloom's Taxonomy cognitive domain	• Develop a simple heuristic • Use a domain-specific protocol • Adopt AOTA clinical practice guidelines • Develop student observation worksheets • Help students connect elements of the occupational therapy process to one another	• Debrief through use of formal debriefing tool (PEARLS Healthcare Debriefing Tool suggested) • Provide performance-specific feedback referencing an example target • Promote Kolb's Learning Cycle using reflective writing, report and progress note writing • Use Fink's Taxonomy of Significant Learning/Bloom's Taxonomy of Affective Learning to explore human dimension of learning

Figure 5-2. Strategies used by FWeds to enhance learning on Level I fieldwork.

Appreciating the human dimension of providing care and one's therapeutic style is also part of the learning, as well as choosing to invest more in some areas of learning than others. Learning how to most effectively gain proficiency in valued areas rounds out Fink's Taxonomy. Table 5-5 provides an overview of the learning domain, the questioning and reflection that might be used by the FWed, and the potential learning results. Although the table illustrates questioning prompts, it could also be used by the FWed as a guide to dialogue. For example, the FWed might discuss how they make connections between commonalities of muscle tone, how they have felt in the past and how they now feel about working with clients who are unable to speak, how this impacts their therapeutic use of self, and what they find interesting or motivating about working with the client population. All or some of these aspects can be explored in back and forth dialogue with the student to promote student reasoning.

Various aspects of reasoning influence one another. Instead of taking a common approach such as "What questions do you have?" at the end of each client session or the end of the day, the FWed can promote clinical reasoning and reflection by utilizing more specific, relevant questions for the situation at hand. Table 5-6 provides an example of open-ended questions that may be used to promote dialogue regarding different types of clinical reasoning. These questions could even be given to the fieldwork student to help them pull the right kind of questions to ask or narrow their focus on as they begin to fully understand the client or setting they are working in.

Active Experimentation

As mentioned earlier in this chapter, opportunities for hands-on learning and active experimentation are critical to the development of clinical reasoning during Level I fieldwork; observation alone is not enough! The FWed plays a critical role in identifying suitable opportunities for students to participate in hands-on learning. An aspect of social constructivism involves the FWed in observing and monitoring the students *zone of proximal development*, or in other words, what they can do independently and what they can do with assistance (McLeod, 2020; Vygotsky, 1978). The FWed should then upgrade the level of challenge as needed according to the student's readiness to engage in additional challenge. The cognitive domain of Bloom's Taxonomy can be a useful tool for determining the student's present abilities and helping students to build on their foundational skills toward further growth. Using this approach is also a tangible way to support a growth mindset, the idea that the student's intelligence or ability to work effectively with clients is

TABLE 5-5
APPLICATION OF FINK'S TAXONOMY OF SIGNIFICANT LEARNING

FINK'S TAXONOMY	FIELDWORK EDUCATOR QUESTION PROMPT	STUDENT BEHAVIOR RESPONSE
Foundational knowledge: Understanding basic information and concepts	"How is muscle tone affected for individuals with neurological disorders?"	Student discusses what they learned in school about muscle tone.
Application: Skill competency; ability to use knowledge in practice	"Can you show me how you might approach range of motion for someone with muscle tone issues?"	Student demonstrates passive and passive assistive range of motion techniques for individual with CVA demonstrating flaccidity.
Integration: The ability to make connections between different people, situations, and ideas	"How would you compare the muscle tone of your client with CVA and your client with a traumatic brain injury? What is your approach to your intervention?"	Student makes connection between commonalities of muscle tone and similarity in neuromuscular interventions.
Human dimension: Learning about self and others, interpersonal interactions, therapeutic use of self, and feelings about encounters	"How did it feel for you to work with your client who had severe dystonia and lack of ability to speak?"	Student expresses anxiety about performance but also concern for well-being of client, noticing more use of therapeutic modes of empathy and encouragement.
Caring: Identifying learning interests and investigating an area of expertise	"What do you find most interesting or motivating in working with clients with neurological disorders?"	Student expresses interest in learning more about the neurological aspects of the disorder and how to apply the task-oriented approach.
Learning how to learn: How to use self-direction and inquiry to become a better student	"How might you learn more about the task-oriented approach? How can I be a resource to you?"	Student learns that they need to use their resources wisely, to ask questions, and read materials outside of class to become proficient in this approach.

not innate, but can benefit from practice. Through review of student knowledge and understanding of a given situation, you can progressively help students to apply skills, analyze the components affecting an intervention, and ultimately, in later Level I experiences, lead students through making clinical decisions that will impact the direction of the therapy process. See Table 5-7 for an example of how Bloom's Taxonomy (Bloom, 1956) might be applied to student learning on Level I fieldwork.

TABLE 5-6
QUESTIONS TO FACILITATE CLINICAL REASONING

ASPECT OF REASONING	QUESTIONS TO ENGAGE A LEVEL I FIELDWORK STUDENT IN CLINICAL REASONING
Narrative	What does this recent change in occupational performance mean to this client?
	How is this change positioned within the client's life history?
	How does the client experience their current condition?
	What vision do I hold for the client in the future?
	What "therapeutic plot" will bring this vision to fruition?
Procedural	What is the diagnosis?
	What symptoms, prognosis, or complications should I be aware of?
	Is there a general protocol associated with assessment or intervention?
	What evidence exists to support chosen interventions?
Interactive	Who is the client?
	What are the client's goals, concerns, interests, and values?
	What are my own preferred therapeutic modes?
	What is the best way to engage with this client?
	How can we most effectively communicate?
Conditional	What contexts are most important to the client?
	What does the future look like when described by the client?
	How can I best engage the client to work toward this imagined future?
Scientific	What information do I need to know to formulate a plan?
	What might a chosen assessment tell me about this client and diagnosis?
	What further information would inform my plan of care?
	How will I confirm whether or not my plan is working?
Diagnostic	Does the problem at hand impact occupational roles or performance?
	Is the pathology or symptoms consistent with expected deficits?
	What cues can I observe that led me to my findings?
	Have I taken the time to interpret those cues and create hypotheses/an alternative hypothesis about the client?
Pragmatic	What organizational supports or barriers exist that may impact the delivery of services?
	Are there physical environmental factors that must be considered?
	How does productivity factor into my ability to manage this client?
	What is my own personal context that may influence the case?
Ethical	How can I ethically use my skills and knowledge to support this client?
	Are there any ethical issues associated with this case?
	Are there any risks associated with the possible outcomes and options for this client?

TABLE 5-7

APPLICATION OF BLOOM'S TAXONOMY COGNITIVE DOMAIN TO STUDENT LEARNING DURING LEVEL I FIELDWORK

BLOOM'S TAXONOMY: COGNITIVE DOMAIN	LEARNING PROMPT FROM FIELDWORK EDUCATOR	STUDENT BEHAVIOR
Remember: Simple recall of facts, memory of concepts from a lecture or lab	"What do you know about one-handed dressing?"	Student reviews knowledge learned in school or takes a pretest before the start of the Level I fieldwork
Understand: Articulate or work with concepts, may involve classifying, locating, translating	"Teach me how you would apply one-handed dressing in your own words."	Student voices, in their own words, the sequential process of one-handed dressing for the upper extremity
Apply: Use previously acquired information in novel circumstances	"Demonstrate how you would apply one-handed dressing for someone with a right CVA."	Student demonstrates how to apply one-handed dressing for a client with a right CVA
Analyze: Make connections or differentiate between ideas, compare or distinguish one case from another	"Why is the affected arm put in the sleeve first? Why would the client need a prompt to pull the garment over their shoulder?"	Student analyzes the components of the dressing process and what effects each component of the process
Evaluate: Appraise or critique process or ideas, argue a position or defend a stand	"What would be the best dressing assessment to use for someone with left weakness, left neglect, and cognitive issues?"	Student compares and evaluates between choices and determines a most effective course of action
Create: Design or develop new plans or activities from distinct and different sources. Create is considered the highest level skill in the cognitive taxonomy.	"How could you combine your knowledge of technology and your experience with clients with neurological disorders to design an adaptive device for cueing the client on steps for dressing?"	Student puts together knowledge from different sources to create a new solution to a problem

Reasoning Out Loud and Therapists Modeling of Practice

An important first step that FWeds can take to help students develop their clinical reasoning is to encourage them to articulate their thinking despite their novice status. To do so, they must create a *safe* place for students to explore their reasoning, understanding that there is often not a *right* answer to many practice situations. Copley et al. (2017) conducted a focus group of experienced pediatric FWeds who routinely modeled this strategy for their students. They reported commonly using different types of knowledge from different sources in their reasoning (assessment results, discussion and observation with clients and others, their own expertise and experience with previous clients, research

---

Box 5-9

CLINICAL REASONING OUT LOUD

Procedural reasoning: "I see we have a new consult for a client 3 days postoperative from a flexor tendon repair. Let's see what the surgeon used as a protocol. So I see the protocol the surgeon is following is for Zones 2 to 5. What do we need to know about these zones? What is the appropriate timeline to follow? Are there any additional questions we need answered from the surgeon prior to starting therapy? We also need to fabricate a splint. Since it's a flexor tendon protocol, we will need a dorsal hood. Let's get to work with starting with the splint, then we will review the protocol and precautions with the client."

Narrative reasoning: "Our first evaluation today is with Jake. He is now 2 weeks status post his spinal cord injury and has just arrived at the rehab center. Before we check in with him, I think we really need to take a look at how he is coping. It's important for us to understand what this change in his occupational performance really means to him. Where does he see his future self? What are the things we might be able to help him adapt with that he loved doing before? Let's be sure to learn as much as we can about what is meaningful to him, in addition to our physical assessment today."

Interactive reasoning: "Mrs. Reyes has told us that she is independent living alone after her most recent stroke. She is now back in the hospital after a fall, and based on the chart review, it seems like this is not the first time she has had an accident. I'm gathering that she gets confused in recalling these incidents as well. I'm starting to think Mrs. Reyes is someone who needs more support than she is letting on ..."

---

and theory, and the practice context), but found that students often viewed their systematic process of *reasoning through action* as simply "trial and error." Therefore, the FWeds realized they needed to talk out loud about their thinking so students would see the complexity of the process. These FWeds created a safe place by making it clear from the beginning of the fieldwork that they would all, FWeds and students alike, be talking out loud about their thinking as a means of encouraging students to verbalize what they were thinking. Although they encouraged students to ask questions, they realized students often struggled with identifying an appropriate question because part of reasoning development is formulating the right question. By emphasizing that it is acceptable to not know something, they aimed to encourage students to verbalize their thinking as a means to help them think through a problem and identify the relevant cues to pay attention to and eventually recognize the overall pattern of a problem. They initially asked students to describe what they saw, as students felt safer answering something concrete. They also encouraged students to talk about problems rather than hide them and modeled openness by telling students stories where things had gone wrong for them.

Familiarity with various types of clinical reasoning will also help you to articulate out loud your own reasoning process and can also be used as a tool to help students identify a focus for their therapy efforts (Box 5-9).

Positive role modeling of practice ideals coupled with explanation of actions is central to learning how to implement client-centered and occupation-based practice. Students learn from modeling by teachers, FWeds, and other employees (Maloney & Griffith, 2013; Ripat et al., 2013). For example, seeing the effectiveness of incorporating occupation into assessment and treatment is motivating to students. However, positive role modeling of such best practices (client-centered and occupation-based practice) is often not available, which is discouraging to students (Copley et al., 2011; Maloney & Griffith, 2013). Copley et al. (2011) identified various turning points in students' learning process. Students gradually recognized the value of using an occupation-centered approach when they saw it successfully modeled and used to elicit assessment data while also positively impacting child motivation and performance.

Role modeling helps the student to visualize the cues that the therapist is attending to, recognize the patterns of cues, and appreciate how the therapist limits the problem and works within available space to both formulate and solve the problem. They also learn to attend to the process of therapy, in other words, the affective components (discussed in Fink's Taxonomy of Significant Learning) that can lead to insights that make therapy meaningful and engaging to the client. Through the modeling provided in Copley's study, students realized they could make their therapy sessions more fun and positively impact child motivation. Early in their learning, they found it helpful when FWeds would jump in when they needed help as this gave them opportunity to closely observe and recalibrate their actions, but later in the placement, they valued the opportunity to experiment on their own.

This finding is consistent with the stages of psychomotor development addressed in Bloom's Taxonomy of Learning discussed in Chapter 2: (1) imitation, (2) manipulation, (3) precision, and (4) articulation. Students first learn to *imitate* the actions of their therapist, and later, with practice, are able to *manipulate* the action, or in other words, complete the same action habitually as they practice with a variety of clients and in a variety of contexts. For example, students may first learn to adjust tubes and lines in acute care by direct modeling, then demonstrate the ability to perform the task without modeling as they practice with different types of tubes and lines across different types of clients. Students on a Level I fieldwork are typically not able to perform with *precision* but may approach this ability if given enough opportunity to practice. They typically are not able to alter skill application to new circumstances on a Level I fieldwork (*articulation*) but would learn to do this during their Level II fieldwork. Modeling is especially important as students learn to incorporate occupation into their intervention process, as it is very difficult for students and novice therapists to direct their thinking away from underlying skills and performance components and toward a contextualized view of occupation (Copley et al., 2011; Mitchell & Unsworth, 2005).

Modeling of best practices, especially when coupled with reasoning out loud, is effective in helping students realize that ideals of practice learned in the academic setting might be applied differently in practice. In other words, when FWeds reason out loud and also model with their actions, students are able to put together both cognitive and affective learning in order to more effectively implement *narrative, interactive,* and, later in the process, *conditional reasoning.* For example, students who were interviewed about their understanding of client-centered practice reported that they eventually understood that client-centered practice was more of a collaborative and inclusive process rather than a need to either relinquish all power or eliminate all risk (Ripat et al., 2013). Opportunities to observe seasoned therapists and benefit from collaboration and consultation with more experienced therapists also provides a context for professional socialization and professional identity development (Ashby et al., 2016; Coker, 2010). While students will first appreciate the affective components of learning that include *receiving* and *responding*, it is apparent that the components of *valuing, organizing,* and *characterizing* impact how the affective experience is internalized to impact development of professional interests and, ultimately, professional identity.

Students especially appreciate seasoned therapists' active application of theories that they learned during their academic education to their professional work with clients (Gat & Ratzon, 2014). Use of the theoretical foundations of the profession may serve to ground affective learning in the language and concepts of the profession, rather than the influence, expertise, or charisma of the supervising therapist. Use of occupational therapy theoretical models helps students structure their reasoning to address the medical condition while also applying best practice ideals (Copley et al., 2011; Kuipers & Grice, 2009a). Use of familiar terminology learned in school may help students to recognize relevant cues and patterns. As an example, Nielsen et al. (2017) describe using the Person-Environment-Occupation Model as a framework for helping students on a Level I fieldwork who worked with a community-based refugee program to identify areas of need for clients and plan for each weekly intervention. Another application of theory as an organizing framework might be using an occupational behavior model to organize and describe the services provided to a population group or within a treatment setting. See Table 5-8 for examples of applying occupational behavior models to a description of services provided in diverse practice settings.

TABLE 5-8

APPLICATION OF
OCCUPATIONAL BEHAVIOR MODELS IN PRACTICE

Model of Human Occupation	In this state psychiatric hospital, we realize that our clients often have a long history of difficulties by the time they come to us. Therefore, we start with an accurate assessment of current skills, but we are also interested in the habits and routines that support their current roles and changes they would need to make to support participation in activities that reflect their values and interests. We know that environment can play a key role, so we look at the influence of the social, physical, and cultural environment on their participation. At the end of the day, we hope to influence their overall competency and sense of identity, so that they are able to adapt well when they leave the hospital setting.
Occupational Adaptation Model	The clients we serve in our outpatient treatment setting want to return to work. They only receive services for a limited amount of time, so it is essential that they learn to take active ownership for addressing their occupational needs. In our programming, we provide the readiness skills they need for their work, including physical ability and their emotional and cognitive aptitudes. We place them in actual work stations early in the rehabilitation process, using our own clinical reasoning to fit them with environments where they can achieve some success but also be challenged. We engage them in problem solving to increase their awareness of what is and is not working for them, encourage them to use the skills they have developed and problem solve changes they might make to be more effective. In that way, we increase their ability to adapt and be successful in their work environments, even though they might not have resolved all of their skill deficits.
Person-Environment-Occupation Model	In this elementary school system, students are most successful when they can engage in the various occupations of education. Some students are disadvantaged in that they lack the cognitive, sensory-motor, and psychosocial skills to effectively perform in the classroom, as well as small group learning. We work collaboratively with the teacher, and in some cases, the paraprofessional to support the student in learning new study and social interaction skills and ways to manage sensory information so as to sustain attention and emotional regulation. We are also attentive to the impact of the environment on student performance and look for the best fit in skills development for educational performance, while simultaneously adapting the social, physical, and cultural environment to impact performance. We also work with the teacher and paraprofessionals to maximize the students educational performance by adapting the educational activities when needed to fit the available environment and skills of the clients.

(continued)

TABLE 5-8 (CONTINUED)

APPLICATION OF OCCUPATIONAL BEHAVIOR MODELS IN PRACTICE

Canadian Model	The bulk of our clients in this outpatient setting have orthopedic concerns or are working with us to extend therapy gains made in the inpatient rehab setting. We are reimbursed through both private pay and insurance. It is critical that our clients are engaged in their therapy process and satisfied with the outcomes achieved. We see a high rate of cancellation or withdrawals from therapy if engagement is not achieved. Therefore, we ensure that they have a good understanding of what we can achieve in occupational therapy from the start. We interview our clients using the Canadian Occupational Performance Measure (COPM) or a similar tool to identify the occupational outcomes they want to achieve, as well as the kind of activities that they will participate in outside of therapy sessions to achieve their goals. We check with them regularly to get their perspectives on their progress and the activities used in the therapy process and revise goals and activities as needed to maintain focus on their occupational priorities.
Ecological Model	Many of our inpatient rehabilitation clients in this veterans hospital have medical issues related to battle injuries, including acquired brain damage, loss of limbs, or severe burns. Our goal in therapy is to return them to the highest quality of life and largest range of tasks that they can participate in. We begin by identifying the tasks of concern to the individual, engage them in skill training for the task, while simultaneously exploring how to alter the task or environment to maximize performance. We also anticipate and prevent obstacles to progress and actively look to engage them in tasks situated in contexts that maximize their strengths. Realizing that they will live with lifelong challenges, in the context of our rehab program, we create opportunities for them to participate in the wider community on an even playing field. For example, through use of adaptive equipment, our clients participate in downhill skiing Olympics.
Kawa Model	In this acute care hospital, many of our clients are immigrants who come to us with cultural differences that impact our ability to engage them in the therapy process. We first strive to understand their perspective on their life story and context, as well as barriers and potential avenues to enhance their occupational performance. The whole team is then engaged in addressing occupational concerns to create the greatest degree of harmony between the client and their cultural context. This may involve efforts by the client to gain skills to enhance performance, but it also may involve intervention with the family, community, or institutional culture to maximize balance and harmony in the life of the individual within their context.

TABLE 5-9
QUESTIONS FOR HEURISTIC DEVELOPMENT

1. What questions would you ask yourself if you faced a challenging clinical scenario?

2. What type of thinking routines would you like your students to develop?

3. What would your students ask if they were engaged in this thinking?

4. What questions can you ask to encourage this thinking?

5. How can you turn these questions and thinking steps into a thinking routine heuristic, a sort of repeatable set of questions or actions that isolates and engages a repeatable pattern of thinking?

Adapted from Delany, C., & Golding, C. (2014). Teaching clinical reasoning by making thinking visible: An action research project with allied health clinical educators. *BMC Medical Education, 14*(20), 2-10.

Chunking Information Through the Use of Heuristics, Domain-Specific Protocols, and Observation Worksheets

Chunking information plays a key role in the process of cue acquisition and pattern recognition as novices learn to create links between data sources so that decision making is based on a sound knowledge of the problem (Roberts, 1996; Schell, 2018). Delany and Golding (2014) engaged FWeds in a problem-solving process to develop a simple **heuristic** to make their expert thinking more visible to students. The idea was to simplify their complex reasoning to a thinking routine that they could easily teach to students. By thinking through the actual steps that they took to solve complex problems, educators were able to group their behaviors into *heuristics*, thinking routines that they could then repeat, model, and encourage students to regularly use.

To do this, educators were asked a series of questions to help them make visible their thinking. These questions are provided in Table 5-9. This helped them to identify and then repackage their thinking steps into thinking routines (repeatable actions) that they could pass on to students to encourage an automatic way of thinking.

For example, when engaging in treatment planning with a client, a therapist might find that they use a simple heuristic of (1) asking the client *why* they are *here*, (2) asking *what* are caregiver or client *goals*, and (3) summarizing *what* you (the therapist) could do to *help*. This simple heuristic might then be summarized as (1) why here, (2) what goals, (3) what helps. By summarizing the heuristic in a repeatable form, they found it could be used as a tool to cue the student while working with a client. The process of developing a heuristic typically had more than one cycle, as therapists would develop heuristics, try them out with students, and then refine them to communicate their thinking steps more precisely. For example, in the heuristic discussed previously, the therapists found that step 2, what are the patient's goals, actually also involved sorting and categorizing the goals into areas of occupation, underlying components contributing to problems, and contextual barriers or supports. Through identifying, developing, and then refining their heuristics, FWeds became more aware of their thinking and made their unobservable thinking accessible to students. In addition, they became more attentive to student learning and improved their teaching effectiveness.

Use of a heuristic with students on Level I fieldwork is particularly helpful as students want to engage in the therapy process and in client interactions but may need cueing to link steps of the therapy process together. Table 5-10 provides examples of heuristics that represent various aspects of the therapy process.

TABLE 5-10
HEURISTICS FOR THE THERAPY PROCESS

CLINICAL ACTIVITY	THINKING ROUTINES
Assessing a patient with a musculoskeletal injury	1. Underlying structures 2. Connecting structures 3. Patterns of pain and symptoms
Reassessment of a child after an initial evaluation	1. What changes occurred in the child's symptoms since last presentation? 2. What is the impact of treatment on their occupational performance? 3. Should you continue or change your treatment?
Client-centered treatment planning	1. Why is the client here? 2. What are this person's goals? 3. Summarize what you could do to help them achieve their goals.

Adapted from Delany, C., & Golding, C. (2014). Teaching clinical reasoning by making thinking visible: An action research project with allied health clinical educators. *BMC Medical Education, 14*(20), 2-10.

The use of a **domain-specific protocol**, defined as "a set of procedures or steps to be followed for the accomplishment of a given task" has been identified as helpful in the development and refinement of clinical reasoning skills. Kuipers and Grice (2009a, 2009b) found that both novices and experts showed subtle changes in the content and structure of their reasoning following exposure to a domain-specific protocol. They conducted individual interviews with 13 novice and 8 expert therapists prior to and following exposure to a domain-specific clinical reasoning protocol. The protocol was designed for use with upper limb hypertonia due to brain injury and defined barriers to upper limb function in three progressively limiting scenarios, and listed potential goals for each of the three clusters, ranging from improving quality and flexibility of grasp and movement, to preventing and reducing muscle or soft tissue contracture, to managing joint changes and maintaining joint integrity.

Following exposure to the protocol, the reasoning of the novice therapists more closely reflected the reasoning of experts to include both a structural approach, as well as a theoretical practice perspective. After learning the protocol, experienced therapists demonstrated greater therapist/client collaboration and use of upper limb–related constructs to structure their reasoning. In a domain-specific protocol, the important cues and patterns have already been identified for the student, and the problem has been isolated making it much easier to enact the steps of solving the problem. In delimiting the problem, the therapist is no longer required to put maximal effort toward the hard work of problem formulation and solution enactment but is able to expand from procedural reasoning to access other aspects of learning and reasoning, in other words, to appreciate the larger picture of the therapy process.

This may explain why Kuipers and Grice (2009a, 2009b) found that when a domain-specific protocol was used, novice therapists expanded their thinking from procedural to also include scientific reasoning, whereas experienced therapists expanded the depth of their narrative, interactional, and scientific reasoning in response to the protocol. Organizational clinical protocols, while helpful, can be built upon further by the adoption of clinical practice guidelines that may be

TABLE 5-11

STUDENT WORKSHEET MODEL OF HUMAN OCCUPATION APPLICATION

Volition: What do you notice about the client's interests, values, and belief in their ability to do things?	
Habituation: What roles seem important to the client? How do their habits and routines impact role performance?	
How does their performance capacity impact their ability to participate in occupations? This would include their motor skills, thinking (processing) abilities, and communication skills.	
How does the client's social and physical environment impact occupational performance?	

more widely utilized by the profession. These guidelines are generally based on systematic reviews or a synthesis of best practice evidence, which can allow for a novice (or expert) practitioner to confidently navigate the clinical reasoning process based on research evidence.

When might a protocol approach be helpful? As mentioned earlier, the sequence of the therapy process is not always visible to the novice and especially to the Level I fieldwork student. Spelling out the sequence of procedures used for a specific occupational therapy procedure, such as assessment, or for use with a given population orients the student to what to observe for if observing a therapy process. Most students, for example, would find the AOTA practice guideline series to be helpful to their learning to work with a specific diagnostic category, such as individuals who have sustained a stroke (AOTA, 2016).

The protocol might also be translated into an **observation worksheet** so that students can direct their observations to better appreciate what the steps of a specific process look like in practice and ask questions about aspects of the process that they did not notice or understand. Observation worksheets are especially helpful on Level I fieldwork placements as observation is often identified as a first step to learning, but without direction, students may miss important details. Observation worksheets can focus on any aspect of the reasoning process and on all types of clinical reasoning. For example, one could ask students to review the clinical reasoning questions posed in Table 5-3 of this chapter and direct student observation to the type of reasoning used in client interactions. Observations might be directed toward specific components of theoretical reasoning, such as the concepts of an occupational behavior model or frame of reference (Table 5-11).

This is helpful for students in keeping perspective of the complementary relationship between the occupational focus of therapy and addressing underlying factors and skills that contribute

TABLE 5-12

STUDENT WORKSHEET FOR CONNECTING THE OCCUPATIONAL THERAPY PROCESS

What screening tool would be best to determine the need for cognitive assessment?	
Based on screening results, what cognitive assessments are indicated?	
Based on results of cognitive testing, what modifications should be made in treatment goals?	
Given cognitive limitations and capacity for change, what occupation-based interventions should be provided?	
Based on client's response to intervention, how will you modify interventions for the next treatment session? Why?	

to occupational performance. In addition, directed attention to connecting various elements of the occupational therapy process to one another helps the students to connect therapist actions, such as assessment, treatment planning, intervention, and outcomes measurement to one another (Table 5-12).

Debriefing, Performance-Specific Feedback, and Reflection on Practice

Debriefing

Using guided discovery and prompting questions during debriefing helps students adjust their practice approach and develop skills in evaluating their own performance (Copley et al., 2011; Maloney & Griffith, 2013). Students who experienced educator/instructor debriefing following treatment sessions reported that it helped them to identify answers for themselves and to develop their problem-solving and analysis skills. To successfully participate in this process, students had to let go of concrete learning strategies and actively participate in a discussion about their level of understanding and reasoning. The guided discovery process challenges the student to reflect on various components of the treatment session and actively notice the effects of various interventions. The PEARLS Healthcare Debriefing Tool, originally published by Bajaj et al. (2018), is commonly cited as a best practice structure for health care students (Figure 5-3). Through review of the components of this debriefing model, you will notice attention to both cognitive and affective learning, components that are addressed in Bloom's Revised Learning Taxonomy.

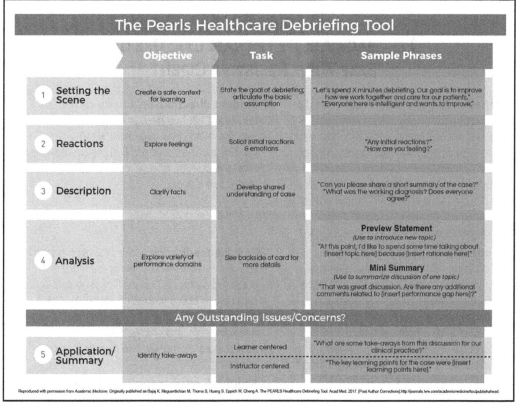

Figure 5-3. Utilizing the PEARLS Healthcare Debriefing Model. (Reproduced with permission from Roberts, L. W. [2022]. Learning to care for patients: A comment on "blind spots." *Academic Medicine, 97*[5], 619. https://doi.org/10.1097/ACM.000000004637.)

Performance-Specific Feedback

Performance-specific feedback is highly valued by students, but especially by students representing Generations Y and Z (DeIuliis & Saylor, 2021). Clynes and Raftery (2008) suggest that feedback begins by providing students with examples from practice that can be viewed as specific targets and standards. Feedback can then be provided relative to the target, focused on evaluating behavior and work performance and not on student character. The best feedback is highly specific and descriptive of what actually occurred. Asking for the students' self-assessment before giving feedback provides insight into the students' ability to evaluate their own practice performance. Students appreciate feedback that confirms effectiveness in applying clinical reasoning skills, as well as corrective feedback letting them know where they are off track (de Beer & Martensson, 2015; Koski et al., 2013; Rodger et al., 2011). This is also consistent with fostering a growth mindset for learning.

Student's clinical reasoning skills are most likely to be improved through corrective feedback if this feedback is accompanied by suggestions on how to improve (Table 5-13). The absence of feedback has negative implications for student learning as students are left to learn through trial and error (Chur-Hansen & McLean, 2006).

TABLE 5-13
FEEDBACK ABOUT THERAPEUTIC USE OF SELF WITH RESISTIVE CLIENT

Behavior target: Client is nonverbal due to multiple disabilities and often refuses therapy involvement. It is difficult to gauge the client's cognitive capacity to engage in activities. Be generous with encouraging mode to engage in therapy. Be specific in instruction so it is clear what you want the client to do. Be ready to adapt the activity up or down as needed.	**Student direction:** *Because the client is nonverbal, you will need to be extra verbal and generous with encouragement. Be specific in your instruction so we can better evaluate their cognitive abilities, and be ready to adapt your instruction if needed.*
Student behavior: Student began interaction with encouraging client to participate, smiling, and noting positive responses. Student was also instructing client in how to position their hand to hold a marker with a built-up handle to color a poster for their room. After 5 minutes, the student fell silent, and then kept asking the client if they liked the activity.	**Positive feedback:** *I noticed that you began your interaction with generous use of the encouraging mode: I noticed that you told Clyde that he was doing a good job of holding his pencil and turning his paper when writing. I also noted that you gave him specific instructions for how to hold his marker, and he was following your direction.* **Feedback observation and question:** *But then I noticed that you stopped talking and started asking questions instead. What happened?*
Student response: *I noticed that Clyde seemed to become more agitated the more that he colored, and I wasn't sure why. I worried that he did not like the activity or found it to be too childish for him.*	**Feedback and suggestion:** *When you started asking questions, I noticed that he quit coloring altogether and was no longer engaged in the project. He cannot answer open-ended questions as he is nonverbal, and so it is likely that your questions had the effect of causing further disengagement. Instead, think about how you could adapt the activity to increase his engagement and continue with an emphasis on encouragement and instruction because you did this very well at the beginning of your session!*
Student response: *That makes sense. I can adapt the activity next time to be a larger poster. I also noticed that he really likes Star Wars, so I will bring a Star Wars poster next time. I do feel more confident in my ability to encourage and instruct and am glad that what I did seemed effective.*	

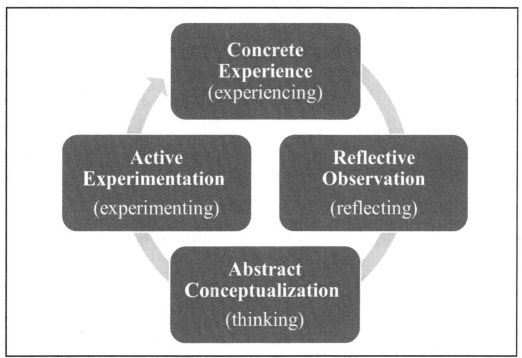

Figure 5-4. Kolb's Learning Cycle. (Adapted from Kolb, A. Y., & Kolb, D. A. [2017]. Experiential learning theory as a guide for experiential educators in higher education. *Experiential Learning & Teaching in Higher Education, 1*[1], 7-44 and Kolb, D. A. [2015]. *Experiential learning: Experience as the source of learning and development.* [2nd ed.]. Pearson Education.)

Reflection on Practice

An important skill for the novice is to learn to juggle the many *doing* aspects of a therapy session and to also use their metacognition to stand back and observe their own participation to see where it could be improved in the future. To adequately do so, there is a need to analyze and break down the elements contributing to the situation in enough detail to see an emerging pattern. Kolb's learning cycle, discussed in Chapter 2, is a helpful framework for the reflection process. As can be seen in Figure 5-4, reflection begins with some kind of *concrete experience*, such as conducting an initial assessment with a client. After the experience, the student will *stand back* from the experience and recall what happened through *reflective observation*, and then through *abstract conceptualization*, the student will analyze the components of the experience to determine what elements contributed to success and what may have detracted from the experience. For example, in an assessment experience, the student may determine that their strong introduction to the assessment process helped the client to focus, while having multiple documents on the table was distracting to the client and seemed to impact their attention span. The final stage in the cycle involves the student in another similar experience, now altering and using *active experimentation* to try to achieve better results. In the scenario discussed, for example, the student would remove all extraneous materials from the table to see if the client had a better attention span. The reflection process described is most effective when the student has multiple opportunities to engage in concrete learning experiences so that the patterns that contribute to success or challenges can emerge.

Reflecting on practice in written form is important to the teaching and learning of professional reasoning. FWeds report that it helps them to know how students are reasoning (Copley et al., 2017; Hanson et al., 2011). A simple and yet effective form of student reflection occurs when students identify a situation that has happened in the treatment context, describe the factor that both positively and negatively affected the situation, and state what might be done in the future to better address the situation. This type of reflection helps students to see the various conditions that

TABLE 5-14
STEPS FOR REFLECTIVE WRITING

Briefly describe the situation.	I conducted a 1-hour interview with a client with a bipolar diagnosis using the COPM. The client was able to complete the entire assessment, but their reporting was not accurate.
What was effective?	I effectively introduced myself and described the purpose of the assessment. I asked questions in each of the categories. I gave clear directions to the client to fill out the self-assessment portion of the tool.
What was not effective?	When I asked open-ended questions, I was not prepared with prompting questions to help the client stay on task. They often rambled, taking extra time, and not providing relevant information. I had a hard time redirecting them once they were off task.
What would you do differently next time?	I will review the client's chart in advance to ensure that their responses were consistent with reality. I will prepare prompting follow-up questions for each area of the COPM. I will review behavioral management strategies for keeping the client on task.

might affect an activity outcome, and also helps them to learn to think on their feet when encountering unexpected responses to their therapy efforts. See Table 5-14 for an example of reflective writing adapted from the work of Hanson et al. (2011).

Also keep in mind that written activities, such as progress notes or reports, force students to commit their clinical reasoning to paper, giving supervisors a clearer idea of their reasoning process. Additional forms of writing, such as case studies, help to gain a clear picture of what students are observing, and how they draw their conclusions. FWeds who were surveyed felt that writing helped students to organize their thoughts and explained that writing provides students with a structure, which can be important when dealing with the messiness of practice (Copley et al., 2017). Modeling the process of writing a report rather than just showing students the finished process was considered useful again to illustrate the messiness of practice and the complexity of the reasoning process.

In addition to use of reflection during the Level I fieldwork experience, it may be helpful to explore the student's overall learning at the conclusion of the Level I learning experience. Earlier in this chapter, Fink's Taxonomy was suggested as a means to facilitate dialogue between the student and FWed, but it also may be a helpful tool for students to reflect on their significant learning experiences on Level I fieldwork, particularly in regard to the impact on their development of therapeutic use of self, appreciation for the human dimension of therapy, development or refinement of values related to health care, and their overall abilities for learning. Table 5-5, presented earlier in the chapter, illustrates this process within a specific element of the therapy process, but it could easily be expanded for a midterm or final reflection.

Bloom's Taxonomy of Affective Development may also be a useful tool for promotion of reflection on the student's experience of refining their values structure and learning to align their values with the values of the profession. See Table 5-15 for an example of a student reflection tool that might be used in preparation for a group discussion of overall learning during Level I fieldwork. The reflection questions explore not only affective aspects of learning, but also the overall impact on professional identity development.

TABLE 5-15

STUDENT REFLECTION OF AFFECTIVE LEARNING AND PROFESSIONAL IDENTITY DEVELOPMENT

BLOOM'S TAXONOMY: AFFECTIVE DOMAIN	CATEGORY DESCRIPTION	REFLECTION QUESTIONS
Receiving	Being sensitive and open to new ideas, concepts, client stories, and situations. Able to tolerate differences encountered.	"What new ideas, concepts, client stories, or situations did you encounter? How did you initially react to the differences you encountered?"
Responding	Beginning to show commitment to new ideas, situations, ways of living by actively responding with words or actions.	"How did your response to new ideas, situations, or ways of living encountered during your Level I fieldwork change over time?"
Valuing	Openly demonstrating stronger commitment to different ideas or ways of living. Communicating new values verbally, in actions, online, etc.	"Have you noticed any differences in how you respond to different ideas and ways of living outside of your fieldwork experience? Please provide an example."
Organizing	Prioritizing some values over others to create one's own value system.	"What shifts in values or priorities have you noticed when you are working with clients? Have you found that you prioritize some values over others? Please explain."
Characterizing	Internalizing values, integrate value system into daily life.	"Has your Level I fieldwork experience affected the way you want to practice or your career interests in any way? If so, please explain how and what actions you plan to take in the future to integrate this learning into your life."
Professional identity	How does what I am learning impact who I want to be as an occupational therapist, and what I would like to do?	"Overall, how does your Level I learning impact who you want to be as an occupational therapist, and what you would like to do?"

SUMMARY

Level I fieldwork offers unique opportunities for students to take what they are learning in the classroom and apply it to practice. Understanding differences in the types of reasoning used in practice and the continuum of clinical reasoning can help FWeds to choose strategies that will meet students at their level of learning and bring them one step beyond.

Although there are challenges to engaging students in clinical reasoning, knowledge of challenges upfront help the FWed thoughtfully choose effective strategies for learning. The fieldwork context plays a key role in the development of clinical reasoning, and orientation at the beginning of the fieldwork helps students conceptualize what to focus on within the fieldwork context. FWeds play a key role in helping students to feel comfortable within the fieldwork context. In addition, they introduce students to the thinking that underlies the therapy process, through their modeling, reflection, talking out loud, engagement of students in active learning opportunities, and through debriefing and questioning processes that make their thinking and actions transparent to students. In addition to a better understanding of the occupational therapy process, opportunities to work directly with clients helps students to gain an understanding of their therapeutic effectiveness, appreciate the affective aspect of practice, discover professional interests, and begin to internalize the values of the profession.

The desired outcome of this chapter is that FWeds feel genuinely prepared to meet the accreditation standard for Level I fieldwork to "provide practice application experiences designed to enrich didactic course work through directed observation and participation utilizing the occupational therapy process…" (ACOTE, 2018, p. 41). We hope you also take advantage of the learning opportunities provided to build upon your fieldwork mentorship skills.

LEARNING ACTIVITIES

1. Clinical Reasoning Contiuum: Where Do You Land?

   To support the fieldwork student, it is important to first understand where we align ourselves in the clinical reasoning continuum. First, where do you believe you fall, in terms of novice to expert? When you think back to your first occupational therapy position, mark where you believe you started, then where you see yourself today.

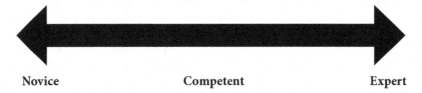

| Novice | Competent | Expert |

   What behaviors or activities caused you to rank yourself where you did? Were there individuals who supported your development? What behaviors or activities did they promote in your own learning?

Now consider a recent client you worked with. Think about all aspects of this case: the client and their factors, the individuals involved in the case, the context, etc. What components of clinical reasoning do you find you use most often? What does it look like when you incorporate narrative reasoning vs. scientific reasoning? Share your thoughts and be as specific as possible!

_____

_____

_____

_____

_____

2. Consider the overview of a clinical reasoning process presented in Table 5-3. Select a client from your caseload with your fieldwork student and ask them to think through this client in terms of the chart. What areas do they struggle to recognize or find easier to determine? How can this process help them to better organize their thoughts around clinical reasoning?

Cue acquisition	
Pattern recognition	
Limiting the problem space	
Problem formulation	
Problem solution	

3. Apply the Model of Context Specific Professional Reasoning to your site by filling in the blanks. Refer to Table 5-4 in the text for an example.

Relationship between practitioner and client	
Organization where therapy is provided	
Influence of legislation and government policy	
Impact of social structures and culture	

4. How can you use the categories of Fink's Taxonomy of Significant Learning (see Table 5-5) to more effectively reflect and dialogue with your next Level I fieldwork student?

5. Identify common skills that you would like to teach students during Level I fieldwork. Apply Bloom's Taxonomy cognitive domain to determine how you could advance students through the domain categories (see Table 5-7).

6. Refer to the example of clinical reasoning questions provided in Table 5-6. Which questions are you most likely to pursue in your own practice? Which are you less likely to ask yourself? How might these questions be helpful in your work with students?

7. Practice clinical reasoning out loud by choosing one of the clinical reasoning types provided in Box 5-9 and providing a narrative from your own practice.

8. Develop a _Student Observation Worksheet_ for your practice setting. See Table 5-11 and 5-12 for examples.

9. Using the PEARLS Healthcare Debriefing Tool from Figure 5-3, develop a debriefing script that you might use with Level I fieldwork students in your practice.

10. Identify a student that you have formerly worked with who did not demonstrate a skill successfully. Use Table 5-13 to identify (1) a target behavior that you would have liked the student to perform, (2) directions you could have provided the student, (3) a positive feedback statement, (4) a feedback observation, and (5) a question you might have asked. What impact might this have made on the student's learning?

11. Use the categories of Table 5-14 to reflect on therapy you provided to a recent client that did not go as you had hoped. What do you gain through this reflection process? In what situations might you share about this experience with your students?

ADDITIONAL RESOURCES

AOTA Clinical Guidelines: https://www.aota.org/Practice/Researchers/practice-guidelines.aspx
Cronin, A., & Graebe, G. (2018). *Clinical reasoning in occupational therapy.* AOTA Press.
Schell, B. A., & Schell, J. W. (2018). *Clinical and professional reasoning in occupational therapy.* Wolters Kluwer.

REFERENCES

Accreditation Council for Occupational Therapy Education. (2018). *2018 accreditation council for occupational therapy education standards and interpretative guide.* https://www.aota.org/~/media/Corporate/Files/EducationCareers/Accredit/StandardsReview/2018-ACOTE-Standards-Interpretive-Guide.pdf

American Occupational Therapy Association. (2016). *Top 10 recommendations from occupational therapy practice guidelines for adults with stroke.* https://www.aota.org/-/media/Corporate/Files/Secure/Practice/EB/Top-10-Recommendations-Practice-Guidelines-Adults-With-Stroke.pdf

Ashby, S. E., Adler, J., Herbert, L. (2016). An exploratory international study into occupational therapy students' perceptions of professional identity. *Australian Occupational Therapy Journal, 63*(4), 233-243. https://doi.org/10.1111/1440-1630.12271

Bajaj, K., Meguerdichian, M., Thoma, B., Huang, S., Eppich, W., & Cheng, A. (2018). The PEARLS health care debriefing tool. *Academic Medicine, 93*(2), 336. https://doi.org/10.1097/ACM.000000000002035

Bartz, D., Thompson, K., & Rice, P. (2017). Maximizing the human capital of millennials through supervisors using performance management. *International Journal of Management, Business and Administration, 20*(1), 1-9.

Berkley Graduate Division. (2021). *Social constructivism.* Graduate Student Instructor Resource Center. https://gsi.berkeley.edu/gsi-guide-contents/learning-theory-research/social-constructivism/

Bloom, B. S. (1956). *Taxonomy of educational objectives: The classification of educational goals.* Longmans.

Carr, M. & Shotwell, M. (2007). Information processing theory and professional reasoning. In B. A. B. Schell & J. W. Schell (Eds.), *Clinical reasoning and professional reasoning in occupational therapy* (pp. 36-68). Williams & Wilkins.

Chipcase, L. S., Buttrum, P. J., Dunwoodie, R., Hill, A. E., Mandrusiak, A. & Moran, M. (2012). Characteristics of student preparedness for clinical learning: Clinical educator perspectives using the Delphi approach. *BMC Medical Education, 12,* 112. https://doi.org/10.1186/1472-6920-12-112

Chur-Hansen, A., & Mclean, S. (2006). On being a supervisor: The importance of feedback and how to give it. *Australas Psychiatry, 14*(1), 67-71. https://doi.org/10.1080/j.1440-1665.2006.02248.x

Claro, S., Paunesku, D., & Dweck, C. S. (2016). Growth mindset tempers the effects of poverty on academic achievement. *Proceedings of the National Academy of Sciences, 113*(31), 8664-8668. https://doi.org/10.1073/pnas.1608207113

Clynes, M. P., & Raftery, S. E. C. (2008). Feedback: An essential element of student learning in clinical practice. *Nurse Education in Practice, 8*(6), 405-411. https://doi.org/10.1016/j.nepr.2008.02.003

Cohn, E. S. (1989). Fieldwork education: Shaping a foundation for clinical reasoning. *American Journal of Occupational Therapy, 43*(4), 240-244. https://doi.org/10.5014/ajot.43.4.240

Coker, P. (2010). Effects of an experiential learning program on the clinical reasoning and critical thinking skills of occupational therapy students. *Journal of Allied Health, 39*(4), 280-286.

Copley, J. A., Bennett, S., & Turpin, M. (2017). Decision-making for occupation-centred practice with children. In S. Rodger & A. Kennedy-Behr (Eds.), *Occupation-centred practice with children: A practical guide for occupational therapists* (pp. 349-372). Wiley-Blackwell.

Copley, J. A., Rodger, S. A., Graham, F. P., & Hannay, V. A. (2011). Facilitating student occupational therapists' mastery of occupation-centered approaches for working with children. *Canadian Journal of Occupational Therapy, 78*(1), 37-44. https://doi.org/10.2182/cjot.2011.78.1.5

Copley, J. A., Rodger, S. A., Hannay, V. A., & Graham, F. P. (2010). Occupational therapy students' experiences in learning occupation-centred approaches to working with children. *Canadian Journal of Occupational Therapy, 77*(1), 48-56. https://doi.org/10.2182/cjot.2010.77.1.7

de Beer, M., & Martensson, L. (2015). Feedback on students' clinical reasoning skills during fieldwork education. *Australian Occupational Therapy Journal, 62*(4), 255-264. https://doi.org/10.1111/1440-1630.12208

DeIuliis, E. D., & Saylor, E. (2021). Bridging the gap: Three strategies to optimize professional relationships with generation Y and Z. *The Open Journal of Occupational Therapy, 9*(1), 1-13. https://doi.org/10.15453/2168-6408.1748

Delany, C., & Golding, C. (2014). Teaching clinical reasoning by making thinking visible: An action research project with allied health clinical educators. *BMC Medical Education, 14*(20), 2-10.

Deloitte. (2016). *The 2016 deloitte millennial survey winning over the next generation of leaders.* https://www2.deloitte.com/content/dam/Deloitte/ global/Documents/About-Deloitte/gx-millenialsurvey-2016-exec-summary.pdf

Dreyfus, H. L., & Dreyfus, S. E. (1986). *Mind over machine: The power of human intuition and expertise in the era of the computer.* Free Press.

Fink, L. D. (2003). *Creating significant learning experiences: An integrated approach to designing college courses.* John Wiley & Sons.

Fink, L. D. (2013). *Creating significant learning experiences: An integrated approach to designing college courses.* [Ebook]. Jossey-Bass.

Gat, S., & Ratzon, N. Z. (2014). Comparison of occupational therapy students' perceived skills after traditional and nontraditional fieldwork. *American Journal of Occupational Therapy, 68*(2), e47-e54. http://doi.org/10.5014/ajot.2014.007732

Graen, G. B., & Schiemann, W. A. (2013). Leadership-motivated excellence theory: An extension of LMX. *Journal of Managerial Psychology, 28*(5), 452-469. https://doi.org/10.1108/jmp-11-2012-0351

Hanson, D. (2011). The perspectives of fieldwork educators regarding Level II fieldwork students. *Occupational Therapy in Health Care, 25,* 164-172.

Hanson, D., Larson, J. K., & Nielsen, S. (2011). Reflective writing in Level II fieldwork. *OT Practice.*

Hills, C., Boshoff, K., Gilbert-Hunt, S., Ryan, S., & Smith, D. R. (2015). The future in their hands: The perceptions of practice educators on the strengths and challenges of "Generation Y" occupational therapy students. *The Open Journal of Occupational Therapy, 3*(4). https://doi.org/10.15453/2168-6408.1135

Hochanadel, A., & Finamore, D. (2015). Fixed and growth mindset in education and how grit helps students persist in the face of adversity. *Journal of International Education Research, 11*(1), 47-50. https://doi.org/10.19030/jier.v11i1.9099

Johnson, C. R., Koenig, K. P., Piersol, C. V., Santalucia, S. E., & Wachter-Schutz, W. (2006). Level I fieldwork today: A study of contexts and perceptions. *American Journal of Occupational Therapy, 60*(3), 275-287. https://doi.org/10.5014/ajot.60.3.275

Kolb, A. Y., & Kolb, D. A. (2017). Experiential learning theory as a guide for experiential educators in higher education. *Experiential Learning & Teaching in Higher Education, 1*(1), 7-44.

Kolb, D. A. (2015). *Experiential learning: Experience as the source of learning and development.* (2nd ed.). Pearson Education.

Koski, K. J., Simon, R. L., & Dooley, N. R. (2013). Valuable occupational therapy fieldwork educator behaviors. *Work, 44,* 307-315. https://doi.org/10.3233/WOR-121507

Kuipers, K., & Grice, J. W. (2009a). The structure of novice and expert occuaptional therapists' clinical reasoning before and after exposure to a domain-specific protocol. *Australian Occupaitonal Therapy Journal, 56,* 418-427. https://doi.org/10.1111/j.1440-1630.2009.00793.x

Kuipers, K., & Grice, J. W. (2009b). Clinical reasoning in neurology: Use of the repertory grid technique to investigate the reasoning of an experienced occupational therapist. *Austalian Occupational Therapy Journal, 56*(4), 275-284. https://doi.org/10.1111/j.1440-1630.2008.00737.x

Lang, J. (2006). *Small teaching.* Jossey Bass.

Liu, K. P. Y., Chan, C. H. C., & Hui-Chan, C. W. Y. (2000). Clinical reasoning and the occupational therapy curriculum. *Occupational Therapy International, 7*(3), 173-183. https://doi.org/10.1002/oti.118

Maloney, S. M., & Griffith, K. (2013). Occupational therapy students' development of therapeutic communication skills during a service-learning experience. *Occupational Therapy in Mental Health, 29*(1), 10-26. https://doi.org/10.1080/0164212X.2013.760288

McLeod, S. (2020). Lev Vygotsky's sociocultural theory. *Simply Psychology.* https://www.simplypsychology.org/vygotsky.html

Mitchell, R., & Unsworth, C. A. (2005). Clinical reasoning during community health home visits: Expert and novice differences. *British Journal of Occupational Therapy, 68*(5), 215-223. https://doi.org/10.1177/0308022605800505

Neistadt, M. E. (1996). Teaching strategies for the development of clinical reasoning. *American Journal of Occupational Therapy, 50*(8), 676-684.

Nielsen, S., Jedlicka, J. S., Hanson, D., Fox, L., & Graves, C. (2017). Student perceptions of non-traditional Level I fieldwork. *Journal of Occupational Therapy Education, 1.* https://doi.org/10.26681/jote.2017.010206

Ripat, J., Wener, P., & Dobinson, K. (2013). The development of client-centredness in student occupational therapists. *British Journal of Occupational Therapy, 76*(5), 217-224. https://doi.org/10.4276/030802213X13679275042681

Roberts, A. E. (1996). Clinical reasoning in occupational therapy: Idiosyncrasies in content and process. *British Journal of Occupational Therapy, 59,* 372-376.

Roberts, L. W. (2022). Learning to care for patients: A comment on "blind spots". *Academic Medicine, 97*(5), 619. https://doi.org/10.1097/ACM.000000004637

Rodger, S., Fitzgerald, C., Davila, W., Millar, F., & Allison, H. (2011). What makes a quality occupational therapy practice placement? Students' and practice educators' perspectives. *Australian Occupational Therapy Journal, 58*(3), 195-202.

Rogers, J. C. (1983). Eleanor Clarke Slagle Lectureship—1983; Clinical reasoning: The ethics, science, and art. *American Journal of Occupational Therapy, 37*(9), 601-616.

Schell, B. (2018). Professional reasoning in practice. In B. Schell & G. Gillen (Eds.), *Willard and Spackman's occupational therapy* (13th ed.). Wolters Kluwer.

Schell, B. A., & Schell, J. W. (2018). *Clinical and professional reasoning in occupational therapy.* Wolters Kluwer.

Seif, G., Coker-Bolt, P., Kraft, S., Gonsalves, W., Simpson, K., & Johnson, E. (2014). The development of clinical reasoning and interprofessional behaviors: Service-learning at a student-run free clinic. *Journal of Interprofessional Care, 28,* 559-564. https://doi.org/10.4276/030802213X3679275042681

Strong, J., Gilbert, J., Cassidy, S., & Bennett, S. (1995). Expert clinicians' and students' views on clinical reasoning in occupational therapy. *British Journal of Occupational Therapy, 58*(3), 119-123.

Turpin, M. J., & Hanson, D. (2018). Learning professional reasoning in practice through fieldwork. In B. A. Schell & J. W. Schell (Eds.), *Clinical and professional reasoning in occupational therapy* (2nd ed., pp. 439-460). Williams & Wilkins.

Turpin, M. J., & Iwama, M. (2011). *Using occupational therapy models in practice: A fieldguide.* Elsevier.

Unsworth, C. A. (2001). The clinical reasoning of novice and expert occupational therapists. *Scandinavian Journal of Occupational Therapy, 8*(4), 163-173.

Unsworth, C., & Baker, A. (2016) A systematic review of professional reasoning literature in occupational therapy. *British Journal of Occupational Therapy, 79*(1), 5-16. https://doi.org/10.1177/0308022615599994

Vygotsky, L. S. (1978). *Mind in society: The development of higher psychological processes.* Harvard University Press.

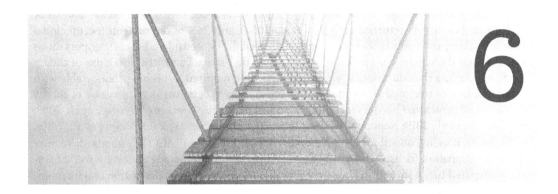

Thinking With Theory

Debra Hanson, PhD, OTR/L, FAOTA
and Jason C. Lawson, PhD, MS, OTR/L

The occupational therapy profession, over the last 4 decades, has made many strides in unifying the language of the profession by developing and articulating theories that explain how use of occupation as intervention can influence health (Lee et al., 2008; Lee, 2010). Occupational behavior models, also known as occupation-focused theories, emerged in the later decades of the 20th century as a tool to not only articulate the unique value of the profession but also provide a foundation for the professional identity of occupational therapy practitioners and a framework for everyday clinical reasoning (Elliott et al., 2002; Ikiugu, 2010; Wimpenny et al., 2010). Examples of occupational behavior models generated include, but are not limited to, the Canadian Model of Occupational Performance and Engagement (CMOP-E), the Kawa Model, the Model of Human Occupation (MOHO), the Occupation Adaptation Model (OAM), the Person-Environment-Occupation (PEO) Model, and the Ecological Model (Cole & Tufano, 2008; Schell & Gillen, 2018; Turpin & Iwama, 2011).

Over the past decade and beyond, examples of occupational therapy practitioners actively using occupation-focused theories in practice have emerged in literature, including use with individual clients, groups, populations, and as a tool for program development in diverse practice settings (Cole & Tufano, 2008; Jack & Estes, 2010; Maclean et al., 2012). Davis-Cheshire et al. (2019) surveyed occupational therapy practitioners in the United States and found that 79% indicated that they used occupation-focused theories in practice, and 77% agreed that they were valuable to their practice. However, other evidence suggests that many occupational therapy practitioners find it challenging to use the language and reasoning of occupational behavior models to guide

Hanson, D., & DeIuliis, E. D. (Eds.).
Fieldwork Educator's Guide to Level I Fieldwork (pp. 143-183).
© 2023 Taylor and Francis Group.

their everyday practice (Ikiugu, 2010; Lee, 2010; Melton et al., 2009, 2010; O'Neal et al., 2007). For example, from 145 surveys returned to O'Neal et al. (2007), only 26% of respondents (occupational therapists working with adults with developmental disabilities) considered theory important as a guide for their daily practice. There are many factors that impact a practitioner's use of theory in practice including the educational preparation and time required to become comfortable with new theories, lack of role models for theory implementation, skepticism as to the value of theory application, and contextual barriers including time and pragmatic concerns (Boniface et al., 2008; Davis-Cheshire et al., 2019; Keponen & Launiainen, 2008; Leclair et al., 2013; Melton et al., 2010).

The Accreditation Council for Occupational Therapy Education (ACOTE) standards require attention to occupation-focused theory in entry-level occupational therapy education so that students are prepared to use theory and occupation-based models to inform evaluation and intervention in practice (ACOTE, 2018). Students spend about 2 years learning the language and customs of the profession but report difficulty in using their knowledge of theory and applying it in practice if their fieldwork educators (FWeds) do not communicate use of theory in practice (Towns & Ashby, 2014). Koski et al. (2013) found that students rate the value of using information about clients' occupational performance in intervention more highly than FWeds, who may be more likely to follow traditional methods dictated by the practice setting or reimbursement requirements. This discrepancy has led to a gap between the educational experience of occupational therapy students and their experiences on fieldwork, which is problematic for student learning (Ikiugu et al., 2009). For example, when working with multiple FWeds, students found that the clinical reasoning of each educator was unique and not shared within the broader professional community (Towns & Ashby, 2014). This impedes student development of reasoning, as students must learn by rote the customs, procedure, and language of each practitioner or facility rather than relying on the clinical reasoning structures anchored to the language of occupation-focused theories learned in their academic education.

Clearly, FWeds play a key role in shaping the attitudes and values of students regarding the value of using theory in everyday practice. This influence may be either positive or negative, dependent on how theoretical knowledge is integrated into the professional reasoning process of the practitioner (Honey & Penman, 2020; Towns & Ashby, 2014). When FWeds value and use occupation-focused models, the students' skills for applying theory to professional reasoning for occupation-based practice are expanded, whereas the depreciation of occupation-focused theory can lead to student development of component-based practice that is not easily distinguished from other professions (Smallfield & Karges, 2009; Towns & Ashby, 2014). Professional practice education, including Level I fieldwork, is expected to be the place where students integrate theoretical knowledge with practice (ACOTE, 2018; Ashby & Chandler, 2010). This can be problematic if practitioners themselves are not comfortable with using occupational therapy models in their own practice.

The purpose of this chapter is to introduce readers to the value of using occupation-focused models to strengthen occupational therapy practice, professional identity, and visibility, and also as a tool to strengthen occupational therapy student clinical reasoning. Recognizing that FWeds may be at various stages of understanding and use of occupation-focused theory, a five-staged model for getting comfortable with theory use in practice will be introduced, and practical strategies for engaging Level I students at the level that best fits the learning stage of the FWed/site will be presented.

KEY WORDS

- **Component-based practice**: Using intervention that targets impairments in body structure or body function with the intent of improving component performance but without attention to client participation in daily life (Smallfield & Karges, 2009; Towns & Ashby, 2014).

- **Frames of reference**: "A system of compatible concepts from theory that guide a plan of action for assessment and intervention within specific occupational therapy domains" (Cole & Tufano, 2008, p. 62). Frames of reference focus on the underlying components contributing to occupational performance. Frames of reference provide specific strategies for addressing elements or components that interfere with occupational performance, such as functional cognition, motor or sensory skills, but do not provide a comprehensive orientation to occupational performance concerns. Common examples include biomechanical and sensory integration frames of reference (Cole & Tufano, 2008).

- **Occupation-focused models**: "Provide an overarching context of occupation that emphasizes the occupational therapists' unique perspective on a client's ability to engage in activities and participate in life" and "attempt to explain the relationship of occupation, person, and environment" (Cole & Tufano, 2008, p. 61). They explain how normative occupational performance is organized and suggest constructs for intervening when challenges in occupational performance are evident.

- **Role-emerging placements**: Designed to promote occupational therapy in a setting where there is not an established occupational therapist role. Students receive direct supervision from a staff member who is not an occupational therapist (Overton et al., 2009).

- **Role-established placements**: Involve direct supervision by an occupational therapist, generally employed within the service, with students practicing skills and performing tasks within an established occupational therapy role (Overton et al., 2009).

- **Scaffolding:** The provision of intentional supports that can be reduced as students incrementally develop independence and mastery (Schell, 2018).

LEARNING OBJECTIVES

By the end of reading this chapter and completing the learning activities, the reader should be able to:

1. Consider the value of adopting a primary occupational therapy occupational behavior model as a conceptual tool to strengthen occupational therapy services and teach clinical reasoning.

2. Become familiar with a five-stage continuum for exploring the use of occupational behavior models in a specific practice setting.

3. Choose strategies that are a best fit for the fieldwork site and educator for engaging students in theory-driven practice.

THE VALUE OF THINKING WITH THEORY

Although occupation-focused theory is often not used in practice, the value of the explicit use of theory in practice is well established. Active theory use in practice has been associated with strong professional identity and resiliency in stressful work environments and a tool to articulate the unique value of services to the public and other health care providers (Ashby et al., 2013; Ikiugu, 2010; Towns & Ashby, 2014). Occupation-focused models are effectively used in program development to organize the delivery of occupational therapy services to a population group in a manner that upholds the unique value of the profession and provides an avenue for application of evidence to practice (Braveman, 2018; Braveman et al., 2008). Use of occupation-focused models in student teaching strengthens the clinical reasoning abilities of students and their likelihood of incorporating occupation into their future intervention (Bonsaksen et al., 2013; Ikiugu & Smallfield, 2015; Leclair et al., 2013; Towns & Ashby, 2014). Each of these value points will be explored in this chapter's next section.

Using Theory to Articulate Unique Value

Occupational therapists provide a unique service in their work with clients, but often struggle to articulate their unique value and contributions to the treatment team (Wilding & Whiteford, 2007). This is a quandary that can lead to a marginalization of services, lack of representation on the treatment team, and/or professional burnout for the occupational therapy practitioner (Edwards & Dirette, 2010; Smallfield & Karges, 2009; Towns & Ashby, 2014). With the broad spectrum of services provided by occupational therapy practitioners, it becomes relatively easy for the practitioner to become derailed from the primary objective of occupational performance (Kielhofner, 2009; Shannon, 1977). In settings where practitioners work with clients with physical disabilities, the emphasis can easily become motor skills, with use of exercise and various biomechanical, neurology-focused, or sensory interventions (Smallfield & Karges, 2009). In mental health practice, attention to the psycho-emotional aspect of services may take priority, and it is tempting for the occupational therapist to align with disciplines of psychology and counseling rather than retain a unique occupation focus (Ashby et al., 2013). Without maintaining a unique focus, the value of occupational therapy services is decreased, and there is an increased risk of role replacement with position vacancy.

Amy Lamb, OTD, OT/L, FAOTA, former President of the American Occupational Therapy Association, spoke often of the need to communicate the unique (distinct) value of occupational therapy to key stakeholders (Lamb, 2016). Through articulation of key concepts, occupational therapy practitioners can better promote their value and achieve *buy in* for services. In addition, they are able to avoid various derailers that lead toward occupational therapy being a profession that *fills in the gaps* from various other professions, since there are many aspects of the profession that overlap with other health care professions. See Box 6-1 for a scenario of therapist burnout related to lack of communication of the unique value of occupational therapy to key stakeholders.

Using theory in practice provides tools to highlight the unique contributions of the occupational therapy profession and to differentiate the professional status of occupational therapy practitioners from that of an activity technician (Ikiugu, 2010; Ikiugu & Smallfield, 2011). The value of theory use is evident in the work of Hanson (2009), who interviewed 12 occupational therapists practicing in physical rehabilitation of adult clients in medical centers across the midwestern states of the United States. She found that all therapists were able to actively incorporate occupation into their therapy, but those who did not use occupation-focused models to orient their work often struggled with incorporating occupation into their definitions of the unique contribution that they made to the treatment team. Hanson (2009) found that occupation was often an "invisible" element that was added to the treatment process to motivate and engage the client but was not visible in the documentation or communications of the occupational therapy practitioner to key stakeholders. On the other hand, those therapists who actively used occupation-focused models to describe their work were readily able to apply occupational concepts to client assessment, treatment planning, goal setting, intervention, and documentation processes required in the medical setting. Similarly, Ashby et al. (2013) found that occupational therapists working in mental health who incorporated occupation-focused theories into their practice were able to differentiate the value of their occupation-focused work from that which was focused on the remediation of psychological process common to mental health settings. Through the process of articulating their

---

BOX 6-1

BURNOUT RELATED TO LACK OF
UNIQUE VALUE OF OCCUPATIONAL THERAPY

Working in physical disabilities, I felt pressure to do the *tried and true* methods of my senior occupational therapist to increase occupational performance. However, when observing them with clients after a shoulder injury next to the physical therapists who were treating patients with shoulder injuries, they were giving the same evaluative measures and following the same treatment protocols. I asked why a physician would order occupational therapy instead of physical therapy (or vice versa) and was told "It depends on who has an opening in the schedule to start treatment." I then asked what the difference between occupational therapy and physical therapy was at this site, and was told "occupational therapists do uppers (referring to upper extremities) and physical therapists do lowers (referring to lower extremities)." My next question was "Well, why do any physical therapists treat shoulders then if occupational therapists treat the uppers?" Candidly, I was told "Go ask the physical therapists." I never did ask a physical therapist and felt uncomfortable every time my clients would ask me what the difference was between physical therapy and occupational therapy, mostly because I didn't know. Similarly, many clients would just refer to me as a physical therapist, and I never bothered to correct them.

Reflection from Chapter Author—Jason C. Lawson, PhD, MS, OTR/L

---

unique contributions within a community of professional practice and avoiding the adoption of activities and roles not central to their work, they were professionally resilient and more able to avoid professional burnout. See Box 6-2 as an example of using an occupation-focused model to articulate the unique contribution of occupational therapy services.

Value of Occupation-Focused Theory to Program Development and Evidence-Based Practice

Why bother using an occupational behavior model when working with a client or when developing a new program? When occupational therapy practitioners provide client programming guided by an occupational behavior model, they are able to ensure that the ideals of the profession for client-centered and occupation-based practice are followed. Use of models is also linked with evidence-based practice (EBP), providing a rationale for intervention that is undergirded with research evidence (Owen et al., 2014). Since every occupational behavior model addresses an aspect of the person, the environment, and occupation, the practitioner can be assured that their practice is firmly grounded in the ideals of the profession. Furthermore, many of the models have built-in assessment tools that can help the practitioner that model ideals are evident, such as the Canadian Occupational Performance Measure (COPM), written for the CMOP-E, and a plethora of assessment tools written for use with the MOHO. When specific assessment tools have not been developed for the model, the practitioner is free to choose tools that represent the concepts, change mechanisms, and outcomes outlined by the model. For example, the COPM has been successfully used to identify occupational performance issues using the OAM for this purpose as it measures the same concept. Similarly, there have been no specific tools developed for use with the PEO Model, but various formal and informal tools might be used to measure model concepts (Box 6-3).

In addition to use of an occupation-focused model to guide occupational therapy intervention for a single client, models have been used to guide program development for a population of clients. When using the occupation-focused model to guide program development, the occupational

Box 6-2
EXAMPLE OF THERAPIST USE OF THEORY TO COMMUNICATE UNIQUE VALUE

Being the only occupational therapist for a contract company and being responsible for the evaluation and treatment of individuals at a skilled nursing facility, outpatient clinic serving both adults and pediatrics, I felt lost and completely overwhelmed shifting focus from one setting/population to the next. I felt many of my treatment plans were scrutinized by administration because they hadn't seen occupation-based goals in an occupational therapy intervention plan before. Their questioning and scrutinizing my intervention plans made me start questioning my years of education and shook my confidence. However, I decided to ground my practice in occupational therapy theory as a means to explain my practice. I chose to use the PEO Model and started to explain how certain aspects of my evaluation were targeting the person and the person's environment, and how my interventions were aimed at maximizing the fit between the person and environment to maximize their occupational performance. Being able to link the evaluation, occupation-based goals, and interventions to a sound, occupational therapy–specific theory gave me the ability and confidence to articulate my rationale to others, thus communicating the distinct value of occupational therapy.

Reflection from Chapter Author regarding practice in rural North Dakota—Jason C. Lawson, PhD, MS, OTR/L

therapy practitioner can ensure that the programming developed is firmly rooted in the ideals of the occupational therapy profession, that occupational performance is highlighted in the programming provided, and the programming is evidence-based. Braveman (2016) provides an excellent overview of the process used to develop programs using both occupation-focused models, as well as related knowledge for the development of occupational therapy programming. Bravemen (2016) also provides examples of programming developed for persons living with HIV/AIDS, as well as a theory-based approach to occupational therapy oncology rehabilitation (Braveman et al., 2018). Further, Lee (2010) provides a review of evidence linked to occupation-focused models and provides examples of programming developed for the CMOP-E, OAM, MOHO, and PEO Model. Examples include medical and community settings with a range of ages and health conditions.

Value of Occupation-Focused Models to Student Professional Reasoning Development

Level I fieldwork is meant to provide students with practical experiences that enrich didactic (academic) coursework. Foundational didactic coursework may include use of theory, models, and frames of references in order to expose students to the profession's language and guide clinical reasoning. **Theory** may include related knowledge from other disciplines, such as psychology or neuroscience. **Occupation-focused models** explain how normative occupational performance is organized and suggest constructs for intervening when challenges in occupational performance are evident. **Frames of reference** provide *specific strategies* for addressing elements or components that interfere with occupational performance, such as functional cognition and motor or sensory skills, but do not provide a comprehensive orientation to occupational performance concerns. The requirements for Level I fieldwork vary considerably and may include site-specific, community Level I fieldworks, faculty-led service learning experiences, and even simulated experiences. Furthermore, Level I fieldwork placements in emerging areas of occupational therapy practice has

Box 6-3
PEO MODEL ASSESSMENT SCENARIO

Client: 9-year-old boy with Down syndrome (Bob)—referred to outpatient occupational therapy services to assess motor coordination. Child's mom (Linda) is present during the occupational therapy evaluation.

Assessment: Occupational Performance

- **Dressing (Information obtained through occupational profile interview and observation)**

Bob typically wakes up at 6 a.m. and comes down to breakfast. Linda gives him cereal, then brushes his teeth and helps him get dressed. Bob takes a long time and gets easily distracted, so Linda usually does his dressing for him so they are not late for school. Clothing typically consists of jeans with zipper, button up shirts with T-shirt, underwear, socks, and tennis shoes that tie. He is unable to don or doff his shirt or jacket, button his shirt, zip his pants, or tie his shoes. He is able to assist with pulling up jeans once they are laid out for him.

Assessment: Person

- **Physical:** The Bruininks-Oseretsky Test of Motor Proficiency Second Edition (BOT-2) assessment is used and focuses on the subtests of: Fine Motor Precision, Fine Motor Integration, Manual Dexterity, and Upper Limb Coordination. Your results indicate a descriptive category of "well-below average" compared to his same-aged peers.

- **Cognitive:** From the occupational profile, and administration of the BOT-2, Bob required additional verbal cues to stay on task or follow directions. An academic consult will be sought for cognitive testing completed within his academic education

- **Sensory:** Bob appears to tolerate hand-over-hand assist when you go to demonstrate some skills needed for the BOT-2. You note that he is overweight and has a low muscle tone quality and observe low muscle tone, endurance, and decreased coordination during BOT activities. Sensory profile demonstrates issues with sensory textures (food, soap, clothing, etc.) consistent with sensory avoidant behavior.

Assessment: Environment (Information obtained through informal interview)

- **Physical:** Bob and his parents live in a ranch style home on a 2-acre lot in a city of 50,000 people. Bob's bedroom is near his parents and clothing is placed in dresser drawers out of his reach. He is bathed by his mother in a walk in shower down the hall from the bedrooms.

- **Social:** Bob lives with his mom and Larry (his dad) with no siblings. Parents work opposite shifts, so that they can be totally responsible for Bob's dressing needs. Mother reports that good family friends occasionally come over for game night, but otherwise, Bob does not participate in any extracurricular or social activities with specific dressing needs.

- **Cultural:** Bob and Linda are White. They are committed to Bob's care and see it as a part of God's plan for them. This Christian family values work and family. They share the caregiving responsibilities equally. Bob's dress is conservative, consistent with family values.

been noted to be on the rise (Hanson & Nielsen, 2016; Nielsen et al., 2017). Not only is each Level I fieldwork placement incredibly unique, but the scheduling of such experiences may range from a block placement at a site for a full week, or intermittent visits over the course of the academic term (Evenson et al., 2015). Level I fieldworks are designed to correspond with curricular content and the student's ability to communicate, observe, and participate in familiar select elements of the occupational therapy process. Since fieldwork is meant to connect the didactic coursework, including theory, models, and frames of references to practice, this should be a focal point of the experience regardless of the population, setting, or elements of the occupational therapy process available for student participation.

In a typical **role-established** Level I fieldwork setting, students may benefit from observing how the occupational therapy process is implemented within the setting. They can apply theoretical concepts learned in their didactic coursework by outlining concepts of an occupation-focused model and then identifying how and in what ways each concept of the model is being reflected in the occupational performance of an individual client or a population of clients. This requires student knowledge of the concepts of an occupation-focused model as they explain occupational performance. It does not require the student to understand how occupational therapists will use model concepts to measure performance and initiate client change, which is much more difficult for the student to identify without guidance from an occupational therapy practitioner. In a **role-emerging** Level I fieldwork setting, the student is able to identify concepts of an occupation-focused model that impact occupational performance. Furthermore, students may use an occupation-focused model as a framework for helping nonoccupational therapy personnel appreciate the role that occupational therapy might play in the practice context.

Occupational behavior models were created to unify the various settings of the profession; therefore, concepts of a given model may be integrated into one's practice without full recognition by the practitioner. However, in most cases, unintentional or implicit use of a model often mixes concepts of occupation-focused models, frames of reference, and models borrowed from other professions. The result is not readily recognizable by the observer. Intentional and explicit model implementation involves use of model concepts to inform all elements of the treatment process, which are assessment, treatment planning, goal setting, intervention implementation, documentation, and outcomes measurement.

There are many different kinds of knowledge used by occupational therapists to make practice decisions. Chapter 5 highlighted some of the kinds of reasoning used to make decisions in practice. When therapists make practice decisions, they should be able to articulate the reasoning behind their action as an important teaching strategy for their Level I fieldwork student. Honey and Penman (2020) interviewed 18 occupational therapy students who had just completed a 1-week placement and found that having access to the therapists' reasoning process and the opportunity to ask questions played a critical role in their learning. Many occupational therapy practitioners have difficulty explaining the theoretical knowledge that underpins their practice (Kinn & Aas, 2009). Box 6-4 has an example illustrating what it must feel like for a fieldwork student who is unable to recognize the language and reasoning of their FWed.

When occupational therapy practitioners draw primarily from nonpropositional knowledge, in other words, the professional craft knowledge they have obtained from practice experience, in explaining their reasoning process, students report difficulty in following the key concepts underpinning their work. Why would this be the case? Towns and Ashby (2014) surmised that in the academic sector, students are expected to learn about and distinguish differences between occupation-focused models and frames of reference as the foundation to clinical reasoning. When they are engaged in fieldwork and their FWeds do not know or use terms associated with theoretical knowledge or try to embed theory into their practice, students report confusion and having reduced confidence in the professionalism of the FWed (Box 6-5).

However, students had a more positive learning experience when they observed their educators trying to embed theory into their practice, even if the educator had difficulty in describing

---

Box 6-4

SCENARIO

Imagine that you are planning to visit a foreign country, somewhere you have never been before. How exciting that would be! You want to be very prepared, and take time to learn the language so that you can converse with the people who live there. You spend 2 years not only learning the language, but also learning about the activities, customs, and traditional ways of doing things in this new country, and finally feel ready to go. The day arrives for your big trip, and before you know it, you are in the very land you have dreamed about for so long. You greet the first people that you see, but they do not appear to know the language you have learned (no matter, they probably do not live here). As you continue to converse in the language that you have learned, you are soon disheartened as it appears that no one knows the language you have learned and not only that, the customs you were taught to expect are not consistently evident! In fact, it seems that everyone in this country seems to speak their own dialect, and it is up to you to decipher the rules of language and customs used by each individual. Imagine your frustration and confusion!

Box 6-5

EXAMPLE OF STUDENT CONFUSION

I was excited and full of energy to complete my fieldwork experience. Yet, as I observed my FWed, it became confusing seeing how we, in occupational therapy, were different than physical therapy or even an aide. We were doing the same arm exercises with most of our clients for every session. I became bored and disappointed. Was all this education really needed to do the same thing day in and day out? I never understood why the FWed was choosing to do all those exercises, and I felt uncomfortable asking because I didn't want to appear stupid, unappreciative, or disrespectful. Many times, the clients shared that they didn't even want to go to therapy, and most never seemed engaged in their sessions.

Reflection from Chapter Author—Jason C. Lawson, PhD, MS, OTR/L

---

how it was used. For students, the FWeds' interest in learning to articulate their actions through the lens of theory was akin to respect for EBP and the need to base practice on more than just personal experience. In addition, the therapists' use of theory helped to connect the reasoning process with language that was understandable to the student (Towns & Ashby, 2014). Table 6-1 provides a comparison of the student's learning experience when theory is used to drive practice, and when its use is not evident.

Dancza et al. (2021) investigated how experienced occupational therapy practice FWeds supported student learning and identified three key focal points for professional reasoning development: (1) guidance of learning by intentionally making connections for students between their university learning and what was applied in the practice context; (2) making visible to students theory-to-practice links through use of two-way dialogue and cognitive apprenticeship instructional methods (Table 6-2); and (3) supportively challenging students to answer questions for themselves, try new ideas, and learn from the consequences with opportunity for reflection and supportive discussion with their FWed.

Intentional reference to the concepts, change mechanisms, and outcomes of occupation-focused theory when addressing client concerns is helpful to student development of clinical reasoning. To make intentional reference to theory, FWeds need to become aware of their own reasoning process and use of theory. By doing so, they are able to intentionally model theory use

---

TABLE 6-1
COMPARING THEORY USE AND NONUSE IN OCCUPATIONAL THERAPY STUDENT LEARNING ON FIELDWORK

LEARNING WITH THEORY-DRIVEN PRACTICE	LEARNING WITHOUT THEORY
Use of terminology common to profession bridges the academic–practice gap.	Student is confused and overwhelmed as concepts seem new and unfamiliar.
Student and FWed understand and can articulate the unique role and value of occupational therapy in the setting.	Student and FWed are unable to identify how occupational therapy differs from other professions; "turf" wars may be evident.
The focus of occupational therapy intervention is on improving occupational performance.	The focus of occupational therapy is use of rote exercises or treatment techniques founded on neurological, motor, or cognitive theory to improve body function.
Collaboration with the client is encouraged to identify meaningful occupations.	Therapist uses the same interventions for everyone despite what the client finds meaningful.
Student is able to learn and generalize best practices in the profession across different types of practice settings.	Student views each occupational therapy setting as unique and different with no unifying themes for the profession.

TABLE 6-2
COGNITIVE APPRENTICESHIP INSTRUCTIONAL METHODS

Modeling	Reflection	Articulation	Questioning
Coaching	Scaffolding	Fading	

---

to students and articulate to students how they use theory in practice. Every occupation-based model explains everyday occupational performance using different concepts, but they all explore some aspect of the person, occupation, and environment. Every model has a unique focus for encouraging occupational performance. For example, working from the perspective of the OAM, immersing the client in occupation to enhance adaptive capacity would be the focus of intervention, whereas the change mechanisms of the PEO Model would emphasize obtaining maximal fit between the domains of the person, environment, and occupation to maximize occupational performance. Unlike OAM, use of PEO may not lead to a change in the individual's abilities, but adaption of the environment and modification of the occupation to achieve the outcome of occupational performance success (Table 6-3).

Nielsen et al. (2017) provide an example of occupation-focused theory to facilitate the clinical reasoning of students. In their study, students completing a community-based fieldwork in pairs provided occupation-based services to assist new immigrants in skills for daily living in a new community. Students met once a week with one another and a faculty preceptor to discuss the occupational needs of their participants and to apply the PEO Model to analyze occupational concerns and the development of assessment and intervention planning. Through this experience,

TABLE 6-3
COMPARISON OF MODEL CONCEPTS, **CHANGE MECHANISMS, AND EXPECTED OUTCOMES**

PERSON-ENVIRONMENT- OCCUPATION MODEL	OCCUPATIONAL ADAPTATION MODEL
Concepts	**Concepts**
Person: Physical, cognitive, sensory, affective, spiritual	Person: Sensory-motor, cognitive, psychosocial
Human occupation: Self-care, productivity/work, leisure, rest/sleep	Human occupation: Occupational challenge in work, play/leisure, or self-care emerging from role expectations
Environment: Physical, social, cultural, institutional, virtual	Environment: Physical, social, cultural
Change Mechanisms	**Change Mechanisms**
When transactional relationships (i.e., "fit" between the key domains) are at their maximum, occupational performance is maximized.	Occupation is used to empower the adaptation process.
Expected Outcomes	**Expected Outcomes**
Obtain maximum fit between the domains of the person, environment, and occupation	Change in adaptive capacity and relative mastery as evidenced by novel adaptations and generalization of adaptions to novel environments
Adapted from Baptiste, D. (2017). The person-environment-occupation model. In P. Kramer, J. Hinojosa, & C. B. Royeen (Eds.), *Perspectives in human occupation: Participation in life* (pp. 137-159). F. A. Davis.	

students were able to analyze person and environmental elements contributing to occupational concerns and to create a balance of interventions aimed at teaching skills, modifying occupations, or addressing environmental issues to address client needs and enhance their client's occupational performance. An example of PEO intervention applied to the earlier case study of Bob (Box 6-3) is provided in Box 6-6. It illustrates the use of the PEO Model to direct intervention focused on the occupational performance issue of dressing. The expected outcome is to optimize performance through finding a best fit between the person, the environment, and the occupation.

GETTING STARTED WITH USING OCCUPATIONAL BEHAVIOR MODELS

Up to this point, we hope you have decided that the time and effort you might put into learning or relearning the concepts of occupational behavior models will be worth the effort for you, your students, and for your overall value and visibility of occupational therapy services within your present setting.

Learning to think with theory does not happen overnight, it is a process that happens over time with intentional actions that support changes in both thinking and behavior. Two different

---

Box 6-6

APPLICATION OF PEO MODEL TO
OCCUPATIONAL THERAPY INTERVENTION WITH BOB

Setting: Outpatient Pediatric Services

Occupational Issue: Dressing

Goal: Donning/doffing a coat, zipping independently, tying shoes with visual cues

Interventions: Targeting each aspect of PEO, described below.

Person: Teach skills for dressing that will increase motor strength and fine motor coordination. Use **fun** activities that look at the **same** skill as pinching a zipper and pulling, pinching shoelaces, initial stages of tying. Maybe play dress up with a Ninja Turtle or create a lacing strip of a Ninja Turtle. Pinching play dough for strengthening, digging little "treasures" out of theraputty to work on the strength of the pincer grasp pattern. Repetition and feedback are key for skill acquisition.

Occupation: Add a zipper pull to make it easier to zip his coat. Use a simplified shoe tying method or paint dots on his laces so he knows where to pinch and wrap the loop.

Environment: Consider a quiet location and blocked practicing of these skills across environments (home and school—again, may need to collaborate with the school-based occupational therapist to reinforce techniques). Set up a visual schedule board for him to see the steps he needs to complete, and practice using this visual board. Ask school paraprofessional to cue him to steps as needed.

---

models for advancing theory use in occupational therapy have informed the development of our five-stage continuum for learning to use theory in practice. Leclair et al. (2013) developed the Theory Advancement Process (TAP) to stimulate application of the CMOP-E with students and occupational therapy practitioners, and through this process, identified pertinent factors and a progression to be considered for therapists learning to apply new theories into their practice. In addition, the Transtheoretical Model of Change (TTM; Prochaska et al., 2009), which is a change model often applied to consumers' adoption of new behaviors to support health, offers a continuum of learning that is applicable to implementation of theory into practice. Each approach will be summarized and then combined to form a continuum for application of theory to practice; ideas for Level I student engagement within this continuum will follow.

Leclair et al. (2013) explored the factors and processes supporting application of theory in daily practice. They found in the literature that a focus on capacity building, context, embedding theory in everyday practice, engagement and identification of stakeholders, power sharing, opportunities for debate and discourse development of relationships, sensitivity to needs of all stakeholders, mutual trust, and the use of participatory approaches were identified as important. They went on to obtain the perspectives of Level II students and their occupational therapists of what was important for theory advancement and developed the TAP. The TAP Model includes attention to (1) contexts (client, professional institutional, and practice); (2) a climate of collaborative relationships depicting four key elements (trust, power sharing, sensitivity, and respect); and (3) essential processes including building capacity, engaging in discourse, collaborating, and using theory with intention. Together, the reflection action aspect of TAP is evident in these processes (Table 6-4).

TABLE 6-4

OUTLINE OF TAP MODEL STRUCTURE

Contexts	Client context
	Professional context
	Institutional context
	Practice context
Climate of Collaborative Relationships	Trust
	Power sharing
	Sensitivity
	Respect
Processes	Building capacity (building knowledge of theory)
	Engaging in discourse (active, respectful exchange of challenges in theory use)
	Collaboration (shared decision making to find solution to client programmatic issues)
	Using theory with intention (to approach client, assess, plan, implement intervention, determine outcomes, and document)

Adapted from Leclair, L. L., Ripat, J. D., Wener, P. F., Cooper, J. E., Johnson, L. A., Davis, E. L., & Campbell-Rempel, M. A. (2013). Advancing the use of theory in occupational therapy: A collaborative process. *Canadian Journal of Occupational Therapy, 80*(3), 181-193. https://doi.org/10.1177/0008417413495182

A FIVE-STAGE CONTINUUM TO PROMOTE THINKING WITH THEORY DURING LEVEL I FIELDWORK

The concepts identified previously in the TAP Model (Leclair et al., 2013) related to context and collaborative relationships provide a rich backdrop for considerations that should be addressed before the student/fieldwork exchange occurs. The processes of the TAP Model provide the foundation to guide how theory might be introduced and effectively used as a tool for student clinical reasoning development during a Level I fieldwork. The TTM (Prochaska et al., 2009) provides further insight as to stages of change the FWed might move through in use of theory including (1) precontemplation, (2) contemplation, (3) preparation, (4) action, and (5) maintenance.

At the level of **precontemplation**, people do not intend to take action in the near future and are unaware that there are negative consequences to their present behavior; they are likely to underestimate the benefits of changing their behavior and overemphasize the cons of behavior change. In the stage of **contemplation**, people are intent to start a new behavior in the foreseeable future and are ready to thoughtfully consider pros and cons of behavior change but still have some ambivalence toward change. Individuals in the **preparation** stage of change are ready to take small steps toward behavior change within a short period of time (30 days) and believe that behavior change will lead to a better outcome. At the **action** stage, people have recently changed their behavior within the last 6 months and intend to keep moving forward. At the **maintenance** stage, people have sustained their behavior change for more than 6 months and want to avoid relapse.

This helpful framework can also be applied to how practitioners move forward in learning to embed theory into their practice. In the **precontemplation** stage, the practitioners may actively voice no interest in learning about occupation-focused models and may downplay their value to practice. In the **contemplation** stage, the practitioner is ready to thoughtfully consider the pros and cons to theory use in practice. In the **preparation** stage, practitioners are ready to take small steps toward actively using theory in practice, such as learning how to administer a specific assessment tool associated with an occupation-focused model. In the **action** stage, the practitioner may put several steps into action, such as implementing a protocol for assessment and goal setting using a model with several of their clients and plan to extend their work to another population. At the **maintenance** stage, the practitioner may be developing processes and procedures that ensure the work will carry into the future.

In the next section, a continuum of learning for practitioner use of occupation-focused theory is proposed and strategies suggested to promote student and FWed engagement with occupation-focused models during Level I fieldwork.

A CONTINUUM OF LEARNING TO INCORPORATE OCCUPATION-FOCUSED THEORY INTO PRACTICE

As suggested in the literature, occupational therapy practitioners are at different stages in regard to incorporation of theory into practice. Box 6-7 provides a visual map of a five-stage continuum for application of theory into practice. For some, there is little interest or perceived need for change or use of models in practice; this is represented by **Stage 1: Precontemplation**. Others see the need for incorporation of models but have had little training on models and lack capacity to apply them to practice. Therapists who identify with this situation are at **Stage 2: Contemplation and Capacity Building**. Some therapists are aware of various models but have not actually gone through the steps of determining which model is best for their unique situation and context as is represented by **Stage 3: Contemplation**. As a part of determining which model to apply, practitioners, students, and other stakeholders need to work collaboratively so that a climate of trust, power sharing, sensitivity, and respect is developed. Once a specific model is identified, **Stage 4: Using Theory With Intention** is launched. A number of preparations need to occur to get students ready to incorporate mechanisms of theory into their own practice including learning new assessments, developing protocols, and other structures to support the theory's application. After preparations are complete, therapists actively begin to apply theory to their work with clients; this might begin with only a few clients or a specific population but increase in breadth and consistency over time. **Stage 5: Maintenance** is ongoing and represents ongoing policies and procedures to ensure best practices in theory use, to measure effectiveness of theory use, and to incorporate procedures for inclusion of new stakeholders into the theory application process. Practitioner questions that might be the focus of each stage are summarized in Box 6-7.

Box 6-7

A FIVE-STAGE MODEL FOR THINKING WITH THEORY
DURING LEVEL I FIELDWORK

Stage 1: Precontemplation: Assessing Change Needs

What are the strengths and needs of occupational therapy services at my site? Is change needed?

Stage 2: Contemplation and Capacity Building

I have decided to change, but how? What do I know about the concepts, change mechanisms, and expected outcomes of key occupational behavior models?

Stage 3: Contemplation

Engaging in Discourse

Is use of a model of value to my practice? Which model is the best for the client, institutional, professional, and practice context?

Contemplation Through Collaboration

How can we work together to figure out which model or models might be best used in a particular context/situation in a climate of trust, power sharing, sensitivity, and respect?

Stage 4: Using Theory With Intention

Preparation

What structures need to be put into place to ensure that therapy and program processes are guided by intentional use of theory? This may involve learning new assessments and intake procedures, examining formats for incorporation of theoretical concepts in treatment planning, goal setting, client protocols, and documentation processes.

Action

How are structures working for incorporating theory into practice? Are assessments and intake procedures efficient and effective? What changes should be made for improvement?

Stage 5: Maintenance

How can I maintain the momentum of using occupation-focused theory to inform practice? How will structures and processes that were introduced be incorporated into facility policy and procedure so that they are adopted by new members to the treatment team? How can the value of using occupation-focused theory be measured? What steps can be taken to ensure currency with theory/model applications and resources?

THINKING WITH THEORY: START WHERE YOU ARE AND BRING STUDENTS WITH YOU

A number of strategies and actions might be taken by occupational therapy practitioners, academic partners, and students to support the use of occupation-focused theory in practice. Appendix A provides a list of learning activities that would be appropriate for occupational therapy practitioners at each stage of the process. Each stage of the continuum will be discussed here in terms of therapist engagement with learning to use theory and strategies that may be used to partner with academic programs and Level I fieldwork students.

Stage 1: Precontemplation

Although the first stage of change, precontemplation, seems primarily passive, it is here that the journey begins. Perhaps you are an individual who does not see the need for incorporating the use of occupation-focused models in your practice, or perhaps you work with others who feel negatively about theory use. *How does the practitioner move from precontemplation to contemplation?* An important movement at this step is to see that the need for change outweighs the inconvenience of change. Sometimes, assessment of strengths and problem areas can prompt a need for change. For example, as an individual therapist, you may be prompted to change because you want to include more occupation in your intervention, and you are looking for a tool or process to accomplish this. You may be dissatisfied with the visibility and value given to you by your treatment team and be looking for a way to distinguish the role of your profession over another or prove your distinct contribution. Your desire to accomplish goals that are valuable to you may prompt you to consider use of an occupation-focused model as a tool to accomplish your goals to more effectively deliver services and communicate with those around you. A potential exercise that may be helpful for practitioners at this stage is to evaluate strengths and challenges in their occupational therapy programming from the perspective of elements of the person and environments routinely addressed, occupations addressed, as well as whether best practice ideals are evident including occupation-based, client-centered, and EBP principles (Table 6-5).

After having completed an honest evaluation of the programming provided, some challenges or weaknesses may emerge. As a practitioner, you may find you consistently address some aspects of the person rather than others. Due to routine protocol or facility expectations or a number of other issues, you may address activities of daily living (ADLs) in your practice but rarely address occupations, such as leisure or rest and sleep, even though these are issues for your clients. You may find that you consistently address the physical environment but may not address the social or virtual environment that may play an active role in client rehabilitation. You may find that many of your therapeutic interventions are based more on tradition than research evidence.

If you identified any element of your present programming that is lacking, you may be ready to hear that occupational behavior models or occupation-focused theories were designed to address those very issues. And you may be ready to consider use of an occupation-focused theory as a tool to assist you in addressing your area of need. However, it is very difficult for occupational therapists busily working in a practice setting to initiate a change process alone (Leclair et al., 2013; Wimpenny et al., 2010), so it is important that you are working in a context that is supportive of learning.

Level I fieldwork students may assist you at this stage by creating conversations about the overall value of theory in practice sites and situations similar to your own. For example, students may help to create conversations about the value of occupation-focused models to ensure occupation-based, client-centered, or EBP references. Alternately, they might bring in resources or examples that show the use of occupation-focused models in changing the sequence of therapy processes to give more attention to occupation or the use of models to highlight the unique contribution of occupational therapy at specific practice settings. It is also helpful for students to hear that practitioners are taking the initiative to identify and address issues to make their practice better. Generally, students appreciate transparency and the opportunity to collaborate with practitioners on locating resources that may be of help to them. The primary purpose of student exchange at this level of the continuum is to promote conversation about the value of occupation-focused models to address the issues that may have been identified as problematic at the site. Academic faculty will be helpful at this stage to assist the student and the FWed to be ready for exchange. See Table 6-6 for examples of student learning activities that might occur at this level of the continuum.

TABLE 6-5

EVALUATION OF OCCUPATIONAL THERAPY PROGRAMMING

STRENGTHS IN OCCUPATIONAL THERAPY PROGRAMMING	WEAKNESSES/CHALLENGES IN OCCUPATIONAL THERAPY PROGRAMMING
Elements of the person adequately addressed (cognition, motor skills, sensory, pyschosocial)	Elements of the person that are not adequately addressed (cognition, motor skills, sensory, psychosocial)
Relevant occupations addressed (ADLs, instrumental ADLs, leisure/play, education, work, rest/sleep, health)	Relevant occupations not being addressed (ADLs, instrumental ADLs, leisure/play, eduction, work, rest/sleep, health)
Relevant environments addressed (physical, cultural, social, institutional, virtual)	Relevant environments not addressed (physical, cultural, social, institutional, virtual)
Relevant environments addressed (physical, cultural, social, institutional, virtual)	Relevant environments not addressed (physical, cultural, social, institutional, virtual)
Occupations are experienced in context of therapy; therapy is client centered	Occupations are not experienced in context of therapy but an end goal; therapy is not client centered or some elements lack client centeredness
Therapy is evidence based	Therapy is primarily based on tradition, not evidence based

Stage 2: Contemplation and Capacity Building

At the contemplation stage, practitioners are ready and willing to learn about occupation-focused models and to consider the pros and cons of their use in their practice setting. It is an important stage but can also be a frustrating experience for practitioners who have already established competence in their practice and may struggle with what might be perceived as "going back" to the kinds of conceptual learning associated with learning about models. Wimpenny et al. (2010) initiated a process with practitioners to learn the MOHO and apply it to their mental health practice setting. One therapist, in reflecting on this process said:

> I've actually felt really negative over the past two or three [sessions]; it has been hard. Oh, the last one I nearly didn't come. It is a learning process, isn't it? It's not all going to be easy, and I do feel the model [MOHO] is beneficial and will work within the teams. It's just getting it going. I've just felt like I've been winging [it] all the time. It's how I felt, and it's been really difficult to be positive about it. (Wimpenny et al., 2010, p. 511)

It is hard to learn new things; it is even harder to learn new things as an adult learner, so consideration of principles of adult learning will be helpful to remember when designing learning activities that will benefit both students and FWeds at this stage.

Adult learners are typically not interested in learning new things unless they need to learn them, unless they are connected to a problem or concern that they already have (Knowles et al., 2011). Learning as an adult is typically a "need to know" situation. Therefore, it is important that students or faculty who assist in this process engage practitioners in what they already know of a concept or how they may already use it in their own practice. Students may have access to PowerPoints (Microsoft), handouts, or various other multimedia tools to teach about a model, but

TABLE 6-6

EXAMPLES OF LEVEL I STUDENT LEARNING ACTIVITIES APPROPRIATE FOR STAGE 1

STUDENT AND ACADEMIC FACULTY COLLABORATION	STUDENT AND FIELDWORK EDUCATOR COLLABORATION
Student meets with academic faculty/ academic fieldwork coordinator to identify common population receiving services at fieldwork site and to determine occupation-focused models most commonly used with population. Student secures professional literature showing application of model to population for personal preparation.	Student observes occupational therapy treatment session with a specific occupation-focused model in mind, noting impact of models' concepts of person, environment, and occupation on client performance. Student and FWed discuss student observations and potential value of model to population or individual; student refers to professional literature and examples as needed.
Student meets academic faculty and other peers completing Level I fieldwork at similar sites with similar populations and reviews example of occupation-focused theory applied to an individual or population similar to fieldwork site. Students discuss benefits to model use discussed in article and potential challenges.	FWed reviews example (provided by academic program) of occupation-focused model applied to an individual or population similar to fieldwork site. FWed reflects on similarities and differences between case example provided and the population or a specific client treated onsite. FWed shares reflections with student, and both discuss potential benefits and challenges to model application onsite.
In advance of Level I fieldwork placement, FWed shares with academic fieldwork coordinator/occupational therapy faculty the strengths and challenges of occupational therapy programming onsite, with particular attention to providing occupation-based and client-centered intervention to clients. Students meet in small groups to discuss common challenges and brainstorm, with academic faculty guidance, how use of an occupation-focused model may be helpful in supporting strengths and addressing challenges.	Student and FWeds meet to discuss common challenges to occupation-based and client-centered intervention onsite. FWed shares tools and strategies used onsite to address challenges. Student shares ideas generated through faculty-led group discussion as to how use of an occupation-focused model may benefit site.

(continued)

Table 6-6 (continued)
Examples of Level I Student Learning Activities Appropriate for Stage 1

STUDENT AND ACADEMIC FACULTY COLLABORATION	STUDENT AND FIELDWORK EDUCATOR COLLABORATION
Academic faculty meet with preselected Level I FWeds in webinar format to discuss challenges to provision of occupation-based and client-centered practice across various practice settings. Academic faculty provide review of two different occupation-focused models and how they have been used to address challenges to occupation-based and client-centered practice. FWeds and faculty collaborate about how model application may be helpful to challenges evident in their setting. Students either attend or watch recordings of webinars and identify elements of the exchange process that are helpful in planning for discussion with their FWeds.	Students meet with FWeds who discuss challenges to provision of occupation-based and client-centered practice in their practice setting. Students share with FWeds about an occupation-focused model that has been used to address similar challenges in similar settings. FWeds reflect on how model application might be helpful to addressing challenges. FWeds then provide feedback to students on their strengths and challenges in regard to their ability to engage in and promote discussion on occupation-focused models (this might be incorporated into the Level I fieldwork evaluation).
Students share with academic faculty the elements of the exchange process that they found helpful in watching the FWed webinar. Academic faculty review with students elements that promote discussion and exchange on occupation-focused models in the precontemplation stage. Students role play with one another, alternating between student and FWed role, and then share with the larger group strategies they found helpful in promoting open discussion and exchange.	Students share with assigned FWeds what they learned about challenges of providing occupation-based and client-centered care and engage FWed in discussion of challenges of applying these practice ideals in their setting. Students share about one occupation-focused model, and how it was used to address challenges and thoughts from webinar on model use, then invite FWed to share perspectives. FWed then provides feedback to student on their strengths and weaknesses in regard to their ability to engage in and promote discussion on occupation-focused models (this might be incorporated into the Level I fieldwork evaluation).

this should be combined with some opportunity for practitioners to translate concepts into their own experiences or to relate to their clients. For example, following a student presentation, the student and educator could brainstorm application of the model to clients on the therapist's caseload, which essentially moves the therapist from precontemplation to contemplation.

It may be helpful for academic faculty to spend some time with students prior to the Level I fieldwork to give them the opportunity to practice incorporating adult learning techniques into their presentations or to the provide feedback in advance of presentations that are to be given in the practice setting. Sometimes students may also be in the position of applying model concepts to clients or various situations that occur during the Level I experience. For example, through the use of observation checklists, students might observe various clients and identify how the concepts of a model apply to that client or to any of the processes already used by the therapist and share their observations with the therapist. Table 6-7 provides further ideas as to what Level I fieldwork student assignments may be appropriate for this stage, types of fieldwork placements suitable for the assignment, and ways in which the assignment can promote building theory capacity for the site and FWed.

Stage 3: Contemplation: Engaging in Discourse and Collaboration

Although getting up to speed with understanding model concepts, learning differences between models, and frames of reference, and gaining terminology to speak in the language of occupation-focused models may have been challenging, it all becomes worth it once the practitioner is at this stage in learning. It is at this stage that the practitioner is able to draw together both their propositional and nonpropositional knowledge to make a conscious decision about which model is the best fit for a situation or practice problem or perhaps for a specific client or population. This stage is particularly fun when discourse can occur related to the stage. This is also the stage where students will find that practitioners actively use model concepts, sequences, and tools when talking about their clients or when brainstorming as to which model is a best fit for the situation. Knowing model concepts, students can more readily engage in the discussion; however, they are at a disadvantage in regard to nonpropositional knowledge. They have not actually worked enough with a client with a traumatic brain injury, for example, to understand what it really involves to teach a routine and for that habit pattern to inform a role that the client can be proud of. However, they do want to hear those stories, and they love to hear the stories through the concepts of the model.

This is the stage where practitioners and key stakeholders are primarily engaging in discourse as to *which* model is a best fit for a given situation. It is an important stage because it occurs on the eve of deciding, as a group or an individual, to actually invest in learning the very specific processes and skills required for carrying out a specific model. Although the conversation at this stage may be somewhat hypothetical for the student, for the practitioner, it is often steeped in practice experience. Braveman et al. (2008) provided a framework and a process for using the occupational behavior model to organize occupational therapy services for unique population groups, which has since been applied to several populations and highlighted in occupational therapy education of best practices in occupational therapy management. The framework includes four steps for determining which model is the best fit for the population. Four questions are suggested to guide selection of conceptual practice models (Box 6-8).

This four-step process also provides a focus for student learning activities. As occupational therapy practitioners consider which model will best fit the needs of the client or client population and provide ideas for encouraging occupational change, the student can contribute by locating examples of model use with a similar population. In addition, students can contribute by locating research evidence that supports use of the types of change mechanisms that are suggested by the

TABLE 6-7

LEVEL I FIELDWORK ASSIGNMENT IDEAS FOR CONTEMPLATION: BUILDING CAPACITY

STUDENT ASSIGNMENT IDEAS TO PROMOTE FIELDWORK EDUCATOR LEARNING OF OCCUPATION-FOCUSED MODEL	TYPES OF LEVEL I FIELDWORK PLACEMENT	IDEAS FOR LEVERAGING ASSIGNMENT VALUE
Students find a journal article about a model of practice and create a simple handout illustrating major concepts of the model. They might also identify the specific sequence of steps suggested by a specific model.	Block Faculty led Simulation	FWeds can collect handouts over time, reflect on main components of the models, and consider which model concepts relate to their area of practice. Handouts can serve as an observational tool for future students and a means to identify how theory can inform various steps of the assessment and intervention process.
Students identify *a population* being served onsite and find a journal article showing how practice model concepts, change mechanisms, and outcomes are applied with the population. They create a simple handout illustrating common population characteristics and the fit for the concepts, change mechanisms, and outcomes of the model.	Block Faculty led Simulation	FWeds can collect handouts over time, reflect on main components of the models, and consider how model concepts, change mechanisms, and outcomes might relate to their area of practice. Handouts can serve as an observational tool for future students.
Students gain background information *on a specific client* at their site and find a journal article on a model that was applied with the same diagnoses in individualized intervention. Students might create a handout showing how model concepts are evident (or could be evident) in the evaluation process, how model change mechanisms are evident in intervention provided, and how model outcomes are reflected in measurement of change.	Block Faculty led Simulation Probono clinic	As students outline how model concepts, change mechanisms, and outcomes apply, they can also identify areas of disconnect and in what ways other aspects of the model might be included. Over time, this will help the FWed or faculty member to integrate more elements of the model to their work with specific clientele or to a specific simulation case or cases.

Box 6-8

Four Questions to Guide Selection of Conceptual Practice Models in Program Planning (Braveman, 2016, p. 391)

1. Does the model specify the underlying mechanisms of action necessary to facilitate the desired type of change?

2. Is there sufficient evidence to support application of the models to the consumer group and the type of change you wish to facilitate?

3. Do the models fit with the social, organizational, cultural, political, professional, and financial contexts in which the program must be implemented?

4. Does implementation of the model have any special requirements for space, equipment, or personnel? (Braveman, 2016, p. 391).

---

model for the population. See Table 6-8 for a comparison of the concepts, change mechanisms, and expected outcomes for the MOHO and OAM. In the example, it is clear that the MOHO attributes the change process to occupational engagement. If using MOHO for a population of individuals with addictions, the student would look for research evidence supporting that concept. If using OAM for the same population, the student would look for research showing that engaging the client in actual occupations followed by reflection about supports and hindrances to performance (reflection of relative mastery) would eventually help the client develop problem-solving skills to maximize adaptation skills to avoid addictive behaviors. By bringing in examples and supportive research evidence, students can contribute to the process of comparing models and engage in conversation with practitioners as to how the concepts, mechanisms of action/change, and outcomes associated with specific models fit with the needs of the clients. For example, Kielhofner et al. (2004) provide a very instructive example of how the concepts of MOHO are used to guide vocational program development for a population of individuals with AIDS. Students may also be directed to bring in research evidence that directly supports application of the model to the consumer group and the type of change/outcomes desired by practitioners. For example, for clients with limited capacity for change, a model that highlights best fit may be more appropriate than a model that suggests change in capacity. Short-term care settings, such as acute care, may also offer limited capacity for change due to the short time frame. A model, such as PEO, would be a better choice to address the immediate occupational needs and has been discussed as an appropriate fit within the acute care setting (Maclean et al., 2012). Contrast this with an outpatient mental health setting and a population of individuals diagnosed with various forms of anxiety and depression. When the programming focus is on development of coping skills, use of cognitive behavioral framework for emotional regulation and self-management of anxiety/depression, there is definitely a focus on changing capacity. Therefore, a model, such as OAM or MOHO, whose outcome is change in occupational adaptation, would be a good fit for this setting.

In steps three and four of the suggested process, the focus turns toward discussion of resources available in the practice context to support model application. This is a very important step of the process which helps students appreciate the importance of considering the impact of context on practice. This principle is also evident in the TAP Model conceptualized by Leclair et al. (2013). Students might first engage by making their own list of context considerations but are likely to

TABLE 6-8

COMPARISON OF MODEL CONCEPTS, CHANGE MECHANISMS, AND EXPECTED OUTCOMES

MODEL OF HUMAN OCCUPATION	OCCUPATION ADAPTATION MODEL
Concepts	**Concepts**
Person: Volition, habituation, performance, capacity	Person: Sensory-motor, cognitive, psychosocial
Human occupation: Skills, performance of a form, participation	Human occupation: Occupational challenge in work, play/leisure, or self-care emerging from role expectations
Environment: Physical, social, cultural	
Change mechanisms	**Change mechanisms**
Driven by clients' occupational engagement; doing, thinking, and feeling under certain environmental conditions.	Occupation is used to empower the adaptation process.
Expected outcomes	**Expected outcomes**
Occupational adaptation achieved through attainment of occupational competence and alignment of occupational identity.	Change in adaptive capacity and relative mastery as evidenced by novel adaptations and generalization of adaptions to novel environments.

Adapted from Kielhofner, G. (2008). *A model of human occupation: Theory and application* (4th ed.). Williams & Wilkins and Grajo, L. C. (2017). Occupational adaptation. In P. Kramer, J. Hinojosa & C. B. Royeen (Eds.), *Perspectives in human occupation: Participation in life* (pp. 137-159). F. A. Davis.

quickly appreciate that practitioner experience within the context unveils factors that the students are not likely to identify.

Although students may feel at a disadvantage, especially in the last steps in this process, due to their relative lack of familiarity with the clientele or programming provided at the site, it is also possible that practitioners will feel intimidated by student knowledge of model concepts or access to research evidence in this process. Therefore, it is very important that a context of mutual learning, trust, and power sharing as suggested by the TAP Model (Leclair et al., 2013) should permeate the learning process. The student should be respectful of the practice experiences of the FWed and the wealth of nonpropositional knowledge that they hold and also sensitive to the difficulty of learning and applying the new language of occupation-focused theory. In the meantime, the practitioner may need to be very encouraging of the student in regard to their awareness, knowledge, or resources that they have in relation to occupation-focused models and the power differential that is held by the FWed in relationship to the student. For some students, for example, it may be difficult to engage in discourse that involves disagreement with their FWed or to provide information that may add to the discussion if they sense that this information may not be welcomed or valued in the discussion. See Table 6-9 for an example of student learning activities that may be appropriate for this stage of the continuum.

TABLE 6-9

STUDENT LEARNING ACTIVITIES TO PROMOTE DISCOURSE AND COLLABORATION

LEARNING ACTIVITY	TYPE OF FIELDWORK	OUTCOME
Using handouts made by previous groups, students might work in small groups to compare and contrast the effectiveness of two different models in evaluating population needs, guiding intervention choices, and enhancing their clinical reasoning skills. Students can identify research studies that support model use with a population or research studies that support application of model concepts to change processes for the population.	Faculty-led experience Block placement	As students identify and compare how each model guides the actions of faculty during the faculty-guided experience, the faculty member also becomes more familiar with each model of practice and applicability to their practice population and site. Research studies supporting model use may be used to propose to administration resources needed for model application.
Several small groups of students could each be assigned one model and told to identify how the model's concepts might guide their interactions with a given case or learning activity. Student groups could compare and contrast how their assigned model guided their clinical reasoning or problem solving. Students could also debrief on what model concepts were not addressed and problem solve around how those concepts/processes could be incorporated in their future case, learning activities, simulations, fieldworks, or practice.	Simulation	Simulations vary greatly on having the student focus on a particular skill or interaction with a client. Educators could use the analysis from students about what was missing from the simulation related to their models to strengthen or add to the simulations for future use.

Stage 4: Using Theory With Intention: Preparation and Implementation

In this stage, practitioners have chosen a model that they wish to use with a client or a client population and are concerned about establishing the structures that need to be put into place to ensure that therapy and program processes are guided by intentional use of theory. This may involve learning new assessments and intake procedures, examining formats for incorporation of theoretical concepts in treatment planning, goal setting, client protocols, and documentation processes. Once the structures have been established, practitioners need time to practice using them and engage in multiple checkpoints for determining how the structures are working. For example, they may need to discuss whether new assessments or intake procedures are efficient and effective, and what changes should be made for improvement.

It is important to understand that preparation and implementation take place over a sequence of time. Melton et al. (2010) suggest that changes in therapist thinking and behavior are required in this process, and they describe this continuum of activity using the analogy of air travel. Stage 1 is identified as *in the hangar*, Stage 2 as *on the runway*, Stage 3 as *take off*, and Stage 4 as *in the air*. Each phase of thinking and behavior is illustrated in Table 6-10.

Keponen and Launiainen (2008) describe a similar five-step process for helping occupational therapists to develop occupation-focused clinical reasoning over time using the MOHO. Their process uses MOHO assessment instruments to both deepen knowledge of this model and apply it to practice in an actual occupational therapy practice setting. Learning takes place both in workshop format and application of workshop content with clients. **Step 1** begins before attending a workshop. Therapists describe in detail a typical client and the client's occupational performance. They then analyze the practice context and existing assessment protocol and identify areas in which assessments might be improved. Finally, they identify an MOHO assessment most suitable for improving the process. **Step 2** includes an interactive lecture where therapists are introduced to key MOHO concepts and encouraged to share examples that pertain to their clients. This is coupled with videotapes of assessment administration, out of class meetings, and practice with the assessment with their chosen client and tutorial groups exploring the instrument's effectiveness. **Step 3** engages the therapist in a problem setting process using the data gathered from the MOHO assessment and incorporating MOHO key concepts in therapeutic reasoning. The focus of **Step 4** is formulating and documenting goals that focus on occupation rather than impairment, in the context of tutorial groups. In **Step 5**, the final step, therapists reflect on the effects of using MOHO-based concepts, assessments, and treatment planning on professional knowledge, skills, practice, and documentation.

Regardless of what approach is used, therapists will engage in an iterative process during this stage of the continuum as they find new insights about their practice and clinical reasoning and learn new information about tools and processes that may support them. Students and practitioners can learn from one another at this stage. At the request of the site, students may be able to bring assessment instruments from their academic program that are consistent with the model/theory that practitioners are learning to use. Students may have case studies and other resources from their academic programs that practitioners would find helpful. Often, other faculty are involved through small group discussion or consultation with the practice site. Ideas for students to contribute to therapist learning at this stage are provided in Table 6-11.

Each type of Level I fieldwork placement may have a different way of supporting student clinical reasoning using concepts of occupation-focused models. Some ideas for strategies that might be employed across different types of Level I fieldwork to support preparation and implementation of model use are found in Box 6-9. In addition, ideas for student involvement at a site that is fully implementing use of an occupation-focused theory in practice is found in Appendix B.

TABLE 6-10

PRACTICE DEVELOPMENT OUTCOME STAGES

THINKING WITH THEORY OUTCOME	STAGE	BEHAVIORAL INDICATOR
Occupational therapist has not: • Attempted to use theory to reason/case formulate in practice • Had the opportunity to undertake training in model concepts • Used model tools knowledgeably or with adequate supervision	In the hangar	Occupational therapist has: • Tried using model assessments but is not adequately trained • Not read model assessment manuals • Has considered and/or tried using model assessments in practice but decided that they were not relevant or useful
Occupational therapist is: • Trying to reason and case formulate using model • In process of training/reading model material	On the runway	Occupational therapist is: • Trying out various model-based assessments with colleagues • Not using the model to report opinion or reasoning for work with clients as of yet
Occupational therapist has: • Started using chosen model to reason/case formulate about client's/population's challenges in practice intermittently	Take off	Occupational therapist has: • Undertaken training in assessments associated with the model
Occupational therapist is: • Able to articulate the client's or population's situation using model concepts • Using model routinely in practice to reason and formulate case planning	In the air	Occupational therapist is: • Using model assessments routinely in practice • Synthesizing knowledge of model concepts to interpret assessment results

Adapted from Melton, J., Forsyth, K., & Freeth, D. (2010). A practice development programme to promote the use of the model of human occupation: Contexts, influential mechanisms and levels of engagement amongst occupational therapists. *British Journal of Occupational Therapy, 73*(11), 549-558. https://doi.org/10.4276/030802210X12892992239350

TABLE 6-11

STUDENT LEARNING ACTIVITIES TO PROMOTE PREPARATION AND THEORY IMPLEMENTATION

FIELDWORK EDUCATOR LEARNING	STAGE 4: USING THEORY WITH INTENTION	STUDENT LEARNING
Occupational therapist: • Attempts to use theory to reason/case formulate in practice • Is learning new assessment tools and therapy sequences consistent with model choice	Stage 4: Preparation	Occupational therapy student: • Asks questions and confirms information and processes associated with therapist reasoning • Practices model assessments in advance of Level I fieldwork with peers and oversight of occupational therapy faculty. Prepares demonstration of model assessment tool during Level I fieldwork
Occupational therapist is: • Able to articulate the client's or population's situation using model concepts • Using the model routinely in practice to interpret assessment results, reason, and formulate case planning	Stage 4: Action	Occupational therapy student is: • Asking FWed questions about model concepts and application to client or populations; actively using texts and other resources to engage in dialogue with FWed about model use • Engaging in interpreting assessment results through model lens with feedback from FWed • Applying the model to formulation of treatment planning

Stage 5: Maintenance

During this stage, the focus of activities for the practitioner shifts from direct patient contact or program planning to identification and development of processes, procedures, and policies that will maintain the application of theory processes for future programming. As discussed in the TAP Model (Leclair et al., 2013), attention is given to the maintenance of theory application in the institutional and practice context. Therefore, the focus of student learning also shifts to an administrative and management perspective, which offers an ideal opportunity to apply

Box 6-9
STUDENT ACTIVITIES TO SUPPORT
PREPARATION AND IMPLEMENTATION

Preparation Phase:
Block Placements

FWeds might begin by asking their Level I fieldwork students to relate the commonly used assessments that are used at the site to the main concepts of the model. When the student makes the connection of which assessments specifically address the concepts of the model, the student will begin to identify how models guide and inform occupational therapy evaluation. This may also introduce some gaps where current assessment tools do not address processes or concepts of the model. This may prompt discussion as to what new assessment tools should be incorporated to support clinical reasoning from the perspective of the chosen model. Students may also check out assessment tools associated with a select model to share with practitioners and possibly provide a workshop demonstrating and engaging clinicians in trying out the assessment tool for addressing needs with their clients.

Together with the FWed, students might review an aspect of documentation to review for consistency with model application (e.g., this could be initial note, progress, or discharge summary, but not likely all three, usually one). Student identifies where it is congruent or not, which is discussed between the student and FWed. FWed notes areas of agreement or additional insights on student perspectives. Student worksheets are collected and summarized, then used for later occupational therapy staff meeting or committee work to identify areas of congruence or dissonance of site procedures with expected model processes.

Faculty-Led Fieldwork Experiences

Faculty may begin by asking students to identify models that they see evident in the clinical reasoning of the faculty member. Faculty might direct students to create a list of currently used assessment tools at the fieldwork site and identify which assessment tool contributes to what concepts of the models. Additionally, students could be tasked with researching and finding assessments that could fit with concepts of the models. Faculty could then choose to explore or assign students to report on the value of using alternative assessments that may help address other components of the models that may not have been addressed before. Faculty might also lead students in learning and practicing use of assessment tools associated with a specific model with one another and eventually with clients at the site to support clinical reasoning using model concepts.

Simulation

Depending on what part of the occupational therapy process the simulation is targeting (evaluation or intervention), students could be tasked with debriefing about how their interactions with the case simulation would have differed based on using concepts from an assigned model and associated assessment tools. Given an assigned model, a group of students may be required to administer an assessment associated with the model to one another, and then discuss how use of the assessment tool would have influenced their clinical reasoning process in the simulation.

(continued)

Box 6-9 (continued)
Student Activities to Support
Preparation and Implementation

Implementation Phase:

Block Placements

Students might be directed to practice using a specific tool prior to the Level I placement and be ready to implement it on a client during their experience. In addition, the FWed can ask the Level I fieldwork student to research and identify other assessment tools (perhaps covered in their program or located in their student resources) that are not currently available at the site that could also address specific concepts of the model. Students could present basic content about a new assessment tool anchored in how and where it assists the therapist to target a particular model concept.

Level I fieldwork students could also track each of the interventions they observe and specify how they contribute to the intervention aspects of the model. Additional, site-specific frames of references may also be added to enhance more specificity and direction to the application of specific interventions. At this stage, the FWed will be able to directly share observations about theory implementation with the student, and the student's role would be to confirm that the therapists clinical reasoning is consistent with what the student learned in school or to raise questions in areas of uncertainty.

Faculty-Led Fieldwork Experiences

Faculty can articulate the rationale for their chosen evaluation and intervention methods in terminology familiar with the student. Faculty could assign students to explore and present on any new assessments that could be implemented or added to the fieldwork site based on concepts of a model. Level I fieldwork students could also track each of the interventions they observe and specify how they contribute to the intervention aspects of the model. Additional, site-specific frames of references may also be added to enhance more specificity and direction to the application of specific interventions.

Simulation

Depending on what the student is demonstrating for the simulation, students could be relating what they are demonstrating by communicating any rationale to the educator by using the model's terminology and concepts. Following the experience, educators can debrief with students regarding how the demonstrated skill targets an aspect of the model concepts.

management skills to theory-driven practice. Occupation-focused theory might be applied to the development of documents describing occupational therapy programming for different program stakeholders, developing therapy protocols that support therapy processes, and data measurement systems to collect outcomes that support the value of occupation-focused practice with foundations in occupation-focused theory. Program descriptions might be written to communicate the role of occupational therapy to consumers and also to other health care professions. See Table 6-12 for an illustration of specific program descriptions that are written to correspond with specific occupation-focused theories.

Therapy protocols generally describe a decision tree or a sequence of actions that will be taken to support client occupational performance. Each occupation-focused theory has a proposed process or sequence of steps. If influenced by occupation-focused theory, the therapy protocol would incorporate steps of the occupational therapy assessment or intervention process suggested by the theory and would include measurement of outcomes associated with theory use. Students might be engaged in evaluating current protocols for their consistency with suggested model processes and suggest changes if needed. In addition, students might apply their knowledge of data collection and research design to engage with practitioners in the development of data collection systems that collect outcomes associated with model use.

Identification and development of processes for training of new therapists or students in theory use will engage students in consideration of personnel management issues, another important aspect of entry-level occupational therapy practice. For example, they might consider whether an interactive workshop, online learning, or periodic testing/assessment should be incorporated in the training process. Similarly, they might be drawn into discussions regarding maintenance of therapist skills in theory application, which demonstrates attention to the professional context (Leclair et al., 2013). Topics might include how to promote continuing education, updating of skills, and recognition of therapist accomplishments regarding theory integration into practice (Table 6-13).

SUMMARY

Occupational therapy practitioners have unique skills in the application of occupation-based treatment to the health care needs of their clients. At the heart of occupation-based practice is the ability to effectively use occupation-focused theory as the organizing construct of service delivery. The FWed is in a strong position to influence occupational therapy students regarding theory use in the future. Students do not expect perfection, but value FWed efforts to advance their practice to align with best practice ideals using theoretical tools of the profession. Many factors influence the ability of the FWed to intentionally apply theory to practice, including their own knowledge and abilities, as well as contextual barriers. Although there are many challenges to the active use of theory in practice, there are also many resources now available to support the interested practitioner. A five-step continuum, using concepts from the TAP Model, proposed by Leclair et al. (2013) and following a process suggested by the TTM (Prochaska et al., 2009), was used to align therapist readiness for theory application with student learning activities appropriate for a Level I fieldwork. The learning activities proposed at the end of this chapter will further assist the student and FWed to communicate with one another using the language of the profession, communicate the value of occupational therapy to key stakeholders, and to enhance clinical reasoning when providing occupational therapy services to individuals, populations, and groups.

TABLE 6-12

APPLICATION OF OCCUPATION-BASED THEORIES TO PROGRAM DESCRIPTIONS

MODEL OF HUMAN OCCUPATION

Concepts:

- Person: Volition, habituation, performance capacity

- Human occupation: Skills, performance, participation

- Environment: Physical, social, cultural, economic, political

   Change: Driven by clients' occupational engagement; doing, thinking, and feeling under certain environmental conditions (Kielhofner, 2008)

   Outcomes: Occupational adaptation stemming from occupational identity and occupational competence

MOHO Program Description: In this state psychiatric hospital, we realize that our clients often have a long history of difficulties by the time they come to us. Therefore, we start with an accurate assessment of current skills, but we are also interested in the habits and routines that support their current roles and changes they would need to make to support participation in activities that reflect their values and interests. We know that environment can play a key role, so we look at the influence of the social, physical, and cultural environment on their participation. At the end of the day, we hope to influence their overall competency and sense of identity so that they are able to adapt well when they leave the hospital setting.

PERSON-ENVIRONMENT-OCCUPATION MODEL

Concepts:

- Person: A unique being with a variety of skills

- Environment: Cultural, socioeconomic, institutional, physical, social considerations

- Occupation: Self-directed, functional tasks/activities over the lifespan

- Occupational performance: Dynamic experience of a person/engaged in purposeful activities/tasks within an environment

   Change: Comprehensive assessment to derive a clear picture of the degree of congruence (or fit) between the person, environment, and occupation.

   Outcome: An improved fit will result in improvements to occupational performance

PEO Model Program Description: In this elementary school system, students are most successful when they can engage in the various occupations of education. Some students are disadvantaged in that they lack the cognitive, sensory motor, and psychosocial skills to effectively perform in the classroom, as well as small group learning. We work collaboratively with the teacher and, in some cases, the paraprofessional to support the student in learning new study and social interaction skills and ways to manage sensory information so as to sustain attention and emotional regulation. We are also attentive to the impact of the environment on student performance and look for the best fit in skills development for educational performance, while simultaneously adapting the social, physical, and cultural environment to impact performance. We also work with the teacher and paraprofessionals to maximize the students educational performance by adapting the educational activities when needed to fit the available environment and skills of the clients.

(continued)

TABLE 6-12 (CONTINUED)

APPLICATION OF OCCUPATION-BASED THEORIES TO PROGRAM DESCRIPTIONS

CANADIAN MODEL OF OCCUPATIONAL PERFORMANCE AND ENGAGEMENT

Concepts:

- Person: Cognitive, affective, physical: spirituality at core

- Environment: Cultural, socioeconomic, institutional, physical, and social considerations

- Occupation: Self-care, leisure, productivity

- Occupational performance and engagement: Health, well-being, occupational justice

    Change: Occupational concerns are addressed through a client-centered process with a central focus on occupational performance

    Outcomes: Enhanced occupational performance, occupational justice, and client empowerment through a client-centered process

CMOP-E Program Description: The bulk of our clients in this outpatient setting have orthopedic concerns or are working with us to extend therapy gains made in the inpatient rehab setting; we are reimbursed through both private pay and insurance. It is critical that our clients are engaged in their therapy process and satisfied with the outcomes achieved. We see a high rate of cancellation or withdrawals from therapy if engagement is not achieved. Therefore, we ensure that they have a good understanding of what we can achieve in occupational therapy from the start. We interview our clients using the COPM or a similar tool to identify the occupational outcomes they want to achieve, as well as the kinds of activities that they will participate in outside of therapy sessions to achieve their goals. We check with them regularly to get their perspectives on their progress and the activities used in the therapy process and revise goals and activities as needed to maintain focus on their occupational priorities.

Adapted from Turpin, M. J. & Iwama, M. K. (2010). *Using occupational therapy models in practice* (pp. 117-134). Churchill-Livingston; Kielhofner, G. (2008). *A model of human occupation: Theory and application* (4th ed.). Williams & Wilkins; and Baptiste, D. (2017). The person-environment-occupation model. In P. Kramer, J. Hinojosa, & C. B. Royeen (Eds.), *Perspectives in human occupation: Participation in life* (pp. 137-159). F. A. Davis.

TABLE 6-13

STUDENT LEARNING ACTIVITIES FOR THE MAINTENANCE STAGE

Processes/protocols/ procedures	The student might engage in discussion with the FWed about common processes/protocols and procedures used by the site and their congruence with a specific occupation-focused theory. A group of students might develop a decision tree or modify an existing decision tree already developed by the site that outlines steps of the intake, assessment, and intervention process following the steps suggested by the theory.
Policies	Policies for client care may be reviewed by the student to discern consistency with processes suggested by occupation-focused theory and modifications needed to ensure client-centered, occupation-based, and evidence-based care.
Program descriptions	Students might review program descriptions already written for internal and external audiences, and modify to reflect concepts, change mechanisms, and outcomes supported by a given occupation-focused model. They might also design patient brochures or other promotional materials for use with the broader community.
Data management	Students might have opportunity to review data already collected by the department to demonstrate efficacy of services and engage in discussion with FWed as to how data support outcomes congruent with a chosen occupation-focused theory. Students might discuss specific data from an assigned assessment tool that might be used to provide evidence of client change. Students might work with data already obtained from a limited number of client records showing *before* and *after* ratings and apply statistics to investigate quality of findings.
Personnel management	Using resources from their management coursework, students might review the orientation process commonly used for integration of new therapists at site and suggest changes to help new therapists become familiar with occupation-focused theory application. In a similar manner, students might consider how ongoing continuing education might look for therapists already engaged in application of occupation-focused service delivery and incentive programs to recognize therapist achievements in this area.

LEARNING ACTIVITIES

1. Review your facility website or other promotional materials for your setting. How are occupational therapy services described? How accurate is this description? How does this effect the overall value given to occupational therapy services by the treatment team?

2. Review Boxes 6-1 and 6-5. What examples of identity confusion might occur in your practice context?

3. Circle the factors that impact your own use of occupation-focused theory: *"... educational preparation and time required to become comfortable with new theories, lack of role models for theory implementation, skepticism as to the value of theory application and contextual barriers including time and pragmatic concerns."* Underline those that especially influence your use of theory at your present practice site.

4. Review Table 6-1 and mark the items that are most reflective of the student's experience at your site. Based on this exercise, what changes would you like to make at your site to strengthen the student's learning experience?

5. What resources do you have in your professional community that may assist you in moving forward with using occupation-focused theory at your site (academic programs, state, regional, and national professional associations, online resources, book and library access, etc.). How might these resources be helpful to you in your work with students?

6. Review Box 6-7 and determine what stage of the continuum you are at in regard to application of occupation-focused theory to practice. Are you at the same or a different stage from that of other therapists at your site? How does this impact your next steps in theory use?

7. Based on the stage you identified in the previous question, what student learning activities suggested for that stage stand out to you as helpful? What additional ideas would you suggest?

REFERENCES

Accreditation Council for Occupational Therapy Education. (2018). 2018 accreditation council for occupational therapy education standards and interpretive guide. *American Journal of Occupational Therapy, 72*(2), 7212410005p1-7212410005p83. https://doi.org/10.5014/ajot.2018.72S217

Ashby, S., & Chandler, B. (2010). An exploratory study of the occupation-focused models included in occupational therapy professional education programmes. *British Journal of Occupational Therapy, 73*(12), 616-624. https://doi.org/10.4276/030802210X12918167234325

Ashby, S., Ryan, S., Gray, M. & James, C. (2013). Factors that influence the professional resilience of occupational therapists in mental health practice. *Australian Occupational Therapy Journal, 60*(2), 110-119. https://doi.org/10.1111/1440-1630.12012

Baptiste, D. (2017). The person-environment-occupation model. In P. Kramer, J. Hinojosa, & C. B. Royeen (Eds.), *Perspectives in human occupation: Participation in life* (pp. 137-159). F. A. Davis.

Boniface, G., Fedden, T., Hurst, H., Mason, M., Phelps, C., Reagon, C. & Waygood, S. (2008). Using theory to underpin an integrated occupational therapy service through the Canadian model of occupational performance. *The British Journal of Occupational Therapy, 71*(12), 531-539. https://doi.org/10.1177/030802260807101206

Bonsaksen, T., Celo, C., Myraunet, I., Grana, K. E., & Ellingham, B. (2014). Promoting academic-practice partnerships through students' practice placement. *International Journal of Therapy and Rehabilitation, 20*(1). https://doi.org/10.12968/ijtr.2013.20.1.33

Braveman, B. (2016). *Leading and managing occupational therapy professional services* (2nd ed.). F. A. Davis.

Braveman, B. (2018). Professional reasoning in occupational therapy management. In B. A. Schell & J. W. Schell (Eds.), *Clinical and professional reasoning in occupational therapy* (pp. 461-476). Williams & Wilkins.

Braveman, B. Kielhofner, G., Belanger, R., & Llerena, V. (2008). Program Development. In G. Kielhofner (Ed.), *The Model of Human Occupation: Theory and Application* (4th Ed., pp. 442-465). Williams & Wilkins.

Braveman, B. Munoz, L. A., Hughes, J. K., & Nicholson, J. (2018). Cancer and oncology rehabilitation. In H. M. Pendleton & W. Schult-Krohn (Eds.), *Pedretti's Occupational Therapy for Physical Dysfunction* (8th Edition, pp. 1134-1141). Elsevier.

Cole, M. B., & Tufano, R. (2008). *Applied theories in occupational therapy: A practical approach*. SLACK Incorporated.

Dancza, K., Copley, J., & Moran, M. (2021). PLUS framework: Guidance for practice educators. *Clinical Teacher, 18*(4), 431-438. https://doi.org/10.1111/tct.13393

Davis-Cheshire, R., Davis, K., Drumm, L., Neal, S., Norris, E., Parker, M., Prezzia, C., & Whalen, C. (2019). The perceived value and utilization of occupational therapy models in the United States. *Journal of Occupational Therapy Education, 3*(2). https://doi.org/10.26681/jote.2019.030211

Edwards, H., & Dirette, D. (2010). The relationship between professional identity and burnout among occupational therapists. *Occupational Therapy in Health Care, 24*(2), 119-129. https://doi.org/10.3109/07380570903329610

Elliott, S. J., Velde, B. P., & Wittman, P. P. (2002) The use of theory in everyday practice: An exploratory study. *Occupational Therapy in Health Care, 16*, 45-62. https://doi.org/10.1080/J003v16n01_04

Evenson, M. E., Roberts, M., Kaldenberg, J., Barnes, M. A., & Ozelie, R. (2015). National survey of fieldwork educators: Implications for occupational therapy education. *American Journal of Occupational Therapy, 69*(Suppl. 2). https://doi.org/10.5014/ajot.2015.019265

Grajo, L. C. (2017) Occupational adaptation. In P. Kramer, J. Hinojosa, & C. B. Royeen (Eds), *Perspectives in human occupation: Participation in life* (pp. 137-159). F. A. Davis.

Hanson, D. J. (2009). The professional identity of occupational therapists: Construction, enactment and valued supports (Order No. 3360663) [Doctoral dissertation, North Dakota State University]. *ProQuest Dissertations and Theses Global*.

Hanson, D., & Nielsen, S. K, (2016). Introduction to role-emerging fieldwork. In Costa, D. (Ed.), *The essential guide to fieldwork education* (2nd ed.). AOTA.

Honey, A. & Penman, M. (2020). 'You actually see what occupational therapists do in real life': Outcomes and critical features of first-year practice education placements. *British Journal of Occupational Therapy, 83*(10), 638-647. https://doi.org/10.1177/0308022620920535

Ikiugu, M. N. (2010). Analyzing and critiquing occupational therapy practice models using Mosey's extrapolation method. *Occupational Therapy in Health Care, 24*(3), 193-205. https://doi.org/10.3109/07380570903521641

Ikiugu, M. N., & Smallfield, S. (2011). Ikiugu's eclectic method of combining theoretical conceptual practice models in occupational therapy. *Australian Occupational Therapy Journal, 58*(6), 437-446. https://doi.org/10.1111/j.1440-1630.2011.00968.x

Ikiugu, M. N., & Smallfield, S. (2015). Instructing occupational therapy students in use of theory to guide practice. *Occupational therapy in health care, 29*(2), 165-177. https://doi.org/10.3109/07380577.2015.1017787

Ikiugu, M. N., Smallfield, S., & Condit, C. (2009). A framework for combining theoretical conceptual practice models in occupational therapy practice. *Canadian Journal of Occupational Therapy, 76*(3), 62-70. https://doi.org/10.1177/000841740907600305

Jack, J., & Estes, R. I. (2010). Documenting process: Hand therapy treatment shift from biomechanical to occupational adaptation. *American Journal of Occupational Therapy, 64*(1), 82-87. https://doi.org/10.5014/ajot.64.1.82

Keponen R., & Launiainen, H. (2008). Using the model of human occupation to nurture an occupational focus in the clinical reasoning of experienced therapists. *Occupational Therapy in Health Care, 22*(2-3), 95-104. https://doi.org/10.1080/07380570801989549

Kielhofner, G. (2008). *A model of human occupation: Theory and application* (4th ed.). Williams & Wilkins.

Kielhofner, G. (2009). *Conceptual foundations of occupational therapy practice*. F. A. Davis.

Kielhofner, G., Braveman, B., Finlayson, M., Paul-Ward, A., Goldbaum, L., & Goldstein, K. (2004). Outcomes of a vocational program for persons with AIDS. *American Journal of Occupational Therapy, 58*(1), 64-72. https://doi.org/10.5014/ajot.58.1.64

Kinn, L. G., & Aas, R. W. (2009). Occupational therapists' perception of their practice: A phenomenological study. *Australian Occupational Therapy Journal, 56*(2), 112-121. https://doi.org/10.1111/j.1440-1630.2007.00714.x

Knowles, M. S., Holton, E. F., & Swanson, R. A. (2011). *The adult learner: The definitive classic in adult education and human resource development* (7th ed.). Elsevier.

Koski, J., Simon, R. L., & Dooley, N. R. (2013). Valuable occupational therapy fieldwork educator behaviors. *Work, 44*, 307-315. https://doi.org/10.3233/WOR-121507

Lamb, A. J. (2016). The power of authenticity. *American Journal of Occupational Therapy, 70*(6), 7006130010p1-7006130010p8. https://doi.org/10.5014/ajot.2016.706002

Leclair, L. L., Ripat, J. D., Wener, P. F., Cooper, J. E., Johnson, L. A., Davis, E. L., & Campbell-Rempel, M. A. (2013). Advancing the use of theory in occupational therapy: a collaborative process. *Canadian Journal of Occupational Therapy, 80*(3), 181-193. https://doi.org/10.1177/0008417413495182

Lee, J. (2010). Achieving best practice: A review of evidence linked to occupation-focused practice models. *Occupational Therapy in Health Care, 24*(3), 206-22. https://doi.org/10.3109/07380577.2010.483270

Lee, S. W., Taylor, R., Kielhofner, G., & Fisher, G. (2008). Theory use in practice: A national survey of therapists who use the model of human occupation. *American Journal of Occupational Therapy, 62*, 106-117.

Maclean, F., Carin-Levy, G., Hunter, H., Malcolmson, L. & Locke, E. (2012). The usefulness of the person-environment-occupation model in an acute physical health care setting. *British Journal of Occupational Therapy, 75*(12), 555. https://doi.org/10.4276/030802212X13548955545530

Melton, J., Forsyth, K., & Freeth, D. (2009). Using theory in practice. In E. Duncan (Ed.), *Skills for practice in occupational therapy* (pp. 9–23). Elsevier.

Melton, J., Forsyth, K., & Freeth, D. (2010). A practice development programme to promote the use of the model of human occupation: Contexts, influential mechanisms and levels of engagement amongst occupational therapists. *British Journal of Occupational Therapy, 73*(11), 549-558. https://doi.org/10.4276/030802210X12 89 2992239350

Nielsen, S., Jedlicka, J. S., Hanson, D., Fox, L., & Graves, C. (2017). Student perceptions of non-traditional Level I fieldwork. *Journal of Occupational Therapy Education, 1*(2). https://doi.org/10.26681/jote.2017.010206

O'Neal, S., Dickerson, A. E., & Hobert, D. (2007). The use of theory by occupational therapists working with adults with developmental disabilities. *Occupational Therapy in Health Care, 21*(4), 71-85.

Overton, A., Clark, M., & Thomas, Y. (2009). A review of non-traditional occupational therapy practice placement education: A focus on role-emerging and project placements. *British Journal of Occupational Therapy, 72*(7), 294-301.

Owen, A., Adams, F., & Franszen, D. (2014). Factors influencing model use in occupational therapy. *South African Journal of Occupational Therapy. 44.* 41-47.

Prochaska, J. O., Johnson, S., & Lee, P. (2009). The transtheoretical model of behavior change. In S. A. Shumaker, J. K. Ockene, & K. A. Riekert (Eds.), *The handbook of health behavior change*. Springer Publishing Company.

Schell, J. W. (2018). Teaching for reasoning in higher education. In *Clinical and professional reasoning in occupational therapy*. Wolters Kluwer Health.

Schell, B., & Gillen, G. (2018). *Willard and Spackman's occupational therapy* (13th ed.). Wolters Kluwer Health.

Shannon, P. D. (1977). The derailment of occupational therapy. *American Journal of Occupational Therapy, 31*(4), 229-234.

Smallfield S., & Karges, J. (2009). Classification of occupational therapy intervention for inpatient stroke rehabilitation. *American Journal of Occupational Therapy, 63*(4), 408-413. https://doi.org/10.5014/ajot.63.4.408

Towns, E., & Ashby, S. (2014). The influence of practice educators on occupational therapy students' understanding of the practical applications of theoretical knowledge: a phenomenological study into student experiences of practice education. *Australian Occupational Therapy Journal, 61*(5), 344-352.

Turpin, M., & Iwama, M. K. (2011). *Using occupational therapy models in practice: A fieldguide*. Churchill Livingstone/ Elsevier.

Wilding, C., & Whiteford, G. (2007). Occupation and occupational therapy: Knowledge paradigms and everyday practice. *Australian Occupational Therapy Journal, 54*(3), 185-193. https://doi.org/10.1111/j.1440-1630.2006.00621.x

Wimpenny, K., Forsyth, K., Jones, C., Matheson, L., & Colley, J. (2010). Implementing the model of human occupation across a mental health occupational therapy service: Communities of practice and a participatory change process. *The British Journal of Occupational Therapy, 73*(11), 507-516. https://doi.org/10.4276/030802210X12892992239152

APPENDIX A

Fieldwork Educator Learning Activities to Promote Use of Occupation-Focused Theory

1. Precontemplation

Occupational therapy practitioner contacts local occupational therapy academic program to get suggestions for article showing example of occupation-focused theory applied to a population and setting similar to their own. Academic faculty or local expert is invited to moderate focus group of FWeds discussing relevance and value of model use to their population and context.

As a follow-up, occupational therapy student completes observation of an occupational therapy treatment session noting impact of model identified concepts of the person, occupation, and environment on client occupational performance and discusses their observations of potential model value with FWed.

2. Contemplation: Capacity Building

Moderator provides information on key concepts of occupation-focused model and leads group discussion on congruence of model concepts, change mechanisms, and outcomes to setting population needs, facility context, and objectives.

Occupational therapy practitioners choose a client case from their own practice and "try on" model concepts to see if they fit client needs. Practitioners compare and contrast change mechanisms suggested by the model with the change mechanisms of their current practice and identify strengths and weaknesses of current practice. Practitioners suggest a course for therapy assessment and intervention for their client case using the concepts and change mechanisms of their chosen model.

Occupational therapy practitioners review an assessment tool associated with a specific occupation-focused model (e.g., COPM is associated with CMOP-E, a number of assessment tools are associated with MOHO), and identify presence of model concepts, change mechanisms, and outcome data obtained through it.

3. Contemplation: Engaging in Discourse and Collaboration

In advance of meeting, occupational therapy practitioners have built capacity to understand and apply at least two different models to their own practice. Supported by a moderator, practitioners choose a population of interest at their site and identify strengths and weaknesses of two different models to client application. A population might include an entire setting, such as all of my clients in acute care, or it might be all of my clients in acute care with orthopedic conditions. When you group clients in common categories, what do those look like? Understanding both similarities and differences in how models work is essential to comparison, which is foundational to choosing a model that best describes the work of occupational therapy in a given setting with a given population.

This might follow the pattern of:

A. Identifying congruence of model concepts, change mechanisms, and outcomes to client needs

B. Identifying research evidence that supports model concepts, change mechanisms, and suggested outcomes as pertinent to client population needs

C. Identifying site-specific factors that are a benefit or drawback to model application

D. Identifying resources (time, money, purchase of equipment/space) needed for model application

After identifying benefits and drawbacks to two different models, practitioners are divided into two groups to consider their own experiences working with the population and discuss the drawbacks of each model, problem solving together to identify how the drawbacks might effectively be addressed. The pairs then share their perspectives with the larger group. Ultimately, a decision is made as to a model that will be used to direct programming with the select population.

4. A. Preparation for Using Theory

At this stage, practitioners will identify the sequence of steps associated with the occupation-focused theory and prepare to carry out those steps in their setting. To do so, they need to become familiar with specific assessments associated with model use, practice them on one another, and practice explaining client issues using the language of the occupational behavior model and the data that are obtained by using the assessment tool.

At this stage, practitioners need to work with one another and participate in homework assignments trying out the tools associated with the model on select clients and within various steps of the occupational therapy process within the facility. As practitioners gain skills in using the tools and steps of the theory, they are also finding place and space to use a theory-driven process within the traditions and restrictions of their practice setting. In some cases, this means setting the tradition aside. For example, if there was a tradition to complete cognitive testing on all new clients, but this is incongruent with the steps of the model, that tradition may be dropped as a new process is found to be effective. Preparation for using theory involves lining up the resources and tools that will be needed to carry out all steps of the therapy process. This will begin with consideration of intake and assessment tools and processes but may then progress to use of data for setting treatment goals, intervention planning, and documentation of progress, as well as setting up systems for collection of outcomes data. Preparation activities may include:

A. Examination of referral processes and forms to reflect expected occupational therapy contributions

B. Identifying and learning how to administer specific assessment instruments and learning how to use the data to discuss needs of the client using the language of the model. May include design of an evaluation framework (a protocol) for specific client populations

C. Learning to use data from model assessment tools to support client treatment goals

D. Learning to identify and practice intervention procedures appropriate for treatment goals and aligned with the change mechanisms of the occupation-focused model

E. Learning to document in a manner that is consistent with reimbursement standards and also congruent with expected outcomes of the identified occupation-focused model. Documentation practice will include all stages of documentation required at the facility, for example, the initial and progress note, as well as discharge note

F. Identifying specific data that will be collected as a measurement of therapy outcomes, a data collection system, or process for data analysis and reporting

4. B. Implementation of Theory

Once preparation is complete, implementation involves testing all processes and procedures, first on a select client group, then expanding to other populations or occupational therapy programming. This stage should include many opportunities to reflect on strengths and weaknesses of the assessment, intervention, documentation, and communication processes to determine the need for revision or changes as needed to meet the needs of new client groups. This stage also includes collection and analysis of outcomes data to support theory implementation. In some cases, depending on outcomes data or new research evidence, the implementation of a given model may revert back to Stage 3 (contemplation, discourse, and collaboration) to determine if use of a different occupation-focused model is indicated.

5. Maintenance of Theory Use

A question for practitioners at this stage is "What structures do we (I) need to put into place so that it becomes routine for us (me) to use theory in practice?" Typically, this will include the development of processes and procedures (at both the individual or group level), and if theory-driven program is agreed upon by a group, policies and procedures that extend to a larger group are needed. To take best advantage of promotional benefits of organizing services from a theoretical perspective, program descriptions, websites, and other promotional materials should be developed/refined highlighting the unique contributions and occupational therapy process used onsite. If theory is used more on the individual level, program descriptions, recording processes, and procedures are important for documentation for publication or presentation or for career advancement. It is important to decide what should/will be done to support:

- Program descriptions
- Therapy processes
- Related policies
- Data management systems
- Personnel management

APPENDIX B
Student Learning Assignments Promoting Occupation-Focused Theory Implementation

1. **What does the student know/remember about the concepts of the model in regard to person, occupation, and environment?**

- Quiz upon arrival
- Assigned reading and worksheets to complete in advance of placement
- Facility focus group discussion on model used and why
- Discussion is on the kind of problems that are identified by the site, and how they are congruent with the concepts of the model in regard to person, environment, and occupation

2. **Can the student identify how each of the person and environment elements is impacting occupational participation (the small segments as well as the occupation as a whole)?**

- Observation handout reviewed with Level II student or Level I preceptor
- Review of key diagnostic groups, case studies where student identifies key elements impacting occupational participation

3. **Demonstration of how facility assessment process is congruent in focus and process to that suggested by identified model.**

- Facility demonstration videos
- Handout outlining assessments used and justifying use in regard to model concepts, expected model outcomes, population needs, and facility objectives
- Student review of key assessments used by agency and verification of having completed five identified key assessments on one other individual
- Facility provides case studies illustrating assessment process that follows suggested steps of identified model. Student completes case study choosing appropriate assessments and providing rationale for choices made

4. **Treatment planning: Demonstrate how facility treatment planning process is congruent in focus and process to identified model.**

- Facility provided case study illustrates a treatment planning process that is reflective of steps of identified model and includes common procedural processes of facility. Any variations from the model outlined process in setting goals are identified/noted and rationale provided. It is evident that mechanisms of change central to the identified theoretical model are addressed in intervention planning
- Key documentation elements are reviewed and congruence with model concepts is evident.

5. **Treatment implementation: Demonstrate how facility treatment implementation process is congruent in focus and process to identified model.**

- Faculty-led team or Level II student leads discussion answering the questions: How do the interventions provided target the underlying factors that contribute to the problem? Are the change mechanisms of the model evident in addressing the problem?

6. **Outcomes/treatment review: Demonstrate how facility outcomes measurement process is consistent in focus and process to identified model.**

- A discussion is held regarding the outcomes expected by the model assessed prior to intervention and reassessed after intervention. Can progress be identified? Are outcomes achieved?

7. **Exercise for helping students to connect the dots: A "bottom-up" approach to thinking with models.**

- Provide students a list of diagnoses, assessments, and interventions commonly addressed at your site. For each diagnosis, students might answer the following questions:

A. What cognitive, motor, sensory, or psychosocial issues may be present given the diagnoses?

B. How might these factors impact the commonly addressed occupations?

C. What assessment tools would you use to find out the client's present abilities in occupational performance? Which areas of occupational performance do you think would be of greatest concern given the setting context?

D. Which assessment tools might you use to find out the impact of cognitive, motor, sensory, or psychosocial issues on occupational performance for your given diagnosis?

E. What interventions (from the list provided by the facility) might be used to address occupational performance issues? For each intervention you list, indicate the *change mechanism* of the intervention. For example, does the intervention change a component in the person, adapting or patterning the occupation, or change a contextual feature of the occupational performance required? Or combination?

8. **Helping students to connect the dots across diagnostic categories.**

- Ask students to compare two clients with two different diagnoses on your caseload. What is similar? Different? How does this impact how you will address the issues?

- They might compare in regard to: treatment planning, intervention, expected outcomes.

- For each diagnostic category, students might compare how two different models might address the occupational performance issues identified:

A. Compare how each model views the concepts of person, environment, and occupation. After doing so, indicate which would be a best fit and why.

B. Compare the change mechanisms of two different models. Which would be most effective and why?

C. Compare the outcomes expected for each model. Which would be most pertinent and why?

- What can you learn?

- How would two different models view concepts of the person, environment, and occupation? Which would be a best fit for your targeted population?

- What research evidence do you have that these concepts, change mechanisms, and outcomes are pertinent to your population?

9. **Student learning scenario (adapt as needed to fit your setting):**

Pat, the Level I FWed, wanted Cynthia to consider which model might be a best fit for assessing the needs of young adults in the acute psychiatric unit who had recently been diagnosed with schizophrenia. She asked Cynthia to compare MOHO and the Ecological Model in regard to (1) the concepts addressed, (2) the assessment tools and process suggested by each model, (3) practical considerations of the setting, and (4) the needs of the population. In doing so, she wanted Cynthia to choose the model she thought was the best fit and provide her rationale for her choice. How would you complete this assignment if you were Cynthia?

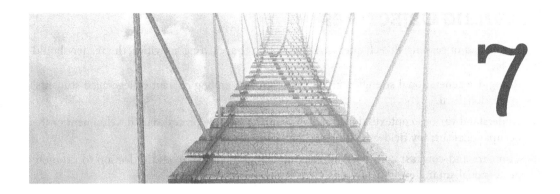

Fostering the Development of Professionalism During Level I Fieldwork

Elizabeth D. DeIuliis, OTD, MOT, OTR/L, CLA

Professional development is an ongoing phenomenon experienced by a health care practitioner throughout their career, especially within the experiential learning process. Educators in the classroom and practice settings play a significant role in helping their students not only to develop the technical skills to be competent in clinical practice but to indoctrinate and socialize to the attitudes and behaviors expected within the profession and the workforce. The latter pertains to what is referred to as *professionalism*. Researchers have indicated that the favored time to initiate views and beliefs about professionalism and professional identity development is *early in the professional training* program (Boyle et al., 2007; Hill, 2000; Schafheutle et al., 2012). Level I fieldwork is an important learning environment to initiate, develop, and refine professionalism in occupational therapy students. This chapter will provide recommendations for the Level I fieldwork educator (FWed) to role model professional behaviors and attitudes, mentorship to fieldwork students in professional development, and strategies to stimulate self-reflection on the professional development process for the Level I fieldwork student.

Hanson, D., & DeIuliis, E. D. (Eds.).
Fieldwork Educator's Guide to Level I Fieldwork (pp. 185-214).
© 2023 Taylor and Francis Group.

LEARNING OBJECTIVES

By the end of reading this chapter and completing the learning activities, the reader should be able to:

1. Recognize generational strengths and areas of growth among current college-aged students' professionalism.

2. Understand various contextual factors that contribute to the professional development of the occupational therapy fieldwork student.

3. Compare and contrast constructs of role modeling, mentorship, and reflection to promote professionalism in Level I fieldwork.

PROFESSIONALISM AS A CORNERSTONE OF OCCUPATIONAL THERAPY PRACTICE

Fieldwork education is an undeniable key component within the "professional preparation" for the occupational therapy student (Accreditation Council for Occupational Therapy Education [ACOTE], 2018, p. 39). While Level I fieldwork is often assumed to serve as a stepping stone to deepen didactic learning and provide introductory technical skill practice, it is also a key learning experience intended to "develop professionalism and competence in career responsibilities" (ACOTE, 2018, p. 39). More recently, in the updated edition of the *Occupational Therapy Practice Framework*, the official document that describes occupational therapy practice, professionalism has been clearly identified as a cornerstone (American Occupational Therapy Association [AOTA], 2020b). A cornerstone signifies a discrete and critical quality that is foundational for the success through the occupational therapy process that is "developed through education, mentorship and experience" (AOTA, 2020b, p. 6). The purpose of Level I fieldwork is to "introduce," "develop," and "enrich" knowledge and skills learned in the classroom in practice settings (AOTA, 1999). Current curriculum requirements in occupational therapy education include teaching knowledge and skills about technical clinical practice, and also key aspects of professional behaviors. With Level I fieldwork being a formal introduction to the occupational therapy process within practice settings, the Level I FWed should be held as a prominent change agent to introduce, develop, and enrich this essential cornerstone of the occupational therapy profession. A starting point is fostering a deeper understanding of what professionalism means.

It was not until recently that a formal definition of professionalism for occupational therapy was proposed: "Professionalism in occupational therapy clinical practice is a dynamic sophistication exemplified by a combination of an individual's personal skill set, knowledge, behaviors, and attitudes, and the adoption of the moral and ethical values of the profession and society" (DeIuliis, 2017, p. 37). Professionalism is a broad construct that involves elements of physicality, with respect to actions and behaviors, as well as core beliefs and mindsets that are internalized as attitudes and values. There are some aspects of professionalism that you can directly observe via a person's facial expressions, body language, handshake, and eye contact. Other aspects of professionalism may be hard to discern by direct observations, such as a person's level of integrity and reliability. In some cases, it may actually be easier to pinpoint what is not professional as opposed to having a clear and succinct characterization of what professionalism is in your practice setting. A more detailed discussion of what professionalism can look like on Level I fieldwork will occur later in this chapter. Although professionalism has just recently been acknowledged as a "cornerstone" of occupational therapy practice (AOTA, 2020b), it is a long-standing desired quality among many professions, inside and outside health care (Table 7-1).

TABLE 7-1

PROFESSIONALISM ACROSS DISCIPLINES INSIDE AND OUTSIDE ALLIED HEALTH

DISCIPLINE	DEFINITION OF PROFESSIONALISM
Medical education	Medical professionals and students are expected to have a specified set of behaviors and attitudes toward patients and society. In 1999, professionalism was listed as a required educational competency via Accreditation Council for Graduate Medical Education (American Board of Internal Medicine, 1994).
	According to the American Board of Internal Medicine (1994), professionalism is defined as "constituting those attitudes and behaviors that serve to maintain patient interest above physician self-interest" (Ludmerer, 1999, p. 881).
Nursing	According to the American Association of Colleges of Nursing (AACN), professionalism is defined as "the consistent demonstration of core values evidenced by nurses working with other professionals to achieve optimal health and wellness outcomes in patients, families, and communities by wisely applying principles of altruism, excellence, caring, ethics, respect, communication, and accountability" (AACN, 2008, p. 26).
Pharmacy	"Professionalism should be the full breadth of skills required to be competent pharmacy practitioners" (American College of Clinical Pharmacy [ACCP], 2009, p. 757). The ACCP (2009) developed a stand-alone document, Tenets of Professionalism for Pharmacy Students, which outlines the essential attitudes and behaviors that signify professionalism, which should be developed and practiced by all pharmacy students.
Physical therapy	In 2000, the American Physical Therapy Association's (APTA's Vision 2020) listed professionalism as one key element for the advancement of the profession. Furthermore, in 2003, the APTA adopted seven core values that are critical elements of professionalism in physical therapy practice, education, and research (APTA, 2019).
Speech-language pathology	The American Speech-Language Hearing Association (ASHA, 2000) refers to professionalism as workplace success skills.
	KASA (an acronym for Knowledge and Skills acquisition) includes a set of knowledge, skills, and competencies that are needed to earn a Certification of Clinical Competence in Speech-Language Pathology, have at least three competencies that specifically address issues of professionalism (ASHA, 2009).

(continued)

	TABLE 7-1 (CONTINUED)
	PROFESSIONALISM ACROSS DISCIPLINES INSIDE AND OUTSIDE ALLIED HEALTH
DISCIPLINE	**DEFINITION OF PROFESSIONALISM**
Teaching	The *Professional Standards for the Accreditation of Teacher Preparation Institutions* (National Council for Accreditation of Teacher Education, 2008) highlights professionalism as a program standard that elementary teachers in training should emulate.
	Scholars within the field of teacher development report that professionalism and how it is to be acquired should be a focus of every teacher education program (Creasy, 2015, p. 23).
Law	Although there is not a specific definition for professionalism for lawyers, the *Model Rules of Professional Conduct* is a list of responsibilities that defines proper conduct of professional disciple and a lawyer's professional role (American Bar Association, 2020).
	The Model Rules have "rules" on the client-lawyer relationship, rules related to the lawyer's role of being a counselor, advocate, maintaining integrity, public service, information about legal services, law firms, and associations/transactions with others (American Bar Association, 2020). These serve as models for the ethics rules of most jurisdictions.

Along with occupational therapy, other allied health professional academic programs, such as physical therapy (APTA, 2019) and speech-language pathology (ASHA, 2000, 2009), pharmacy (ACCP, 2009), nursing (AACN, 2008), and medical education (Ludmerer, 1999), also emphasize the importance of professionalism during didactic and experiential education. While classroom learning and experiential education are essentially designed to prepare college students to enter their chosen career, there is a significant disparity between what current college students vs. employers' perceptions of proficiencies in career ready skills and qualities. For instance, the National Association of Colleges and Employers (NACE) Class of 2020 survey found gaps in key areas of employability, specifically graduating students overreporting competency in skills required to be successful and effective in the workforce (Table 7-2). The gap between the two groups was greatest when it came to students' *professionalism and work ethic*; more than 95% of current college-aged students considered themselves proficient in this area, but less than half of employers agreed (NACE, 2020b).

While a justification of this gap between employers and college students is not completely clear in the literature, excessive confidence, narcissism, or limited self-awareness are hypothesized stereotypes of this generation that can be further explored (Stewart et al., 2020). Limited or a lack of self-awareness is a known growth area for current college-aged students and young professionals (DeIuliis & Saylor, 2021). The use of *self-reflection*, more *direct teaching*, and *role modeling* on key aspects of professionalism can be useful approaches to heighten awareness of these disparities. Some strategies of how to infuse these interventions to develop professionalism during Level I fieldwork will be discussed later in this chapter.

TABLE 7-2
ESSENTIAL VERSUS PROFICIENT CAREER READINESS

	CONSIDERED ESSENTIAL (%)	RATED PROFICIENT (%)	GAP (%)
Professionalism/work ethic	95.1	46.5	48.6
Oral/written communication	93.2	49.0	44.2
Critical thinking/problem solving	99.0	60.4	38.4
Leadership	56.3	30.4	25.9
Career management	37.9	20.6	17.3
Information technology application	53.4	68.6	15.2
Teamwork/collaboration	98.0	85.1	12.9
Global/multicultural fluency	22.3	25.3	3.0

Adapted from National Association of Colleges and Employers. (2020b). *Job outlook 2020*. https://www.vidteamcc.com/stadistics/2020-nace-job-outlook%20(1).pdf

GENERATIONAL PERSPECTIVES ON PROFESSIONALISM

Entitled, lazy, high maintenance, and overly confident are some of the words used to describe current college-aged graduates (van der Wal, 2017). While this is an unfortunate portrayal, this is reflected in the current literature describing current college-aged students and new professionals in the workforce. In generational theory, it is not uncommon for each generation to be described with stereotypical traits, including both positive and negative qualities. A generation is simply a group of people born in the same general time span who collectively share life experiences, such as historical events, formative memories, and societal trends (Weston, 2001). Several generational theorists (e.g., Blythe et al., 2008) argue that shared life experiences generate shared assumptions, attitudes, and beliefs, as well as a cohesive group identity. There is longstanding literature that describes each generation with positive and negative stereotypical traits based upon their formative years. Impactful historical events, parenting styles, and even trends in pop culture all influence a person's identity, attitudes, and belief system (Table 7-3). The youngest generations in the workforce include Generation Y or the Millennials (born between 1981 and 2001), Generation Z (born after 2001; Pew Research Center, 2019), followed by the rising future cohort of college-aged students in the Alpha Generation (born after 2009; McCrindle & Fell, 2020).

Each generation has unique viewpoints and expectations on workplace cultural norms, such as preferred communication style, approach to managing conflict, sense of work ethic, preference for leadership and authority, etc. For example, some older generations (Baby Boomers) prefer a face-to-face conversation to exchange important information vs. an email memo or a phone call conversation to converse vs. a text message. Some (Generation X) may resent coworkers who have a wavering or uncommitted work ethic and struggle to value the importance of work-life balance. Older generations may be more motivated by intrinsic rewards for a job well done, such as gaining respect and recognition from authority, whereas younger generations seem to be more motivated by extrinsic rewards, such as merit raises, promotions, and securing the corner office with the

TABLE 7-3
GENERATIONAL STEREOTYPES

GENERATION	POSITIVE STEREOTYPICAL TRAITS	NEGATIVE STEREOTYPICAL TRAITS
Generation Y	• Curious • Energetic • Tech savvy • Civil minded • Multitaskers • Adaptable to change	• Lack of self-esteem • Lack of self-confidence • Lack of maturity • Require more coaching • Casual view of the workplace
Generation Z	• Confident • Optimistic • Impact oriented • Innovators	• Tech dependent • Overachievers • Sense of entitlement • Lack of self-awareness
Alpha Generation	While there is not a lot of literature yet on this future generation that will enter college and the workforce in a decade, it can be hypothesized that they will have an upbringing that has been technology-supplied like no other, which may significantly impact key aspects of professionalism such as: • Lack of communication skills • Decreased ability to read and interpret social cues • Limited social capital	

Adapted from Deluliis, E. (2017). Definitions of professionalism. In E. Deluliis (Ed.), *Professionalism across occupational therapy practice* (pp. 3-42). SLACK Incorporated and Deluliis, E. D., & Saylor, E. (2021). Bridging the gap: Three strategies to optimize professional relationships with generation Y and Z. *The Open Journal of Occupational Therapy,* *9*(1), 1-13. https://doi.org/10.15453/2168-6408.1748

view. All of these diverse beliefs can contribute to a generational gap in the workforce. Navigating these diverse generational viewpoints, as well as other workplace cultural norms, can be challenging yet yield important learning for students during early experiential opportunities such as Level I fieldwork.

A key aspect in the professional development process for current college-aged students is learning how to bridge this generation gap, as well as align with the workplace norms of their fieldwork site and still meet the expectations of the academic program (Gravett & Throckmorton, 2007). To do this, it involves a discovery of and implementation of strategies and solutions that can build connections (bridges) between generations (DeIuliis & Saylor, 2021). Table 7-3 indicates that self-awareness is a known growth area among current college-aged students and new professionals in the workforce, which adds further support to the known disproportion of "readiness for the workforce" among college graduates and employers. Specific role modeling and direct teaching in professionalism are critical to their success in this area. Strategies and recommendations for the FWed to build upon a Level I fieldwork student's generational stereotypes, including strengths and growth areas, will be presented in the upcoming section of this chapter.

BOX 7-1

NATIONAL ASSOCIATION OF COLLEGES AND EMPLOYERS DEFINITION OF CAREER READINESS

NACE defines career readiness as "the attainment and demonstration of requisite competencies that broadly prepare college graduates for a successful transition into the workplace" (NACE, 2020a).

PROFESSIONALISM AS GROUNDWORK FOR CAREER READINESS

Over recent years, the demands of the workforce have increased, particularly in the health care industry. Pragmatic constraints include but are not limited to high caseloads, low staffing patterns, evolving changes to reimbursement (such as patient driven payment models), and in-demand health care delivery models, such as telehealth. These demands are resulting not just in a push for an increase in clinical skill preparation but rather a necessity for a skill set that is now being characterized as *practice ready* or *employability*. What is also referred to as *soft skills*, the terms practice readiness or workplace readiness are becoming hot catchphrases in the description of ideal career-ready graduates who enter the workforce across disciplines (Barry, 2012; Mattila, 2019; Missen et al., 2016; Murphy, 2015). In some light, this idea of practice readiness can be viewed as a way to modernize familiar terminology used by employers to describe the desired make-up of an employee, such as *hard and soft* skills. Hard skills are often defined as the technical skills to carry out a job or task (Deepa & Seth, 2013). Within occupational therapy, hard skills include competencies to implement the occupational therapy process (AOTA, 2020b), which may include administration of assessment tools, skills to fabricate an orthosis, or the ability to document a thorough progress note in a timely manner. Soft skills are often harder to define and usually align with interpersonal behaviors and attitudes. Being reliable, a good problem solver, and a team player are examples of soft skills (DeIuliis, 2017). Some may argue that softs skills are often more impressionable in the workplace and during the job interview process. It may be a person's hard skills that get their foot into the door of an interview, but in most cases, it is a person's soft skills that demonstrate their ability to be successful and, in some cases, long-term potential in the workforce. Deepa and Seth (2013) even go as far as describing soft skills as *survival skills*, indicating a criticality of workplace success. The value and importance of soft skills are now being relabeled as practice readiness or career readiness skills. See Box 7-1 for career readiness definition.

So, *what are these desired skill sets or competencies of graduates entering the workforce? What does it take to be employable and practice ready regardless of the profession or industry?* Although this list is not specifically aligned for the occupational therapy profession, desired skill sets of all graduates entering the workforce include the following (NACE, 2020c):

- Solid problem-solving skills
- Ability to work in a team
- Strong work ethic
- Analytical/quantitative skills
- Communication skills (written and verbal)
- Leadership
- Initiative
- Detail oriented

For a more detailed definition of how NACE defines these competencies, please visit the official NACE website at https://www.naceweb.org/career-readiness/competencies/career-readiness-defined/.

The Society for Human Resource Management (SHRM, 2019), a professional organization that serves the human resource management and talent development industries, uses the term *applied skills* to identify nonknowledge-based skills desired by employers, which include:

- Dependability/reliability
- Integrity
- Respect
- Teamwork
- Customer focus

Responding to the concerns from employers, allied health educators and researchers are doing more research in this area. In a recent study, O'Brien et al. (2020) investigated characteristics related to work readiness in allied health students in Australia; occupational therapy was represented in the participant sample. The researchers aimed to understand: *What characteristics were considered to be most important ahead of joining an allied health career?* While the research study (O'Brien et al., 2020, p. 4) yielded over 100 qualities aligned with workplace readiness in allied health, a summarized list of the top 10 are:

1. Insight and self-awareness, ability to self-reflect
2. Resilience
3. Communication skills
4. Organization skills
5. Commitment to lifelong learning
6. Professionalism
7. Emotional maturity
8. Adaptability/flexibility
9. Empathy
10. Ability to cope/handle stress

As a construct, participants in the study discussed professionalism broadly, such as adhering to a code of conduct and ethics, as well as through a narrower lens, such as how a person maintains their physical presentation, for example, nail and hair hygiene/care and clothing choices (O'Brien et al., 2020).

In reviewing these lists of attributes by NACE (2020c), SHRM (2019), and O'Brien et al. (2020), there are some patterns regarding desired attributes, as well as characteristics that are reported to be missing or lacking. Employers are expressing frustration in the lack of preparation in the college classroom on career readiness. The top **missing** soft skills in current college graduates include problem solving, critical thinking, innovation, and creativity; the ability to deal with complexity and ambiguity; and communication (SHRM, 2019). Personality characteristics consistent with practice readiness can impact success on fieldwork and overall professional preparation (Skodova et al., 2017). It is recommended that didactic curricula include specific interventions designed to develop coping and interpersonal skills. In response, many rigorous professional degree programs, such as occupational therapy, are beginning to make positive changes in the required preparation of their students. Helping to address these missing soft skills should also be an essential focus of the Level I FWed.

Box 7-2

ACOTE STANDARDS FOR PROFESSIONAL BEHAVIORS

Professional behaviors (evaluation of, advising in) **is now being required by ACOTE** in occupational therapy/occupational therapy assistant curricula (ACOTE, 2018).

ACOTE Standard A.3.5

Evaluation must occur on a regular basis and feedback must be provided in a timely fashion in the following areas:

- Student progress
- **Professional behaviors**
- Academic standing

ACOTE Standard A.3.7

Advising related to professional coursework, **professional behaviors**, and fieldwork education *must be* the responsibility of the occupational therapy faculty

---

ADDRESSING CAREER READINESS AND PROFESSIONALISM IN THE OCCUPATIONAL THERAPY CLASSROOM

Based on the new needs and expectations of the workforce, the development of employability skills has been increasingly important in the training of health care professional students. Educators in the classroom and the clinic need to have a heightened level of awareness to effectively role model and mentor students in professional behaviors and attitudes. Because of these factors, it is not surprising that newly adopted accreditation standards for occupational therapy now require academic programs to advise and evaluate professional behaviors of occupational therapy students regularly (ACOTE, 2018; Box 7-2).

Due to these new accreditation standards, FWeds can anticipate classroom learning and advisement to involve more direct and indirect teaching on professionalism. Situational learning via the use of role play and simulation can be used to mimic real world issues, such as time management, including but not limited to punctuality and managing deadlines and other aspects of professional behaviors, such as interpersonal skills (Brown et al., 2020; Fidler, 1966; McDonald et al., 2013). Using direct instruction, students can be provided specific learning objectives relative to themes around professionalism (Babola & Peloquin, 1999). Examples of direct teaching of professionalism in the classroom by occupational therapy faculty may include:

- An assignment that requires the student to explore knowledge about professionalism in occupational therapy

- An individual lecture, course, or sequence of courses with a specific focus on professional behaviors

- Specific policies and procedures on syllabi and handbooks that clearly outline expectations regarding dress/attire, time/attendance, engagement in class, use of electronic devices, etc.

- Implementation of rubrics to measure professional behavior in the classroom

- Professional behaviors being a percentage of their overall grade in a course (Box 7-3)

Direct instruction in professionalism can be a useful approach to address the self-awareness limitations of current college-aged students. However, there are also indirect teaching approaches that can be done in the academic environment, which may involve an unspoken agenda designated to exemplify or role model desired professional behaviors competencies. Indirect instruction

---

BOX 7-3

FIDLER'S VISION FOR PROFESSIONALISM
AND PROFESSIONAL BEHAVIORS

The scholarship of Gail S. Fidler, a pioneer occupational therapy practitioner, researcher, mentor, and educator, provided important groundwork for professionalism to be viewed as a necessary, yet complex construct within the teaching–learning process. In her paper titled "Developing a Repertoire of Professional Behaviors," Fidler (1996) provided a comprehensive outline for educators and students to broadly consider professional behaviors, and described that competency in with professionalism is an iterative process.

Self-awareness and **becoming more aware** were identified as core areas in Fidler's vision for professionalism and professional behaviors more than 25 years ago.

---

methods include reflective discussion and guided inquiry. Evidence indicates that exposure to more direct confidence-building and problem-based learning in the classroom can enhance students' preparation for real world scenarios in fieldwork (James & Musselman, 2006). Educational theories, such as problem-based learning and case-based learning, can boost independent thought and problem-solving skills (McDonald et al., 2013), which are noted to be desired qualities by employers in the workforce and missing in current college-aged students. When indirect instruction is used, the role of the instructor shifts to that of facilitator, supporter, and guide. A key aspect of indirect teaching is that the student is actively engaged in the learning process, which in turn strengthens their personal connection to the topic area. For instance, during the use of case studies and reflective discussion, educators can facilitate a discussion in how key aspects of professionalism can have a direct impact on future fieldwork success and employability. Here is an example. Academic fieldwork coordinators (AFWCs), faculty members, and even FWeds are often requested to serve as a professional reference for students/recent graduates during the job search process. Whether performed over the phone during a conversation or a response to a questionnaire or survey, employers usually ask questions that target a student/prospective employee's level of professionalism. *Is the student reliable? Were they consistently punctual? Rate and describe their communication and problem-solving skills ... How do they handle stressful situations? Would you hire this student?* These are the characteristics that employers want to vet before they invest in hiring a candidate. When students have a better grasp on the real world impact of their attitudes, behaviors, and actions, it can help improve their self-awareness in this area. Indirect instruction methods may include:

- Active role play or simulations that involve challenging situations experienced on fieldwork or in the workforce, such as how to respond to constructive feedback, managing conflict, etc.

- A faculty/student mentorship system that builds a professional development plan

- Faculty and staff portraying a professional image by their dress and overall presentation

- Faculty and staff role modeling how to formulate professional emails to students using professional language, tone, and style

- Faculty and staff demonstrating appropriate nonverbal, interpersonal skills, such as body language and eye contact during interactions with students and colleagues

While a FWed can anticipate that more direct and indirect teaching on professional behaviors is occurring in the classroom, Level I fieldwork is a crucial learning context to help reinforce application of these skills and close the gap between the classroom and the real world.

PRACTICE SETTING	WORKPLACE NORM
School system	While rubber sole sneakers may not be an acceptable footwear in other settings, due to the dynamic role of the school-based occupational therapist, it may be a requirement of the workplace attire.
	Another example of school-based practice may be that it is acceptable and even encouraged to engage in dress up costumes during holidays, such as Halloween. This may not be an acceptable workplace norm in other settings such as a medical environment.
Trauma clinic in an orthopedic physician office	The use of scrubs may not be acceptable. The physician in charge may expect the staff to wear professional attire such as a business suit or lab coat.
Community practice site at a nonprofit organization	Due to the culture of the site and clients served in the community, casual attire, such as jeans, may be acceptable. Jeans may not be acceptable form of dress in other occupational therapy practice sites such as a hospital.

TABLE 7-4

EXAMPLE OF WORKPLACE NORMS WITHIN DIFFERENT PRACTICE SETTINGS

WHAT DOES PROFESSIONALISM DURING LEVEL I FIELDWORK LOOK LIKE?

Professionalism is "imperative for fieldwork success in occupational therapy," particularly when the FWed holds students to these high standards (Hackenberg & Toth-Cohen, 2018, p. 1). As fieldwork is a bridge between the classroom and the clinic, the Level I FWed is challenged to uphold the expected attitudes, actions, and behaviors established by the academic program, while also socializing the student to the expectations at the fieldwork site. Although there are overarching principles surrounding professionalism that are promoted by official organizations within all occupational therapy practice settings (such as the *Code of Ethics* [AOTA, 2020a] and the *Standards of Practice* [AOTA, 2015]), an important quality of professionalism is that it is context specific (Sullivan & Thiessen, 2015). Various characteristics of professionalism, for instance, appropriate dress code, can be different within a school-based practice setting compared to a hand therapist who works alongside a hand surgeon in a physician's office setting. See Table 7-4 for further examples in this area.

To ensure consistency in expectations, strong communication between the AFWC and the FWed is beneficial (James & Musselman, 2006). Outside of the value of strong rapport between the fieldwork site and the academic program, the AFWC should also empower fieldwork students to take initiative to clarify workplace norms and professional expectations ahead of their fieldwork placements. Furthermore, the FWed should also be encouraged to seek out and request information from the academic program about expected behaviors in key areas, such as time/attendance, dress code, use of electronic devices, etc. Each academic program may have different expectations. For example, some fieldwork programs may provide a certain number of excused days for the

---

Box 7-4

EXAMPLE OF STUDENTS IN ROLE-EMERGING FIELDWORK SITES

For example, students who are placed in **role-emerging fieldwork sites** have increased confidence in their competency and enhanced professional identity. Although the research in the United Kingdom pertains to a final experiential experience, such as Level II, specific aspects of their professional development that were enhanced by the fieldwork experience include autonomous working, problem solving, communication, teamwork, marketing, decision making, and clinical reasoning. These competencies are also known to "ease the transition" of fieldwork students entering clinical practice (Clarke et al., 2015).

---

fieldwork students, whereas other programs have a strict zero tolerance policy for absenteeism. There is emerging literature that discusses how the type of practice site can impact the professional identity development of the occupational therapy student (Box 7-4).

As described earlier in this chapter, professionalism is a *sophisticated combination of skills, knowledge, behavior, and attitudes* (DeIuliis, 2017). One approach to understanding this combination is classifying these aspects of professionalism into intrinsic and extrinsic attributes. Intrinsic qualities refer to those components of being a professional that is related to a person's internal character and overall morality, which can be externalized by their belief system and attitude. Extrinsic qualities include observable behaviors and actions (DeIuliis, 2017). Table 7-5 provides a model of how to conceptualize what professionalism looks like for a Level I fieldwork student. In addition to clearly defining what professionalism looks like at your site, it is critical to self-reflect on the current functioning of you and your team members. Students learn from example. Is the culture and functioning of your site serving as an exemplar for the student? If you are asking your student to arrive on time and comply with dress code policies, are you and your team consistently demonstrating these behaviors and actions too?

Table 7-5 broadly suggests key competencies that a fieldwork student should emulate, as well as some reflective prompts for the Level I FWed to consider in order to promote the student to take ownership of professionalism development in these areas. While the student's technical skill set and clinical performance are certainly a significant part of the fieldwork learning experience, key competencies noted by FWeds of successful students connect closer to professional behaviors.

Although their study was completed within the K to 12 education sector, Tichenor and Tichenor (2009) reported examples of certain unprofessional behaviors that should NOT be exhibited among faculty and preceptors, which included:

- Improper attire/untidy appearance
- Disrespect of students, faculty, staff, clients, etc.
- Tardiness
- Late submission of student feedback/evaluations
- Embarrassment of students within practice setting
- Gossip between faculty/team members with students
- Use of cellphone at practice site
- Absence of or lack of professional development in teaching strategies
- Use of profanity in the educational or practice environment

TABLE 7-5

UNDERSTANDING THE QUALITIES OF PROFESSIONALISM DURING LEVEL I FIELDWORK

	QUALITIES OF PROFESSIONALISM	LEVEL I FIELDWORK STUDENT COMPETENCY	FIELDWORK EDUCATOR REFLECTION
Intrinsic	Self-management	Student exhibits self-discipline and self-awareness and can handle unanticipated or stressful situations on fieldwork.	*During high-volume days, do you maintain your cool and appropriately ask for help or delegate?*
	Critical reasoning skills	Student is able to use logic and deductive reasoning learned in the classroom and apply to clinical scenarios on fieldwork.	*In a novel situation (e.g., a consult for a diagnosis you have never treated before), do you exhibit initiative and take appropriate steps to seek out information?*
	Integrity/honesty	Student exhibits attitudes that are rooted in strong morals and ethics.	*Do you accurately reflect your direct treatment time with clients in your billing and productivity measures?*
	Dependability/reliability	Student arrives on time to fieldwork placement daily.	*Do you and your team role model arriving to work daily on time?*
	Generational and cultural sensitivity	Student is aware of being respectful of different values and belief systems among the health care team.	*Do you and your team demonstrate inclusiveness and welcome students into your workplace culture?*
Extrinsic	Professional image: manners, etiquette, dress code	Student complies with site's dress code policies.	*Do your fieldwork student policies and onboarding materials clearly reflect the dress code of your site?*
	Time management	Student completes daily documentation at fieldwork on time.	*Do you and your team role model complete documentation in the expected time consistently?*
	Adaptability and organizational skills	Student uses a planner/calendar to keep track of assignments and responsibilities.	*Do you suggest and use caseload management strategies to demonstrate effective triage and prioritization skills?*

(continued)

TABLE 7-5 (CONTINUED)

UNDERSTANDING THE QUALITIES OF PROFESSIONALISM DURING LEVEL I FIELDWORK

	QUALITIES OF PROFESSIONALISM	LEVEL I FIELDWORK STUDENT COMPETENCY	FIELDWORK EDUCATOR REFLECTION
	Interpersonal skills	Student uses and maintains eye contact and active listening skills when interacting with patients and the health care team.	*Do you provide your undivided attention and demonstrate mutual respect via verbal and nonverbal communication skills during interdisciplinary team meetings?*
	Teamwork	Student seeks out and collaborates with other students and professionals on the team.	*What are the characteristics of an effective team, and do you and your team demonstrate strong teamwork skills?*
	E-professionalism	Student portrays self professionally online including during email correspondence and maintenance of social media profiles.	*Expect your future fieldwork student to google you or perform a search on social media! Do a social media account check! What are your privacy settings? Is your profile picture providing an impression of you as a professional?*

Adapted from Deluliis, E. (2017). Definitions of professionalism. In E. Deluliis (Ed.), *Professionalism across occupational therapy practice* (pp. 3-42). SLACK Incorporated.

- Disclosure of confidential student information to other students, clients, or team members
- Indecent social media interactions with students/clients
- Provision of inaccurate information to clients or other health care workers

    (Adapted from Akiyode, 2016; Tichenor & Tichenor, 2009)

    In occupational therapy, researchers have noted several factors that can be linked to an unsuccessful fieldwork experience, resulting in student failure, and —SPOILER ALERT— these factors **are not** connected to academic performance such as grade point average. While some of these studies pertain to Level II fieldwork, failure of fieldwork generally is more closely associated with a lack of career readiness and professionalism such as:

- Inability to handle stress (Mitchell & Kampfe, 1990)
- Emotional intelligence (Gutman et al., 1998)

Box 7-5

EVIDENCE ON PROFESSIONALISM
FROM ROLE-EMERGING FIELDWORK

There is emerging research that reports a difference among first- and second-year occupational therapy student's understanding of professionalism. Sullivan and Thiessen (2015) found that **first-year students (i.e., Level I fieldwork students) relied on explicit examples when attempting to understand professional behaviors.** For example, professional image and outer appearance, involvement in professional organizations, advocacy, and community education were important aspects of professionalism viewed by first-year occupational therapy students. Additionally, second-year students (i.e., Level II fieldwork students) emphasized professionalism as being socially constructed (learned over time and through observations), varied across contexts, and made up by ethical and intrinsic factors, possibly drawn from their prior extensive fieldwork experiences.

A key takeaway from Sullivan and Thiessen's (2015) research is that professionalism is a construct that develops and is understood over time.

- Interpersonal skills (Sands, 1995; Tickle-Degnen, 1998)

- Professional behavior (Scheerer, 2003)

- Poor problem-solving and organizational skills, difficulty responding to constructive feedback, lack of initiative (James & Musselman, 2006)

These factors that contribute to poor fieldwork outcomes can be traced back to the desired attributes by employers in the current workforce (NACE, 2020c; SHRM, 2019).

To summarize, an important first step in promoting professionalism in Level I fieldwork is clearly identifying the expectation early in the learning experience. Student onboarding processes, such as initial mailings, emails, fieldwork student handbooks, or even site-specific learning objectives, should clearly stipulate the desired attitudes, behaviors, and actions expected from the fieldwork student (Box 7-5).

After expectations of professionalism and professional behaviors have been clearly identified for the fieldwork student, the FWed can also employ direct and indirect teaching approaches to help the student refine and polish their performance in these areas.

INTERVENTIONS TO ADDRESS PROFESSIONAL BEHAVIORS IN LEVEL I FIELDWORK

Students gain knowledge from role models and mentors through observation, imitation, practice, and guided reflection (Cruess et al., 2015). This section will highlight tips and strategies for the FWed to help develop and refine professional skill sets in occupational therapy students, via role modeling, mentorship, and self-reflection.

Role Modeling

In simplistic terms, a role model is a person looked to as an example. Role models are defined as "individuals admired for their ways of being and acting as professionals" (Cruess et al., 2015, p. 721). The role of a Level I FWed is a prominent role model for the occupational therapy student, both for clinical skill development and how to portray themselves as a professional. As a role model, a FWed emulates what success as a practitioner in their work site looks like. A role model leads by example and should expect that their fieldwork student is always watching, receiving, and interpreting cues, which is supported by Albert Bandura's (1977) social learning theory. Bandura's (1997) research postulates that people learn through observing and imitating others behaviors, attitudes, and actions. Some food for thought … *How do you behave during interdisciplinary meetings? What is your body language during team huddles? Do you role model active listening for your Level I fieldwork student by maintaining eye contact and avoid interrupting other team members when they are speaking?*

A key factor is recognizing that role modeling as a FWed goes beyond clinical practice. For instance, *Is your email style of communication with your fieldwork students professional? Do fieldwork students observe you, the FWed, seek out and attend continuing education and professional development opportunities as a lifelong learner? Are students observing you engaged in servant leadership roles and actively participate in process improvement groups, or with professional organizations (such as AOTA, American Occupational Therapy Political Action Committee, or your State Occupational Therapy Association)? Do you demonstrate openness and willing serve in the role of FWed?* See Figure 7-1 for the components of role modeling.

A further connection to Bandura's (1977) social learning theory shows us that errors or maladaptive responses can be prevented if a person learns a behavior through *observation first*. In addition to being aware of your own attitudes and actions as a role model, a Level I FWed should also be observing their occupational therapy student's imitation or ability to replicate some aspects of professionalism (Box 7-6). *Is your fieldwork student demonstrating appropriate verbal and nonverbal interpersonal skills during interdisciplinary collaboration meetings?* If the answer is no, it is vital that you reflect on the performance of you and your team. Are you effectively role modeling professional behaviors? Educators, including Level I FWeds, need to be aware of the "conscious and unconscious" aspects from role modeling (Cruess et al., 2008, p. 718).

Mentorship

Mentoring is more of a mutual process that involves a mentor (an individual with more experience) and the mentee (a person with less experience) engaging in a formal relationship designed to provide influence and guidance toward goal achievement. Mentors are defined as "experienced and trusted counselors" (Cruess et al., 2015, p. 721). Mentors can have greater impact on learner's professional identity since they have closer and more prolonged contact with the learner (Cruess et al., 2015). Rice and Perry (2013) suggest that mentors "should be good role models" and therefore intentionally demonstrate the "behaviors and style they hope to see in their mentees" (p. 62). As a FWed, mentoring requires you to actively work to build rapport with your student and provide support and advisement to support the success of the student. For example, ahead of a Level I fieldwork experience, a FWed might proactively seek out what learning areas the student wants to explore, based upon prior learning experiences and their unique needs. A formal mentorship plan or learning success plan may be used to solidify goal areas, identify strategies to accomplish goals, and hold the mentor and the mentee accountable. From here, the Level I FWed, as a mentor, provides support and guidance, which may be specific resources or experiences, and keeps the mentee's best interest in mind. One specific strategy that can be used to build rapport and take genuine interest in your Level I fieldwork student is to obtain an occupational profile of the student (DeIuliis, 2011). To effectively learn about your fieldwork student and to begin to establish a mentor and mentee relationship, ask open-ended questions (Rice & Perry, 2013) such as: *Who is your student as a person and occupational being? What is important to them? What motivates them? How do they learn best?* As practitioners, we know the value that therapeutic use of self and

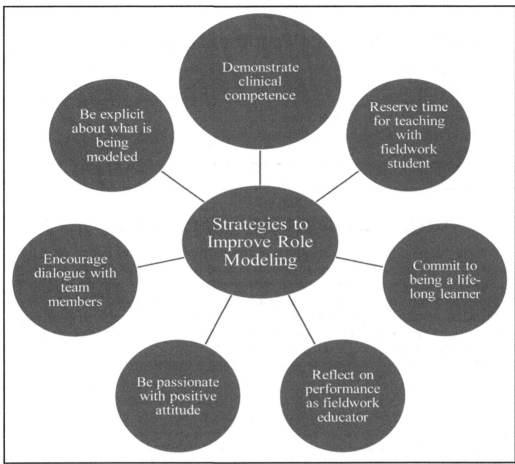

Figure 7-1. Key components of role modeling. (Adapted from Cruess, S. R., Cruess, R. L., & Steinert, Y. [2008]. Role modelling—making the most of a powerful teaching strategy. *British Medical Journal, 336*[7646], 718-721. https://doi. org/10.1136/bmj.39503.757847.BE and Mohammadi, E., Shahsavari, H., Mirzazadeh, A., Sophrabpour, A. A., & Hejri, S. M. [2020]. Improving role modeling in clinical teachers: A narrative literature review. *Journal of Advances in Medical Education & Professionalism, 8*[1], 1-9. https://doi.org/10.30476/jamp.2019.74929)

Box 7-6

THE IMPACT OF ROLE MODELING PEDAGOGY

A recent study by Chien et al. (2020) investigated the impact of role modeling pedagogy on the understanding and awareness of professionalism in occupational therapy students in Hong Kong. Students in the study were required to interview an expert in the field who was considered to be a strong role model and participate in guided reflective activities, including creating an action plan focused on their own professional development. The researchers found that the role modeling pedagogy experience enhanced the students' perceived understanding of professionalism and their awareness of specific professionalism attributes modeled by the experts.

Designing Level I fieldwork learning activities that require occupational therapy students to interview and observe professional role models can be a useful strategy to support the development of professional behaviors and a student's overall professional development.

BOX 7-7

IMPACT OF MENTORSHIP WITH YOUNGER GENERATIONS

Mentorship is a preferred supervision style of younger generations, such as Generations Y and Z. Younger generations dislike authoritative governance that merely prescribes rules and constraints yet seek out an environment and organizational culture to guide, inspire, and mentor them (Bartz et al., 2017; Deloitte, 2016).

Instead of "fieldwork supervisor" or "clinical instructor" as a FWed, view yourself as a mentor.

BOX 7-8

GETTING CREDIT FOR SERVING AS A MENTOR

Outside of earning professional development units (PDUs) for serving as a FWed, did you know that both mentors and mentees can earn PDUs recognized by the NBCOT? Verification documentation includes documented goals, objectives in collaboration with the mentor, and analysis of mentee performance. The mentor MUST be currently certified with NBCOT.

Therefore, engaging in a formal mentor-mentee relationship may be a strategy to enhance your own professional development as a FWed and occupational therapy practitioner. Further details can be found at www.nbcot.org.

---

client centeredness has on client outcomes. These same principles can be viewed through the lens of the FWed and fieldwork student professional relationship. See Box 7-7 to see what generations prefer the mentorship supervision style. An interesting aspect of mentorship is that it can lead to improvements in both professional and personal development. Box 7-8 shows how engaging in a mentor-mentee relationship can earn you PDUs that might be recognized by credentialing groups, such as the National Board for Certification in Occupational Therapy (NBCOT). Mentoring is proven to improve professional practice, such as patient care skills, work relationships, confidence, job satisfaction, and leadership skills (Steven et al., 2008). See Figure 7-2 for components for an effective mentoring relationship.

In contrast, the mentor-mentee relationship and outcomes can be negatively impacted when the mentor fails to be of help and does not meet the unique needs of the mentee (Billings, 2008). Understanding the significance of mentorship within the FWed role is an important factor in being a student-centered FWed.

Self-Reflection

Reflection is a critical component of learning, particularly in higher education (Brookfield, 2015) and experiential learning (Barker et al., 2016; Kolb, 1984). Reflection involves deep thought and intentional scrutiny to analyze one's performance in situations and improve future performance. Described in transformative learning frameworks, experiences play a prominent role in shaping an individual's beliefs, knowledge, and skill (Mezirow, 1997). While designed to be introductory in nature, Level I fieldwork is an essential opportunity for occupational therapy students to purposefully explore and find meaning in their role as an occupational therapy student professional. Research in occupational therapy has indicated that students perceived reflection as a helpful approach in developing goals in professional behaviors (Howard & Barton, 2019). In the fieldwork setting, professional reflection is a vital component in fostering personal growth and

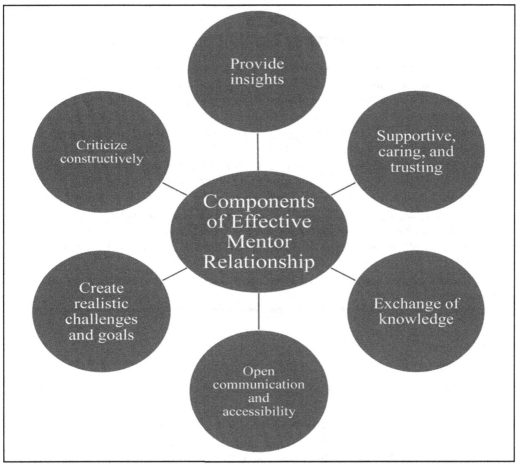

Figure 7-2. Key components of an effective mentorship relationship. (Adapted from Eller, L. S., Lev, E. L., & Feurer, A. [2014]. Key components of an effective mentoring relationship: A qualitative study. *Nurse Education Today, 34*[5], 815-820. https://doi.org/10.1016/j.nedt.2013.07.020 and Rice, J. A., & Perry, F. [2013]. Mentoring and leadership development. In J. A. Rice & F. Perry [Eds.], *Health care leadership excellence: Creating a career of impact* [pp. 57-69]. Health Administration Press.)

strengthening a sense of purpose that emphasizes the importance of using effective and respectful verbal and nonverbal communication with colleagues. It is also a key constituent for active engagement in discussions and meetings and in responding appropriately to team dynamics (Brown et al., 2020). The use of reflection is important to develop critical thinking skills. A systematic review conducted in Australia showed findings that reflection played a prominent role in the development of professional behaviors in occupational therapy and physiotherapy students (Adam et al., 2013). Some occupational therapy students may be required by their academic program to maintain a journal during fieldwork and respond to particular prompts to channel self-reflection in certain areas. A FWed could also design intentional prompts of their own to stimulate reflection during feedback sessions or evaluation with the Level I fieldwork student. Open-ended journal or discussion prompts to stimulate self-reflection can include:

- *What did you observe? What was particular about it? How did you feel about that?*
- *Did you learn anything new or clarify a misconception through this experience?*
- *What struck you differently with this scenario?*
- *What might the client's experience of the session have been?*

Box 7-9
Quick Overview of Work Readiness Scale

The WRS was developed to be used by college-aged students to measure key competencies that employers are looking for. The self-rating tool includes 64 items that present work readiness as a multidimensional phenomenon made up of personal work characteristics, organizational acumen, work competence, and social intelligence (Caballero et al., 2011). The intrinsic aspects of professionalism, particularly emotional intelligence and psychological capital, have been found to predict work readiness (Masole & van Dyk, 2016).

The WRS has been adapted for health care, specifically for nursing students (Walker et al., 2013, 2015) to help identify and provide support for attributes of workplace readiness in health care arenas of practice. The adaptation is referred to as the *Work Readiness Scale–Graduate Nursing* and includes nine new health care relevant items (Walker et al., 2015).

A FWed or occupational therapy faculty member could use the WRS as a starting point to evaluate student's workplace readiness and from there, establish professional development goals.

Additional evaluation strategies on key aspects of professionalism will be discussed later in this chapter.

- *In what capacities did you stretch outside your comfort zone today?*
- *What would you do differently if you could do this again?*
- *How can you apply this learning into a future experience?*

Another approach that may stimulate dialogue and guide self-reflection is the implementation of the *Work Readiness Scale* (WRS; Caballero et al., 2011; Box 7-9).

Role modeling, mentoring, and self-reflection can be useful singular or combined approaches to promote professionalism. Using the desired attributes noted by NACE (2020c) and SHRM (2019), examples of how to nurture and promote student success in these desired workplace readiness areas is depicted in Table 7-6.

EVALUATION OF PROFESSIONALISM DURING LEVEL I FIELDWORK

In addition to specific instruction in professional behaviors, evaluation of student performance is also key. Evaluation in the area of professional behaviors should include summative and formative assessment. *Summative assessment* is considered to be more formal and structured. This may be occurred at formal intervals such as midterm (halfway through the fieldwork experience) and at final, whereas formative assessment is a bit more of an informal diagnostic tool and is ongoing. *Formative assessment* allows the student to receive feedback in an area and then modify their performance. This can take place informally after a patient encounter or during regular feedback meetings. Early identification and intervention (James & Musselman, 2006) on professionalism is important. A Level I fieldwork student should not just learn about performance concerns or problematic issues surrounding professional behaviors during the final evaluation period of the experience. Two examples of formative Level I fieldwork evaluations will be discussed next.

In 2017, the AOTA published *Level I Fieldwork Competency Evaluation for OT and OTA Students* (AOTA, 2017). This tool includes five categories of performance competencies, which include professional behaviors. Within the professional behavior section, there are 12 items. Although this is not a required evaluation for occupational therapy programs to use, the tool

(continued)

TABLE 7-6

HOW TO PROMOTE PROFESSIONALISM AND WORKPLACE READINESS AS A FIELDWORK EDUCATOR

DESIRED ATTRIBUTE OF PROFESSIONALISM	ROLE MODELING	MENTORSHIP	SELF-REFLECTION
Problem-solving skills	"Think aloud" and explicitly verbalize your clinical reasoning to a student	Give your student opportunities to role play and complete problem-solving activities prior to interacting with a patient	To adequately solve a problem, you must first understand it Prompt students to articulate their reasoning and rationale by asking them "Why?" often
Teamwork	Demonstrate respectful, collegial relationship skills with other team members	Offer advice and give feedback on student's ability to work with others	After a team meeting or huddle, have a debrief with your student to call attention to key attributes of interprofessional collaboration and communication that occurred
Work ethic	Model the way Comply to daily tasks with consistent, high-quality work by putting your client first	Help students to find opportunities to imagine themselves as a future occupational therapist	Request that your student journals about what a job well done means as an occupational therapist in your setting. *What does work ethic look like?*
Communication skills (verbal and nonverbal)	Exhibit positive body language during interactions with others and appropriate language in written communications	Give tips and strategies to best communicate with other disciplines For example: *Did you know that genuine smiling while you are talking changes the pitch of your voice to be perceived as more warm and friendly?*	Provide opportunities for the student to have their written documentation peer-reviewed and engage in a discussion about the feedback received

TABLE 7-6 (CONTINUED)

HOW TO PROMOTE PROFESSIONALISM AND WORKPLACE READINESS AS A FIELDWORK EDUCATOR

DESIRED ATTRIBUTE OF PROFESSIONALISM	ROLE MODELING	MENTORSHIP	SELF-REFLECTION
Leadership	Appear confident and speak articulately during team meetings	Encourage your student to attend relevant process improvement team meetings and committees alongside you	Ask your student to seek out and interview a leader in the fieldwork practice setting and write a reflection or journal entry that aligns their findings to a leadership theory
Initiative	Praise your student on completing tasks and responsibilities without being told/directed to	Allow your student autonomy and time to initiate asking questions	Have your student reflect on the following questions: *Am I achieving the goals I have set for myself? What barriers are in my way? What steps can I take to work around the barriers?*
Detail oriented	Provide a checklist or script to help students monitor their effectiveness in obtaining a complete occupational profile during the evaluation process	Guide students to observe how other team members maintain order in their workplace	Have your student reflect on the following questions: *Would I rather focus on the details of work instead of the bigger picture? How do I keep myself organized?*
Dependability/reliability	Model thinking and actions of a team member, not just as an employee	Make yourself accessible and allow open communication so that your student can depend on you to answer questions and seek advice	Share a story with your student about how another team member was more spontaneous than reliable and how it impacted you. Have the student come up with examples for how the coworker could have been more dependable

(continued)

TABLE 7-6 (CONTINUED)

HOW TO PROMOTE PROFESSIONALISM AND WORKPLACE READINESS AS A FIELDWORK EDUCATOR

DESIRED ATTRIBUTE OF PROFESSIONALISM	ROLE MODELING	MENTORSHIP	SELF-REFLECTION
Integrity/respect	Complete documentation for sessions accurately and honestly	Give credit where credit is due and mentor students to take responsibility for their own actions	After a family meeting, have your student debrief the key actions and behaviors of how respect and integrity was displayed during the interaction
Adaptability	Be transparent to the student about how you are modeling adaptability	Be flexible in using teaching strategies that are student-centered to fit the needs of the learner	Have your students journal their successes and challenges on their ability to be flexible in a clinical setting
Self-awareness and insight	Place value in your own teaching identity as an educator	Actively demonstrate self-reflection into your own areas of strength and growth as a FWed Seek out feedback from your student on what is working and what can be improved	Allow students to observe behaviors, self-reflect, and give time to convert observations into actions

Data sources: Cruess, R. L., Cruess, S. R., Boudreau, J. D., Snell, L., & Steinert, Y. (2015). A schematic representation of the professional identity formation and socialization of medical students and residents: A guide for medical educators. *Academic Medicine, 90*(6), 718-725. https://doi.org/10.1097/ACM.0000000000000700; Eller, L. S., Lev, E. L., & Feurer, A. (2014). Key components of an effective mentoring relationship: A qualitative study. *Nurse Education Today, 34*(5), 815-820. https://doi.org/10.1016/j.nedt.2013.07.020; Silva, L. C., Troncon, L. E. A., & Panuncio-Pinto, M. P. (2019). Perceptions of occupational therapy students and clinical tutors on the attributes of a good role model. *Scandinavian Journal of Occupational Therapy, 26*(4), 283-293. https://doi.org/10.1080/11038128.2018.1508495; and Wilkins, E. B. (2020). Facilitating professional identity development in health care education. *New Directions for Teaching and Learning, 2020*(162), 57-69. https://doi.org/10.1002/tl.20391

TABLE 7-7

A REVIEW OF THE AOTA LEVEL I FIELDWORK COMPETENCY EVALUATION AND THE PHILADELPHIA REGION FIELDWORK CONSORTIUM LEVEL I FIELDWORK EVALUATION

AOTA (2017) LEVEL I FIELDWORK COMPETENCY EVALUATION SECTION III: PROFESSIONAL BEHAVIOR	PHILADELPHIA REGION FIELDWORK CONSORTIUM LEVEL I FIELDWORK STUDENT EVALUATION (2ND ED)
Time management skills	Time management skills
Organization	Organization
Engagement in fieldwork experience	Engagement in fieldwork experience
Self-directed learning	Self-directed learning
Reasoning and problem solving	Reasoning and problem solving
Written communication	Written communication
Initiative	Initiative
Observation skills	Observation skills
Participation in the supervisory process	Participation in the supervisory process
Verbal communication and interpersonal skills with patients/clients/staff and caregivers	Verbal communication and interpersonal skills with patients/clients/staff and caregivers
Professional and personal boundaries	Professional and personal boundaries

does clearly indicate that professional behaviors are identified as "mandatory" and "applicable to all practice settings" (AOTA, 2017, p. 1). The AOTA also identifies the purpose of this tool to evaluate skills that "build a foundation" for future success (AOTA, 2017, p. 1). Level I fieldwork is an important developmental milestone ahead of more progressive experiential education, such as Level II fieldwork. Therefore, the Level I FWed is a vital component within an occupational therapy student's professional development. Fieldwork consortiums, which are groups of academic programs and/or AFWCs in a geographic region, have also published evaluation forms to promote standardization in the evaluation of Level I fieldwork. For example, the Philadelphia Region Fieldwork Consortium created the Philadelphia Region Fieldwork Consortium Level I Fieldwork Student Evaluation, Second Edition (PRFC-L1). This tool is endorsed and used by all occupational therapy programs within the consortium, which includes over 10 academic programs. A side-by-side view of these two evaluations is quite similar (Table 7-7).

If a student requires intervention to address aspects of professional behavior, it is important to keep the academic program (via the AFWC) informed:

- Proactively notify the AFWC with any performance concerns.

- Consult with the AFWC regarding any additional resources they may be able to provide to support student success and various teaching approaches.

- Document! Document! Document! Keep objective (not subjective) documentation about the student's performance including performance challenges, as well as performance progress. For example, instead of documenting *"The student has been tardy,"* write *"The student has been tardy 2 times per week for the past 2 weeks."*

- If necessary, use a learning contract or a performance improvement plan to formalize a plan to address the problematic areas, as well as hold the student accountable.

In addition to the FWed providing specific and ongoing evaluation of professional behaviors, incorporating self-assessment by the Level I fieldwork student is also important. Table 7-8 outlines some additional instruments from occupational therapy that a Level I FWed can implement to better understand a fieldwork student's self-assessment of their own professionalism.

SUMMARY

Professional development is an ongoing and complex process, typically initiated in classroom learning, yet emerges as a prominent focus during experiential education. It is through introductory experiential experiences, such as Level I, where occupational therapy students explore and find value and meaning in their role as a representative of the occupational therapy profession and transform from being a student to a future practitioner that is workplace ready. Fieldwork students learn through experiences and observations. Watching others, retaining the information they received, and then imitating the behaviors they observed can have a profound impact on an occupational therapy student's professional development. As occupational therapists, we are trained to adapt our therapeutic approach and use of self to align with the individual needs of our clients in clinical practice. As FWeds, we also need to adapt our teaching approaches and be more mindful of the current needs of the occupational therapy students. Intentional role modeling, guided mentorship, and self-reflection are effective approaches that can help support the development of professionalism in occupational therapy students.

LEARNING ACTIVITIES

Scenario 1: You are a Level I FWed in a school-based setting. You currently have a student that is scheduled to attend fieldwork with you, each Tuesday morning for 10 weeks. It is week 3, and you notice that your fieldwork student's wardrobe is inconsistent with the dress code policy of the site. Furthermore, you have directly observed the student discretely using their smartphone instead of completing self-reflection activities that were assigned.

- As a FWed, what actions should you take to address these unprofessional concerns? Think through an action plan that involves role modeling, mentoring, and self-reflection to address these performance concerns.

Scenario 2: Envision that you are an occupational therapy practitioner who has been practicing for over 10 years and hold a senior position in your department at a skilled nursing facility. You routinely accept Level I fieldwork students, primarily to satisfy your licensure competency requirements. You occasionally arrive late to work in order to pick up your morning coffee but are also frequently observed staying after shift hours to complete documentation requirements. You are well-respected among the novice staff due to your seniority, but you are known to partake in breakroom gossip about other team members and patients.

- Reflect on the consequences of these behaviors and your ability to serve as a role model. Think through an action plan that involves role modeling, mentoring, and self-reflection to address the performance concerns.

TABLE 7-8

TOOLS FOR FIELDWORK STUDENTS TO PROMOTE SELF-EVALUATION OF PROFESSIONALISM ON LEVEL I FIELDWORK

TOOL	DESCRIPTION
AOTA Professional Development Tool (PDT) (AOTA, 2003)	Created by the AOTA, the PDT is used to assess individual learner needs, create a professional development plan, and document professional development activates.
	To facilitate reflection and guide goal setting, the PDT requires the learner to engage in self-assessment.
Philadelphia Region Fieldwork Consortium Level I Fieldwork Student Evaluation, Second Edition (Koenig et al., 2003)	The PRFC-L1 consists of 12 professional behavior items with objective definitions (see Table 7-7).
	FWeds can use this tool to provide formative evaluation of occupational therapy and occupational therapy assistant student professional behaviors during Level I fieldwork, which can improve students' awareness of expected appropriate professional behaviors.
	Students can also be expected to use this tool to self-evaluate their professional behaviors.
Professional Development Evaluation (Randolph, 2003)	The occupational therapy faculty at Saint Louis University help determine students at risk of displaying unsatisfactory professional behaviors in the fieldwork setting. The professional development evaluation evaluates 28 classroom and laboratory behaviors related to six fieldwork and practice goals. Assessment is completed using a 0-to-5 Likert assessment scale.
University of Indianapolis School of Occupational Therapy Student Self-Assessment of Professional Behaviors Tool (Carroll et al., 2002)	The University of Indianapolis School of Occupational Therapy developed this tool to promote self-reflections of professionalism, and it consists of nine professional behaviors that students self-assess. The tool can be used in the classroom or fieldwork setting.
Student Professional Behavior Questionnaire (SBPQ; Yuen et al., 2016)	The SBPQ is a 28-item tool developed by the Occupational Therapy program at the University of Alabama at Birmingham for students to self-assess their behaviors during their academic training. The SPBQ includes three focus area including (1) learning tasks, (2) dealing with others, and (3) dealing with oneself.

REFERENCES

Accreditation Council for Occupational Therapy Education. (2018). *Standards and interpretative guide.* https://www.aota.org/~/media/Corporate/Files/EducationCareers/Accredit/StandardsReview/2018-ACOTE-Standards-Interpretive-Guide.pdf

Adam, K., Peters, S., & Chipchase, L. (2013). Knowledge, skills, and professional behaviours required by occupational therapist and physiotherapist beginning practitioners in work-related practice: A systematic review. *Australian Occupational Therapy Journal, 60*, 76-84. https://doi.org.10.1111/1440-1630.12006

Akiyode, O. (2016). Teaching professionalism: A faculty's perspective. *Currents in Pharmacy Teaching and Learning, 8*(4), 584-586. https://doi.org/10.1016/j.cptl.2016.03.011

American Association of Colleges of Nursing. (2008). *The essentials of baccalaureate education for professional nursing practice.* https://www.aacnnursing.org/Portals/42/Publications/BaccEssentials08.pdf

American Bar Association. (2020). *Model rules of professional conduct.* https://www.americanbar.org/groups/professional_responsibility/publications/model_rules_of_professional_conduct/

American Board of Internal Medicine. (1994). *Project professionalism.* https://medicinainternaucv.files.wordpress.com/2013/02/project-professionalism.pdf

American College of Clinical Pharmacy. (2009). Tenets of professionalism for pharmacy students. *Pharmacotherapy: The Journal of Human Pharmacology and Drug Therapy, 29*(6), 757-759. https://doi.org/10.1592/phco.29.6.757

American Occupational Therapy Association. (1999). *Level I fieldwork.* https://www.aota.org/Education-Careers/Fieldwork/LevelI.aspx

American Occupational Therapy Association. (2003). *Professional development tool.* http://www.aota.org/pdt

American Occupational Therapy Association. (2015). Standards of practice for occupational therapy. *American Journal of Occupational Therapy, 69*(3), 6913410057p1–6913410057p6. https://doi.org/10.5014/ajot.2015.696S06

American Occupational Therapy Association. (2017). *Level I fieldwork competency evaluation for OT and OTA students.* https://www.aota.org/~/media/Corporate/Files/EducationCareers/Educators/Fieldwork/LevelI/Level-I-Fieldwork-Competency-Evaluation-for-ot-and-ota-students.pdf

American Occupational Therapy Association. (2020a). Occupational therapy code of ethics. *American Journal of Occupational Therapy, 74*(Suppl. 3), 1-13. https://doi.org/10.5014/ajot.2020.74S3006

American Occupational Therapy Association. (2020b). Occupational therapy practice framework: Domain and process. *American Journal of Occupational Therapy, 74*(Suppl. 2):7412410010. https://doi.org/10.5014/ajot.2020.74S2001

American Physical Therapy Association. (2019). *Core values for the physical therapist and physical therapist assistant.* https://www.apta.org/apta-and-you/leadership-and-governance/policies/core-values-for-the-physical-therapist-and-physical-therapist-assistant

American Speech-Language Hearing Association. (2000). *Responding to the changing needs of speech-language pathology and audiology students in the 21st century: A briefing paper for academicians, practitioners, employers, and students.* http://www.asha.org/academic/reports/changing.htm#5

American Speech-Language Hearing Association. (2009). *Knowledge and skills acquisition (KASA) summary form for certification in speech-language pathology.* https://www.hhs.k-state.edu/ahs/academics/csd/ugrad/KASASummaryFormSLP.pdf

Babola, K. A., & Peloquin, S. M. (1999). Making a clinical climate in the classroom: An assessment. *American Journal of Occupational Therapy, 53*, 373-380. https://doi.org/10.5014/ajot.53.4.373

Bandura, A. (1977). *Social learning theory.* General Learning Press.

Barker, D. J., Lencucha, J., & Anderson, R. (2016). Kolb's learning cycle as a framework for early fieldwork learning. *World Federation of Occupational Therapists Bulletin, 72*(1), 28-34. https://doi.org/10.1080/14473828.2016.1162373

Barry, M. M. (2012). Practice ready: Are we there yet?. *Boston College Journal of Law & Social Justice, 32*, 247. https://heinonline.org/HOL/LandingPage?handle=hein.journals/bctw32&div=15&id=&page=

Bartz, D., Thompson, K., & Rice, P. (2017). Maximizing the human capital of millennials through supervisors using performance management. *International Journal of Management, Business, and Administration, 20*(1), 1-9.

Billings, D. M. (2008). Developing your career as a nurse educator: The importance of having (or being) a mentor. *The Journal of Continuing Education in Nursing, 39*(11), 490-491. https://doi.org/10.3928/00220124-20081101-09

Blythe, J., Baumann, A., Zeytinoglu, I. U., Denton, M., Akhtar-Danesh, N., Davies, S., & Kolotylo, C. (2008). Nursing generations in the contemporary workplace. *Public Personnel Management, 37*(2), 137-159. https://doi.org/10.1177/009102600803700201

Boyle, C. J., Beardsley, R. S., Morgan, J. A., & de Bittner, M. R. (2007). Professionalism: A determining factor in experiential learning. *American Journal of Pharmaceutical Education, 71*(2), 31. https://doi.org/10.5688/aj710231

Brookfield, S. D. (2015). Critical reflection as doctoral education. *New Directions for Adult and Continuing Education, 2015*(147), 15-23. https://doi.org/10.1002/ace.20138

Brown, T., Yu, M., Hewitt, A. & Etherington, J. (2020). Professionalism as a predictor of fieldwork performance in undergraduate occupational therapy students: An exploratory study. *Occupational Therapy in Health Care, 34*(2), 131-154. https://doi.org/10.1080/07380577.2020.1737896

Caballero, C. L., Walker, A., & Fuller-Tyszkiewicz, M. (2011). The work readiness scale (WRS): Developing a measure to assess work readiness in college graduates. *Journal of Teaching and Learning for Graduate Employability, 2*(2), 41-54. https://doi.org/10.21153/jtlge2011vol2no1art552

Carroll, V. A., Castro, E. R., DeFranco, K. M., Fazio, R. M., Williams, L. L., & Barton, R. A. (2002). Test-retest reliability of a student self-assessment of professional behaviors. *Occupational Therapy in Health Care, 16*(2-3), 1-19. https://doi.org/10.1080/J003v16n02_01

Chien, C. W., Mo, S. Y. C., & Chow, J. (2020). Using an international role-modeling pedagogy to engage first-year occupational therapy students in learning professionalism. *American Journal of Occupational Therapy, 74*(6). https://doi.org/10.5014/ajot.2020.039859

Clarke, C., Martin, M., de Visser, R., & Sadlo, G. (2015). Sustaining professional identity in practice following role-emerging placements: Opportunities and challenges for occupational therapists. *British Journal of Occupational Therapy, 78*(1), 42-50. https://doi.org/10.1177/0308022614561238

Creasy, K. L. (2015). Fostering a culture of professionalism in teacher preparation programs. *Journal of Education and Human Development, 4*(4), 26-31.

Cruess, R. L., Cruess, S. R., Boudreau, J. D., Snell, L., & Steinert, Y. (2015). A schematic representation of the professional identity formation and socialization of medical students and residents: A guide for medical educators. *Academic Medicine, 90*(6), 718-725. https://doi.org/10.1097/ACM.0000000000000700

Cruess, S. R., Cruess, R. L., & Steinert, Y. (2008). Role modelling—making the most of a powerful teaching strategy. *British Medical Journal, 336*(7646), 718-721. https://doi.org/10.1136/bmj.39503.757847.BE

Deepa, S., & Seth, M. (2013). Do soft skills matter? Implications for educators based on recruiters' perspective. *IUP Journal of Soft Skills, 7*(1), 7-20.

DeIuliis, E. D. (2011). Using the occupational profile for student-centered fieldwork education. *OT Practice.*

DeIuliis, E. (2017). Definitions of professionalism. In E. DeIuliis (Ed.), *Professionalism across occupational therapy practice* (pp. 3-42). SLACK Incorporated.

DeIuliis, E. D., & Saylor, E. (2021). Bridging the gap: Three strategies to optimize professional relationships with generation Y and Z. *The Open Journal of Occupational Therapy, 9*(1), 1-13. https://doi.org/10.15453/2168-6408.1748

Deloitte. (2016). *The Deloitte millennial survey 2016 winning over the next generation of leaders.* https://www2.deloitte.com/al/en/pages/about-deloitte/articles/2016-millennialsurvey.html

Eller, L. S., Lev, E. L., & Feurer, A. (2014). Key components of an effective mentoring relationship: A qualitative study. *Nurse Education Today, 34*(5), 815-820. https://doi.org/10.1016/j.nedt.2013.07.020

Fidler, G. S. (1996). Developing a repertoire of professional behaviors. *American Journal of Occupational Therapy, 50*(7), 583-587. https://doi.org/10.5014/ajot.50.7.583

Gravett, L., & Throckmorton, R. (2007). Building a bridge across the generations. In L. Gravett & R. Throckmorton (Eds.), *Bridging the generation gap: How to get radio babies, boomers, gen Xers, and gen Yers to work together and achieve more* (pp. 167-176). Career Press.

Gutman, S. A., McCreedy, P., & Heisler, P. (1998). Student Level II fieldwork failure: Strategies for intervention. *American Journal of Occupational Therapy, 52*(2), 143-149. https://doi.org/10.5014/ajot.52.2.143

Hackenberg, G. R., & Toth-Cohen, S. (2018). Professional behaviors and fieldwork: A curriculum based model in occupational therapy. *Journal of Occupational Therapy Education, 2*(2), 1-14. https://doi.org/10.26681/jote.2018.020203

Hill, W. T, Jr. (2000). White paper on pharmacy student professionalism: What we as pharmacists believe our profession to be determines what it is. *Journal of the American Pharmaceutical Association, 40*(1), 96-102. http://file.cop.ufl.edu/studaff/forms/whitepaper.pdf

Howard, B. S., & Barton, R. (2019). Self-reflection and measurement of professional behavior growth in entry-level occupational therapy students. *Journal of Occupational Therapy Education, 3*(1), 1-20. https://doi.org/10.26681/jote.2019.030103

James, K. L., & Musselman, L. (2006). Commonalities in Level II fieldwork failure. *Occupational Therapy in Health Care, 19*(4), 67-81. https://doi.org/10.1080/J003v19n04_05

Koenig, K., Johnson, C., Morano, C. K., & Ducette, J. P. (2003). Development and validation of a professional behavior assessment. *Journal of Allied Health, 32*(2), 86-91.

Kolb, D. A. (1984). *Experiential learning: Experience as a source of learning and development.* Prentice-Hall.

Ludmerer, K. M. (1999). Instilling professionalism in medical education. *Journal of American Medical Association, 282*(9), 881-882. https://doi.org/10.1001/jama.282.9.881

Masole, L., & van Dyk, G. (2016). Factors influencing work readiness of graduates: An exploratory study. *Journal of Psychology in Africa, 26*(1), 70–73. https://doi.org/10.1080/14330237.2015.1101284

Mattila, A. (2019). Role-emerging fieldwork at community agencies: An exploration of self-efficacy, personal transformation, and professional growth. *American Journal of Occupational Therapy, 73*(Suppl. 1). https://doi.org/10.5014/ajot.2019.73S1-PO8024

McCrindle, M., & Fell, A. (2020). *Understanding generation alpha.* https://generationalpha.com/wp-content/uploads/2020/02/Understanding-Generation-Alpha-McCrindle.pdf

McDonald, G., Jackson, D., Wilkes, L., & Vickers, M. H. (2013). Personal resilience in nurses and midwives: Effects of a work-based educational intervention. *Contemporary Nurse, 45*(1), 134-143. https://doi.org/10.5172/conu.2013.45.1.134

Mezirow, J. (1997). Transformative learning: Theory to practice. *New Directions for Adult and Continuing Education, 74*, 5-12.

Missen, K., McKenna, L., Beauchamp, A., & Larkins, J. (2016). Qualified nurses' rate new nursing graduates as lacking skills in key clinical areas. *Journal of Clinical Nursing, 25*(15-16), 2134-2143. https://doi.org/10.1111/jocn.13316

Mitchell, M. M., & Kampfe, C. M. (1990). Coping strategies used by occupational therapy students during fieldwork: An exploratory study. *American Journal of Occupational Therapy, 44*(6), 543-550. https://doi.org/10.5014/ajot.44.6.543

Mohammadi, E., Shahsavari, H., Mirzazadeh, A., Sophrabpour, A. A., & Hejri, S. M. (2020). Improving role modeling in clinical teachers: A narrative literature review. *Journal of Advances in Medical Education & Professionalism, 8*(1), 1-9. https://doi.org/10.30476/jamp.2019.74929

Murphy, J. E. (2015). Practice-readiness of U.S. pharmacy graduates to provide direct patient care. *Pharmacotherapy: The Journal of Human Pharmacology and Drug Therapy, 35*(12), 1091-1095. https://doi.org/10.1002/phar.1667

National Association of Colleges and Employers. (2020a). *What is career readiness?* https://www.naceweb.org/career-readiness/competencies/career-readiness-defined/

National Association of Colleges and Employers. (2020b). *Job outlook 2020.* https://www.vidteamcc.com/stadistics/2020-nace-job-outlook%20(1).pdf

National Association of Colleges and Employers. (2020c). *Key attributes employers want to see on students' resumes.* https://www.naceweb.org/talent-acquisition/candidate-selection/key-attributes-employers-want-to-see-on-students-resumes/

National Council for Accreditation of Teacher Education. (2008). *Professional standards for the accreditation of teacher preparation institutions.* http://www.ncate.org/~/media/Files/caep/accreditation-resources/ncate-standards-2008.pdf?la=en

Noble, C., Coombes, I., Shaw, P. N., Nissen, L. M., & Clavarino, A. (2014). Becoming a pharmacist: The role of curriculum in professional identity formation. *Pharmacy Practice, 12*(1), 380. https://doi.org/10.4321/s1886-36552014000100007

O'Brien, M., Troy, K., & Kirkpatrick, J. (2020). The allied health work readiness study: Identifying personal characteristics signaling work readiness in allied health students. *Internet Journal of Allied Health Sciences and Practice, 18*(1), 5.

Pew Research Center. (2019). *Defining generations: Where millennials end and generation z begins.* https://www.pewresearch.org/fact-tank/2019/01/17/where-millennials-end-and-generation-z-begins/

Randolph, D. S. (2003). Evaluating the professional behaviors of entry-level occupational therapy students. *Journal of Allied Health, 32*(2), 116-121

Rice, J. A., & Perry, F. (2013). Mentoring and leadership development. In J. A. Rice & F. Perry (Eds.), *Health care leadership excellence: Creating a career of impact* (pp. 57-69). Health Administration Press.

Sands, M. (1995). Readying occupational therapy assistant students for Level II fieldwork: Beyond academics to personal behaviors and attitudes. *American Journal of Occupational Therapy, 49*(2), 150-152. https://doi.org/10.5014/ajot.49.2.150

Schafheutle, E. I., Hassell, K., Ashcroft, D. M., Hall, J., & Harrison, S. (2012). How do pharmacy students learn professionalism? *International Journal of Pharmacy Practice, 20*(2), 118-128. https://doi.org/10.1111/j.2042-7174.2011.00166.x

Scheerer, C. R. (2003). Perceptions of effective professional behavior feedback: Occupational therapy student voices. *American Journal of Occupational Therapy, 57*(2), 205-214. https://doi.org/10.5014/ajot.57.2.205

Silva, L. C., Troncon, L. E. A. & Panuncio-Pinto, M. P. (2019). Perceptions of occupational therapy students and clinical tutors on the attributes of a good role model. *Scandinavian Journal of Occupational Therapy, 26*(4), 283–293. https://doi.org/10.1080/11038128.2018.1508495

Skodova, Z., Lajciakova, P., & Banovcinova, L. (2017). Burnout syndrome among health care students: The role of Type D personality. *Western Journal of Nursing Research, 39*(3), 416-429. https://doi.org/10.1177/0193945916658884

Society for Human Resource Management. (2019). *The global skills shortage: Bridging the talent gap with education, training and sourcing.* https://www.shrm.org/hr-today/trends-and-forecasting/research-and-surveys/Documents/SHRM%20Skills%20Gap%202019.pdf

Steven, A., Oxley, J., & Fleming, W. G. (2008). Mentoring for NHS doctors: Perceived benefits across the personal–professional interface. *Journal of the Royal Society of Medicine, 101*(11), 552-557. https://doi.org/10.1258/jrsm.2008.080153

Stewart, C., Marciniec, S., Lawrence, D., & Joyner-McGraw, L. (2020). Thinkuibator approach to solving the soft skills gap. *American Journal of Management, 20*(2), 78-89.

Sullivan, T. M., & Thiessen, A. K. (2015). Occupational therapy students' perspectives of professionalism: An exploratory study. *The Open Journal of Occupational Therapy, 3*(4), 9. https://doi.org/10.15453/ 2168-6408.115

Tichenor, M., & Tichenor, J. (2009). Comparing teacher and administrator perspectives on multiple dimensions of teacher professionalism. *SRATE Journal, 18*(2), 9-18.

Tickle-Degnen, L. (1998). Working well with others: The prediction of students' clinical performance. *American Journal of Occupational Therapy, 52*(2), 133-142. https://doi.org/10.5014/ajot.52.2.133

van der Wal, Z. (2017). Managing the new work (force). In Z. van der Wal (Ed.), *The 21st century public manager: Challenges, people and strategies* (pp. 112-130). Macmillan International Higher Education.

Walker, A., Storey, K. M., Costa, B. M., & Leung, R. K. (2015). Refinement and validation of the Work Readiness Scale for graduate nurses. *Nursing Outlook, 63*(6), P632-P638. https://doi.org/10.1016/j.outlook.2015.06.001

Walker, A., Yong, M., Pang, L., Fullarton, C., Costa, B., & Dunning, A. M. T. (2013). Work readiness of graduate health professionals. *Nurse Education Today, 33*(2), 116-122. https://doi.org/10.1016/j.nedt.2012.01.007

Weston, M. (2001). Coaching generations in the workplace. *Nursing Administration Quarterly, 25*(2), 11-21. https://doi.org/10.1097/00006216-200101000-00005

Wilkins, E. B. (2020). Facilitating professional identity development in health care education. *New Directions for Teaching and Learning, 2020*(162), 57-69. https://doi.org/10.1002/tl.20391

Yuen, H. K., Azuero, A., Lackey, K. W., Brown, N. S., & Shrestha, S. (2016). Construct validity test of evaluation tool for professional behaviors of entry-level occupational therapy students in the United States. *Journal of Educational Evaluation for Health Professions, 13*(22), 1-6. https://doi.org/10.3352/jeehp.2016.13.22

8

Developing the Level I
Fieldwork Learning Plan

Marsena W. Devoto, MSOT, OTD, OTR/L

Considering the already-described aspects of fieldwork, this chapter will address the practical application of developing and implementing an effective Level I fieldwork plan. Often there are false assumptions about Level I fieldwork experiences that impact the quality of the student learning experience. One example is that some fieldwork educators (FWeds) believe that Level I fieldwork is observation only. This is an incorrect assumption. Many students have already observed occupational therapists prior to attending occupational therapy/occupational therapy assistant schools. Other FWeds embrace the *go with the flow* perspective. In this example, the educator has the student follow them but does not scaffold the student in their learning. Another example may be someone who takes the approach that the student is a *volunteer*. In this model, the student may end up organizing closets, cleaning the treatment space, etc. and is not learning the occupational therapy process. They are not exploring or learning the role of occupational therapy in that setting—they are just performing volunteer work. Another example may be the *extra pair of hands* model, where the student may be treated more like a tech or aide vs. as a learning/growing occupational therapy practitioner.

According to the Accreditation Council for Occupational Therapy Education (ACOTE, 2018) standards, Level I fieldwork is not meant to be observation only. Level I fieldwork is an active process where the student is engaged in their learning. The purpose of Level I fieldwork experiences is to link academic coursework with occupational therapy practice in a real world scenario. The Level I fieldwork experience follows the learning theories and sequence of the academic program

Hanson, D., & DeIuliis, E. D. (Eds.).
Fieldwork Educator's Guide to Level I Fieldwork (pp. 213-265).
© 2023 Taylor and Francis Group.

and connects with what the student is learning in class/labs to practice. In addition, the Level I fieldwork experience should address the student's individual learning needs and professional growth. This chapter aims to provide a roadmap for FWeds and academic fieldwork coordinators (AFWCs) to develop a learning plan for Level I fieldwork students. The hope is to enable the FWed and AFWC to create a manageable and effective Level I experience that (1) meets the needs of the ACOTE, (2) is consistent with the design of the academic curriculum, (3) corresponds to the learning objectives and learning assessment of the fieldwork coursework, and (4) is reflective of the practice experience of the FWed and the learning experiences available at the site.

LEARNING OBJECTIVES

By the end of reading this chapter and completing the learning activities, the reader should be able to:

1. Understand the relationship between ACOTE standards and Level I fieldwork expectations.

2. Appreciate the impact of the academic curriculum on the development of student learning experiences for Level I fieldwork.

3. Understand how the academic learning objectives and student assessment associated with fieldwork coursework influence the design of site-specific student learning activities.

4. Reflect on current practice experience and learning experiences available at the fieldwork site when developing site-specific learning activities.

5. Develop a sequential learning plan for the Level I fieldwork experience.

A ROADMAP FOR THE LEVEL I FIELDWORK LEARNING PLAN

There are multiple variables that need to be considered when developing a fieldwork learning plan. Level I fieldwork experiences are rooted in the accreditation standards for occupational therapy education maintained by the ACOTE. The mission and curriculum of the academic program are developed to align with ACOTE standards but are unique for each program. The philosophy of the curriculum includes learning theories (how people learn) and areas of emphasis that influence the focus and sequence of Level I learning experiences. Didactic and fieldwork coursework must reflect the academic curriculum, and this, in turn, must align with the ACOTE standards. Figure 8-1 provides a broad overview of the variables to consider when developing a learning plan for students at a site.

In this chapter, each consideration for the development of Level I fieldwork learning experiences will be explored including (1) the influence of ACOTE standards on curriculum design, (2) the impact of curriculum design on selection of Level I fieldwork sites and fieldwork course learning objectives, (3) alignment of fieldwork course objectives with site learning opportunities, and (4) developing the learning plan, which includes sequencing of student learning opportunities to accomplish learning objectives. The expected outcome is that the Level I FWed will have the resources needed to develop a site-specific sequential learning plan for Level I fieldwork students.

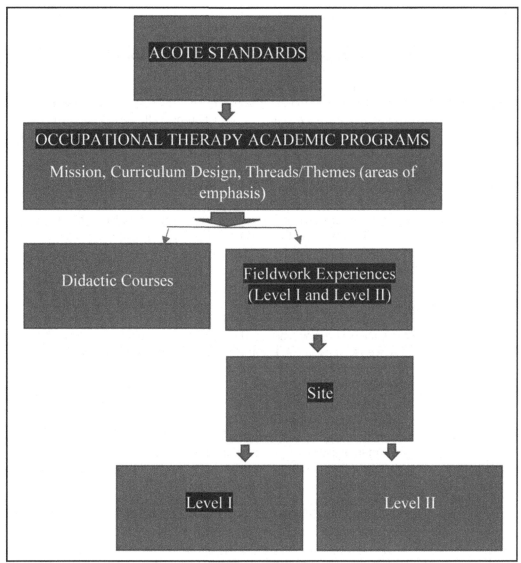

Figure 8-1. Overview of the pathway to developing the learning plan.

THE INFLUENCE OF ACOTE STANDARDS ON CURRICULUM DESIGN

As a FWed, it is important to have a basic understanding of the ACOTE (2018) standards in order to gain perspective on the format, expectations, and overall curricular picture of fieldwork. The main overarching emphasis of the profession and the expected outcome of every curriculum is knowledge about human occupation and the ability to intervene in occupational challenges of everyday life (American Occupational Therapy Association [AOTA], 2017b; Hooper et al., 2018). In the ACOTE standards, fieldwork is viewed as an extension of the academic program curriculum. This means that fieldwork is considered a class within the program's curriculum. The FWed is the instructor, and the fieldwork site is the classroom. Thus, the requirements in the classroom (i.e., the site) and of the instructor (i.e., the FWed) are the same as all other classes or courses. Since fieldwork is regarded as a course in the curriculum, the instructor needs to be qualified to

TABLE 8-1

ACOTE (2018) STANDARDS AND LEVEL I FIELDWORK

Contractual relationship	A documented contract (or affiliation agreement) protects all parties involved in the relationship: clients, students, the site, and the academic institution. It also creates an official relationship with the fieldwork site as an arm of the occupational therapy program.
Fieldwork is part of the curriculum	Fieldwork is part of the curriculum, and thus, the fieldwork site is an extension of the classroom. The importance of developing a strong connection/link between the occupational therapy/occupational therapy assistant academic program and the fieldwork site is stressed in the ACOTE standards. Just as a faculty member needs to understand how their course fits within the curriculum, the FWed needs to have a general understanding of the course sequences and other didactic classes being taught.
The value of teaching and learning	The value of teaching and learning in the classroom, as well as in fieldwork experiences, is evident throughout the ACOTE standards. The FWed has the unique and valuable role of understanding practical application of occupational therapy practice. The students learn about theory and ideal practice. However, the role of the FWed is to teach and model patient/ practitioner interaction/relationships and help students learn to apply theory to practice.
Communication of course expectations and student progress	The communication of expectations and measuring progress in the classroom and in fieldwork is a part of learning and practice. The ACOTE standards require that expectations and student progress be documented via written objectives and evaluation forms. The same forms are not expected to be used by all occupational therapy/occupational therapy assistant programs. The majority of programs look at professional behaviors and possibly some basic technical skills. A *Level I Fieldwork Competency Evaluation for OT and OTA Students* has been designed to assess performance skills that build a foundation for Level II fieldwork (AOTA, 2017). However, this form is not consistently used across all occupational therapy or occupational therapy assistant programs.
Consideration of psychosocial/ mental health factors	The importance of considering psychosocial/mental health factors in every occupational therapy practice setting is reflected in the ACOTE standards. Occupational therapists/occupational therapy assistants consider the whole person—their roles, support system, and environment—when working with individuals. Practitioners consider psychosocial, emotional, and mental health factors when working with clients. However, practitioners do not always discuss this aspect of their reasoning out loud with students. This standard ensures these factors are emphasized in student experiences.

(*continued*)

TABLE 8-1 (CONTINUED)	
ACOTE (2018) STANDARDS AND LEVEL I FIELDWORK	
AFWC and FWed as co-teachers in facilitating student learning	The AFWC is the liaison between the didactic part of the curriculum and the fieldwork sites and experiences. The AFWC communicates the curriculum and collaborates with the FWed on expectations, objectives, and the fieldwork experience as a whole and is responsible to ensure that ACOTE standards related to Level I fieldwork are met.

Adapted from Accreditation Council for Occupational Therapy Education. (2018). *2018 Accreditation Council for Occupational Therapy Education standards and interpretive guide*. https://acoteonline.org/wp-content/uploads/2020/10/2018-ACOTE-Standards.pdf

teach and demonstrate effectiveness in teaching. Just as with other courses, the instructor must understand how their course fits within the curriculum as a whole. A critical aspect of supporting student learning is the ability to intentionally make connections for students between their university learning and its application in the practice context (Dancza et al., 2021). In order to do this, the FWed must understand something about what the student is learning in the curriculum. The instructor must provide documentation of student's progress and learning. Lastly, ACOTE emphasizes the importance of considering psychosocial/mental health factors in every occupational therapy setting. See Table 8-1 for an overview of the influence of ACOTE (2018) standards on Level I fieldwork.

The AFWC is the primary link to the academic program curriculum. They have a good understanding of the curriculum and sequence of the academic program and can communicate this to the FWed (Hanson et al., 2016; Stutz-Tanenbaum et al., 2015). The FWed is the link to occupational therapy practice. This is a two-way relationship where the AFWC and FWed collaborate to develop experiences that support the student's learning within occupational therapy practice. In fact, AFWCs have reported that they find significant professional reward in the opportunities that they have for collaboration and education with FWeds (Stutz-Tanenbaum et al., 2017). To facilitate the collaboration process, FWeds may use the prompts in Tables 8-2 through 8-5 to reflect on the relationship of specific ACOTE standards to their Level I fieldwork context. These questions may facilitate an understanding of the relationship between the academic institute and the fieldwork site. Furthermore, the questions guide the FWed in reflecting on their own practice.

The discussion of ACOTE standards and how they influence Level I fieldwork is a starting place for FWeds. It provides the educator with the underlying academic education foundation of the experiences they will create. This builds a bridge between the educator's practice and the academic program. It provides a common platform from which to communicate with the AFWC. An overview of reflection questions regarding ACOTE standards as they relate to Level I fieldwork is provided in Appendix A.

TABLE 8-2
ACOTE STANDARD C.1.1

STANDARD C.1.1	REFLECTIVE QUESTIONS FOR THE FIELDWORK EDUCATOR	PROMPTS FOR INITIATING DIALOGUE WITH ACADEMIC PROGRAM/AFWC
"Ensure that the fieldwork program reflects the sequence and scope of content in the curriculum design, in collaboration with faculty, so that fieldwork experiences in traditional, nontraditional, and emerging settings strengthen the ties between didactic and fieldwork education" (ACOTE, 2018, C.1.1).	1. Do I know the academic institution's program sequence and scope of content in the curriculum design? (i.e., What courses do the student's take throughout the occupational therapy program? Where in the program do they take pediatrics, mental health, and adult related courses?) *The syllabus for the Level I fieldwork course is a great help here.* 2. Does my site's mission and roles match up with the academic program mission? 3. Is my site/program able to meet the academic program's fieldwork objectives? 4. Can my site/program measure the student's progress with the fieldwork evaluation form the school/academic institute is using?	1. Tell me about your program. 2. Does your program's mission have a specific focus? 3. Tell me about your intervention classes. 4. What is the sequence of your classes? 5. What are your goals for each of your Level I fieldwork experiences? 6. What do you use to measure student progress for Level I fieldwork?

Adapted from Accreditation Council for Occupational Therapy Education. (2018). *2018 Accreditation Council for Occupational Therapy Education standards and interpretive guide.* https://acoteonline.org/wp-content/uploads/2020/10/2018-ACOTE-Standards.pdf

TABLE 8-3
ACOTE STANDARD C.1.3

STANDARD C.1.3	REFLECTIVE QUESTIONS FOR THE FIELDWORK EDUCATOR	PROMPTS FOR INITIATING DIALOGUE WITH ACADEMIC PROGRAM/AFWC
"Document that academic and FWeds agree on established fieldwork objectives prior to the start of the fieldwork experience and communicate with the student and FWed about progress and performance throughout the fieldwork experience. Ensure that fieldwork objectives for all experiences include a psychosocial objective" (ACOTE, 2018, C.1.3).	1. Have I communicated and collaborated with the academic institute and AFWC regarding my own and the site's expectations and roles? 2. Have I collaborated with the AFWC and reached agreement regarding the objectives provided? 3. Am I communicating with my AFWC on my student's progress and performance throughout the fieldwork? 4. How am I incorporating psychosocial/mental health components in my practice?	1. Tell me about your expectations for your Level I students. 2. How do you envision my site in meeting these expectations? 3. What are your fieldwork objectives? 4. Can we collaborate on developing objectives specific to my site? 5. How would you like me to communicate your student's progress (via email? weekly?)? 6. Do you use a form to help students tease out their reasoning? 7. Do you use a specific form or document to help guide students in considering psychosocial/mental health factors in treatment?

Adapted from Accreditation Council for Occupational Therapy Education. (2018). *2018 Accreditation Council for Occupational Therapy Education standards and interpretive guide.* https://acoteonline.org/wp-content/uploads/2020/10/2018-ACOTE-Standards.pdf

TABLE 8-4

ACOTE STANDARD C.1.7

STANDARD C.1.7	REFLECTIVE QUESTIONS FOR THE FIELDWORK EDUCATOR	PROMPTS FOR INITIATING DIALOGUE WITH ACADEMIC PROGRAM/AFWC
"At least one fieldwork experience (either Level I or Level II) must address practice in behavioral health or psychological and social factors influencing engagement in occupation" (ACOTE, 2018, C.1.7).	1. How do I address/ take into consideration how behavioral health, psychological, and social factors affect a person's function and participation in occupations? 2. What does this look like at my site? 3. What factors do I consider when treating patients? 4. How does this influence my practice? 5. How do I teach my student about these factors?	1. Is there an objective related to psychosocial/ mental health factors in the fieldwork I am supervising? 2. How are you measuring the student performance with this objective? 3. How can I support your expectations of this objective at my site?

Adapted from Accreditation Council for Occupational Therapy Education. (2018). *2018 Accreditation Council for Occupational Therapy Education standards and interpretive guide.* https://acoteonline.org/wp-content/uploads/2020/10/2018-ACOTE-Standards.pdf

THE ACADEMIC PROGRAM CURRICULUM DESIGN AND LEVEL I FIELDWORK

All occupational therapy/occupational therapy assistant programs have the same ultimate goal. They all want to develop entry-level generalist occupational therapy and occupational therapy assistant practitioners. Each academic program has their own unique curriculum, philosophy, and proposed sequence of learning, which is influenced by both external and internal factors, based on learning theories, the program's view of progression, and pragmatic elements (AOTA, 2009). It is helpful to understand the academic program sequence in order to see how the FWed's practice supports the courses students are taking.

For example, the curriculum design for some academic programs may follow a human developmental model. In this model, the courses follow the different life stages (pediatrics, adult, and older adult). Another program may divide up their intervention courses in categories of psychosocial, physical disabilities, and wellness across the lifespan. Yet another program may follow the progression of the occupational therapy process (assessment/evaluation, intervention, discharge planning). The focus of the Level I fieldwork is consistent with the sequence of the coursework

TABLE 8-5
ACOTE STANDARD C.1.9

STANDARD C.1.9	REFLECTIVE QUESTIONS FOR THE FIELDWORK EDUCATOR	PROMPTS FOR INITIATING DIALOGUE WITH ACADEMIC PROGRAM/AFWC
"Document that Level I fieldwork is provided to students and is not substituted for any part of the Level II fieldwork. Ensure that Level I fieldwork enriches didactic coursework through directed observation and participation in selected aspects of the occupational therapy process and includes mechanisms for formal evaluation of student performance. The program must have clearly documented student learning objectives expected of the Level I fieldwork. Level I fieldwork may be met through one or more of the following instructional methods: • Simulated environments • Standardized patients • Faculty practice • Faculty-led site visits Supervision by a FWed in a practice environment All Level I fieldwork must be comparable in rigor" (ACOTE, 2018, C.1.9).	1. Am I substituting or overlapping the Level I and II experiences I provide to students? 2. What does the occupational therapy process look like at my site? 3. Am I showing my student what the occupational therapy process looks like at my site? 4. Do I have an evaluation form to assess my student's performance (this is usually provided by the academic institute)? 5. Does the occupational therapy Level I fieldwork experience at my site fall under one of these instructional methods? • Simulated environments • Standardized patients • Faculty practice* • Faculty-led site visits • Supervision by a FWed in a practice environment	1. What evaluations do you use for your Level I fieldwork experiences? 2. Are there specific expectations/tasks you would like your student to perform in the experience? 3. What are some different ways I can accomplish fieldwork at my site? 4. What are the different supervision models other than one-on-one supervision? 5. Am I allowed to take more than one student at a time?

(continued)

TABLE 8-5 (CONTINUED)
ACOTE Standard C.1.9

STANDARD C.1.9	REFLECTIVE QUESTIONS FOR THE FIELDWORK EDUCATOR	PROMPTS FOR INITIATING DIALOGUE WITH ACADEMIC PROGRAM/AFWC
	6. Are there different ways to provide fieldwork experiences at my site? (Brainstorm with your coworkers and the AFWC) a. Can I set up a group experience for several students at the same time where they observe, process, and practice occupational therapy with patients or simulated with each other? b. Can I create an experience where a faculty member comes onsite and guides the student in an experience?	

*Faculty-led practice may be a faculty run clinic where students participate in evaluation and treatment of clients alongside faculty. Some of these practices are probono.

Adapted from Accreditation Council for Occupational Therapy Education. (2018). *2018 Accreditation Council for Occupational Therapy Education standards and interpretive guide.* https://acoteonline.org/wp-content/uploads/2020/10/2018-ACOTE-Standards.pdf

(AOTA Commission on Education, 1999). For example, in the first Level I fieldwork experience, students may focus on learning the process of assessment and interpretation. Then, in the second Level I fieldwork, they may focus on intervention and applying information from assessment and implementing the results into developing and practicing treatment. The third Level I fieldwork in the sequence may focus on having the students participate in the complete occupational therapy process (evaluate, treat, document, reevaluate, and discharge). Other curriculums may place a huge focus on community-based practice. When an academic program curriculum focuses on community, a sequence of Level I fieldwork may focus on serving their local community and individuals. The first Level I may start with the students being paired with a community partner with a disability. In this scenario, the student gets to know the individual as a person first vs. learning about the condition first. They meet weekly for several weeks and talk about the community partner's perspective of navigating their world. The second Level I experience in this curriculum may have the students participate in a probono clinic with occupational therapy supervisors. The third Level I experience may have the student go into the community setting and complete a needs assessment on the organization, develop a program, and implement the program. Cumulatively, these level fieldwork experiences provide students with skills needed to support individuals in the community.

It is up to the Level I FWed to determine whether they are able to provide learning experiences that meet the objectives of the academic institution (AOTA Commission on Education, 1999). Knowing the academic program sequence of courses will help the FWed (or even a new AFWC) discern whether the learning experiences available at the site can support the focus of the curriculum and the coursework that is emphasized at the time of the Level I fieldwork placement. Tables 8-6 through 8-9 provide examples of alignment and lack of alignment between curriculum course sequences and fieldwork sites.

Fieldwork is a learning experience embedded in the curriculum, and fieldwork coursework objectives influence the learning that occurs during fieldwork. As mentioned earlier in this chapter, fieldwork is considered a class, and the FWed is considered the instructor. ACOTE (2018) requires evidence of the process of learning in all courses. ACOTE requires academic programs to explain and document how, why, and what the student learns. Student learning is a process of growth and development. Therefore, FWeds (instructors) use learning objectives to guide them in teaching the course. These objectives are based on the emphasis of the course and identifies what the student needs to do and accomplish in order to demonstrate what they have learned in the course. The course must align with the curriculum. Thus, the objectives for the course support the big picture of the curriculum.

ACOTE emphasizes the value of fieldwork being a course vs. an observation experience. ACOTE (2018) requires that expectations and student progress be documented via written objectives and evaluation forms. As a course, fieldwork has academic program learning objectives. Each occupational therapy/occupational therapy assistant academic program is required to develop fieldwork learning objectives. As mentioned in Chapter 3, the academic program objectives are rooted in the learning theories the program has adopted for their curriculum. Thus, academic programs may have different learning objectives due to their own philosophy and sequence of courses. However, the fieldwork learning objectives are similar because all occupational therapy/occupational therapy assistants are working toward the same goal of developing entry-level practitioners (Box 8-1).

Embedded in these objectives is the emphasis the occupational therapy program has placed on excellence in occupational therapy practice. The program fieldwork course Level I objectives show that the student needs to be able to understand how occupational therapy practice occurs in the setting in which the student is placed. Table 8-10 displays several examples of how learning experiences in different settings may apply to the previously mentioned objective.

Examples of how a student may identify and discuss the rationale for potential occupational therapy assessments relevant to the setting are provided in Table 8-11.

TABLE 8-6

EXAMPLE ONE OF ALIGNING FIELDWORK EXPERIENCE WITH CURRICULUM

OCCUPATIONAL THERAPY CURRICULUM EMPHASIS	TYPE OF SITE	CAN THE SITE PROVIDE AN EXPERIENCE THAT ALIGNS WITH THE ACADEMIC PROGRAM?	HOW DOES THE FIELDWORK EXPERIENCE SUPPORT THE ACADEMIC PROGRAM AND SEQUENCE?
Program emphasis: 1. Evidence-based practice 2. Professionalism and occupational across the lifespan Semester focus: 1. Pediatric assessment, intervention, and practice	General outpatient pediatric facility	Yes	Site matches with semester (pediatrics) and program emphasis (evidence-based practice and professionalism). Occupational therapists practicing in this setting perform assessment/intervention, which matches semester emphasis and program emphasis.
	Skilled nursing facility	No	It does not align with developmental stage (pediatrics). *However, if the semester focus included a course on assessment and evaluation throughout the lifespan or a course in adult/older adult conditions, a skilled nursing facility might support the student's learning sequence.
	Pediatric daycare	Yes	Site matches with semester emphasis (pediatrics). Experience may include occupational therapy/occupational therapy assistant students working with typical developing children in order to gain context of age norms.

TABLE 8-7

EXAMPLE TWO OF ALIGNING FIELDWORK EXPERIENCE WITH CURRICULUM

OCCUPATIONAL THERAPY CURRICULUM EMPHASIS	TYPE OF SITE	CAN THE SITE PROVIDE AN EXPERIENCE THAT ALIGNS WITH THE ACADEMIC PROGRAM?	HOW DOES THE FIELDWORK EXPERIENCE SUPPORT THE ACADEMIC PROGRAM AND SEQUENCE?
Program emphasis: 1. Excellence and innovation 2. Addressing the needs of the underserved in their local community	Adolescent brain injury camp	Yes	Experience reinforces learning in the neuroscience applications and conditions. Students may work alongside campers to better understand their level of function, abilities, and challenges.
Semester emphasis: 1. Mental health and psychosocial evaluation, intervention, and documentation 2. Neuroscience applications and adult conditions	Inpatient psychiatric facility with no occupational therapy	Yes	Experience compliments student learning about adults with psychiatric conditions. Experience may include students working alongside an activity therapist or social worker. The students may observe and run groups and activities. Experience allows students to gain context of challenges and abilities for individuals in this population.

TABLE 8-8

EXAMPLE THREE OF ALIGNING FIELDWORK EXPERIENCE WITH CURRICULUM

OCCUPATIONAL THERAPY CURRICULUM EMPHASIS	TYPE OF SITE	CAN THE SITE PROVIDE AN EXPERIENCE THAT ALIGNS WITH THE ACADEMIC PROGRAM?	HOW DOES THE FIELDWORK EXPERIENCE SUPPORT THE ACADEMIC PROGRAM AND SEQUENCE?
Program emphasis: 1. Occupation and practice Semester emphasis:	Adolescent psychiatric treatment program with occupational therapists on staff	No	Does not match population or types of conditions/types of intervention assessment of the semester.
1. Adult and older physical/cognitive conditions (assessment, intervention, and documentation) 2. Wellness in the aging population	Retirement communities	Yes	Matches population and courses (wellness in the aging population). Student may work with the residents to explore strategies to support older adults again in place.

TABLE 8-9

EXAMPLE FOUR OF ALIGNING FIELDWORK EXPERIENCE WITH CURRICULUM

OCCUPATIONAL THERAPY CURRICULUM EMPHASIS	TYPE OF SITE	CAN THE SITE PROVIDE AN EXPERIENCE THAT ALIGNS WITH THE ACADEMIC PROGRAM?	HOW DOES THE FIELDWORK EXPERIENCE SUPPORT THE ACADEMIC PROGRAM AND SEQUENCE?
Program emphasis: 1. Occupation and practice Semester emphasis:	Adult acute care	Yes	Matches assessment course. Student may observe and practice basic parts of assessments.
1. Pediatrics (assessment, intervention, and documentation) 2. Assessment across the lifespan	Private pediatric school	Yes	Matches population discussed during the semester. Students could screen preschool children for prehension patterns and recommend activities to facilitate growth in these areas.

Box 8-1

SAMPLE OCCUPATIONAL THERAPY/ OCCUPATIONAL THERAPY ASSISTANT PROGRAM MISSION AND LEVEL I FIELDWORK OBJECTIVES

Mission: "To produce graduates who excel in professional practice, scientific inquiry, and advocacy" (Brenau University College of Health Sciences, 2020, p. 13).

The occupational therapy program's Level I fieldwork objectives reflect excellence in practice. The following objectives demonstrate components needed to develop excellence in practice (evaluation and treatment of individuals).

Level I Fieldwork Program Objectives:

1. "Describe to relevant stakeholders occupation and discuss how it relates to occupational therapy/occupational therapy assistant practice and its relationship to health and well-being" (Devoto, 2020, p. 2).

2. "Discuss potential occupational therapy assessments appropriate to the setting and/ or population (including relevant social, cultural, and economic factors that my impact client outcomes) with direction from FWed" (Devoto, 2020, p. 2).

TABLE 8-10

EXAMPLE ONE OF LEARNING EXPERIENCES ACROSS SETTINGS

Academic Program Level I Fieldwork Objective #1

"Describe to relevant stakeholders occupation and discuss how it relates to occupational therapy/occupational therapy assistant practice and its relationship to health and well-being" (Devoto, 2020, p. 2).

FIELDWORK SETTING	LEARNING EXPERIENCE BASED ON OBJECTIVE
School system: The roles for occupational therapy in this setting may be direct and indirect services including consultation with the teacher, as well as working individually with the children.	In this setting, the student might be asked to explain the role of occupational therapy to a new teacher or to a parent in an individualized education program meeting.
Outpatient adult rehabilitation: The role of occupational therapy is focused on provision of direct care to clients and education of families.	In this setting, the student might be asked to explain the role of occupational therapy to a caregiver or to a student in a different discipline.
Community setting: The role may be collaborative, where the occupational therapist works with the other employees to help develop activities that foster independence of consumers.	In this setting, the student might be asked to explain to other employees, students (from a different discipline), or volunteers the role of occupational therapy in this setting.

TABLE 8-11

EXAMPLE TWO OF LEARNING EXPERIENCES ACROSS SETTINGS

Academic Program Level I Fieldwork Objective #2

"Discuss potential occupational therapy assessments appropriate to the setting and/or population (including relevant social, cultural, and economic factors that may impact client outcomes) with direction from FWed" (Devoto, 2020, p. 2).

FIELDWORK SETTING	LEARNING EXPERIENCE BASED ON OBJECTIVE
School system	The FWed might orient the student to available assessment tools and discuss a recent student evaluation and their reasoning for their assessment tool choices. The fieldwork student might be directed to two to three different assessment tools and asked to choose the most appropriate tool based on reasoning articulated by the FWed. The student may also identify how and why they might assess a class or a student in a class without actually performing an assessment on the child.
Outpatient adult rehabilitation	After a student observes the occupational therapist for a day or two to understand the population that is being served, the student might read a patient's chart and discuss with the occupational therapist what assessments they might use to evaluate the client and why.
Community-supported employment setting	Students may observe the members and the different operations within the organization. They may implement (or identify) screens or assessments to help identify member interests and skills. The students could assess different job skills/operations and make recommendations to support the members in their jobs or recommend different roles and responsibilities.

Just as in other academic courses, the Level I fieldwork experience must use some form of measurement of student learning (AOTA, 2019). In didactic coursework, this may be papers, tests, midterm assessments, final assessments, or lab practical assessments. The tool that is used for measuring student progress in Level I fieldwork is a Level I fieldwork evaluation. This form is also based in an academic program's learning theories, curriculum, sequence, etc. Not all occupational therapy/occupational therapy assistant academic programs use the same Level I fieldwork evaluation tool. However, just like with the academic program fieldwork objectives, there are many similarities in Level I fieldwork evaluation forms across different academic programs. The majority of programs assess professional behaviors, and some academic programs assess basic clinical skills as well. The AOTA developed the AOTA *Level I Fieldwork Competency Evaluation for OT and OTA Students* (AOTA, 2017a), which includes skills and professional behaviors. Chapter 13 will go into greater depth on the evaluation process in Level I fieldwork. However, it is important to mention the Level I fieldwork evaluation because it directly ties to the objectives of the fieldwork course, and the FWed needs this information to develop learning activities.

Along with the academic program fieldwork learning objectives and Level I student evaluation, it is important for the FWed to collect information from the student in order to better understand their perspective of their experience and skills as it relates to those needed at your site. A student skills assessment is a tool the educator may use to gather some of this information on the student. For example, some fieldwork sites provide a form that has a list of common functions that they perform as an occupational therapist at their site. They have the student check off their level of experience and comfort. The skills assessment or inquiry gives the educator information about the student's comfort level and experience in different skills. Please see Appendix B for an example of a skills assessment/inquiry.

In addition to a student skills assessment, you might simply have a conversation with your assigned Level I student to understand what they hope to gain from participation in the Level I fieldwork experience from their perspective. Using a focus group format, Honey and Penman (2020) interviewed eight occupational therapy students who had just completed a 1-week learning fieldwork to understand what they wanted to learn from the experience. Students reported that they primarily wanted confirmation that they were in the right profession, and secondly, they wanted experiences [of the occupational therapy process] that they could reflect back upon as they engaged in the remainder of their academic learning. They also valued opportunities to understand the unique needs and complexity of working with clients. They identified eight critical experiences to their learning, including (1) observing an occupational therapy practitioner in action to see how the theory and skills they had learned in the classroom might be applied; (2) seeing the positive impact of therapist work on a client and within an organization; (3) seeing how what an occupational therapy practitioner did at one stage of health care fit into the bigger picture of health care; (4) having access to the therapist's reasoning process and opportunity to ask questions; (5) opportunity for hands-on doing to develop skills, confidence, and an understanding of their capabilities (Table 8-12); (6) getting feedback on their skills; (7) being challenged to think analytically and reflectively about clients; and (8) being challenged to think analytically and reflectively about their own performance. When developing your learning plan, it will be wise to keep these overall student perspectives in mind, and how you might make small adjustments to your learning plan to accommodate individual student learning interests.

ALIGNMENT OF FIELDWORK OBJECTIVES AND SITE RESOURCES: TAKING INVENTORY

The next part of this chapter will focus on how the FWed and site resources fit into this big picture. Figure 8-2 provides a visual representation of educational components contributing to fieldwork design.

The FWed's role is that of a teacher. The FWed is expected to "effectively evaluate and share knowledge in the form of new materials, literature, and educational materials relating to fieldwork that enhance the lifelong learning of future occupational therapy practitioners" (AOTA, 2006, p. 650). The FWed specializes in the area in which they practice (neurology, outpatient pediatrics, school systems, etc.). The FWed works within the parameters of their organization, including the overall role/purpose of the setting, the goals and mission of the program, and the services provided to clients. The "classroom" could be a patient's room, a kitchen, a classroom, a rehab gym, in a patient's home, etc. The FWed needs to consider not only the big picture of their setting but the tools they have access to within their space. In summary, the FWed needs to reflect on themselves, their setting, and the resources they have available at their site. These resources will allow the educator to consider what experiences/opportunities they have available to create a complementary fieldwork to the academic program curriculum. Box 8-2 illustrates examples of site and educator resources.

TABLE 8-12

EXAMPLES OF HANDS-ON LEARNING ACTIVITIES DESIRED BY STUDENTS

Having informal conversations with clients
Writing progress notes
Explaining roles, such as assessment or intervention roles of occupational therapy, to other health care providers and clients
Gathering and assisting with equipment use
Assisting with moving and handling and/or functional transfers
Taking measurements
Contributing to group sessions

Adapted from Honey, A., & Penman, M. (2020). "You actually see what occupational therapists do in real life." Outcomes and critical features of first-year practice education placements. *British Journal of Occupational Therapy, 83*(10), 638-647. https://doi.org/10.1177/0308022620920535

It might be easiest to look at this from a big picture view of the organization and then look at how occupational therapy fits within the picture. From a *big picture* perspective, the FWed needs to consider the program's overarching goal and how the organization serves its clients/consumers. The educator should reflect on their role within the organization and the relationship with their clients. Thinking about the philosophical aspects of the organization and what expertise and knowledge is available to support student learning is helpful (Box 8-3).

These questions are a starting point for FWeds. The questions are meant to help the educator start looking at their site, their role, and their resources from a teaching perspective. As mentioned earlier in this chapter, the site is a classroom, and as a teacher, the FWed needs to look at their environment, processes/system, and resources to determine what tools they have available to use.

Next, the FWed needs to reflect on the role of occupational therapy, and how it fits within the organization. This helps the educator understand how to develop fieldwork experiences within the parameters of that specific setting. The role of occupational therapy can look differently in various settings. For example, in adult outpatient rehab, an occupational therapist may be a stand-alone service and provide direct patient care. In a school setting, occupational therapy may provide direct and indirect services. They may provide direct services to students and consultative services to teachers. In a school system, the team of professionals collaborate with each other, the teacher, and the family to develop an individualized education plan for the student. All disciplines work with the student to facilitate progress toward this plan. In a day program for adults with intellectual disabilities, the occupational therapist may be a part of a team who helps set up the experiences/activities/environment to facilitate participation and optimal independence of participants. Understanding the role of occupational therapy in the site allows the educator to identify learning experiences that may help a student understand the role in that setting. See Box 8-4 for questions that may help the FWed reflect on their practice roles.

In addition, the educator needs to think about the pragmatic components of their job. Think about what happens on a daily basis. The educator needs to think about how their space is set up, what equipment and supplies are available, and their own available time to allocate to the student. In addition, the educator needs to consider the pragmatic operations of the organization as whole. Things to consider might be the flow and culture of the organization, the other employees and

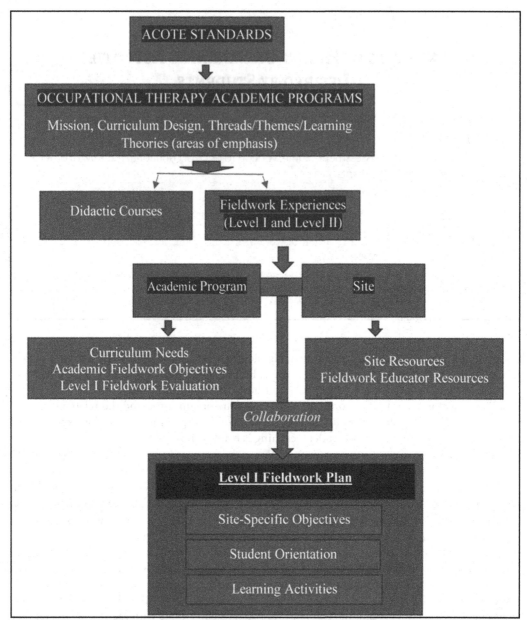

Figure 8-2. Visual representation of the educational components of fieldwork.

consumers in the organization, the routines of the facility, and the overall space. Box 8-5 provides the FWed with probing questions to help determine the available resources, opportunities, and challenges in the setting.

The FWed needs to reflect on the naturally occurring experiences that happen in their setting that might support a student's learning and understanding of the occupational therapy process. These experiences should also support the student's learning in the classroom. See Table 8-13 for examples of naturally occurring experiences that can support student classroom learning.

Reflection on the role that occupational therapy plays within the larger role of the facility/site may also be helpful to identify further available learning experiences. See Box 8-6 for an example of the role of occupational therapy in a fieldwork setting.

Box 8-2

SITE AND EDUCATOR RESOURCES

Site Resources	**Educator Resources**
• Mission/purpose of organization	• Knowledge/experience
• Client population	• Role of educator (individually and how it fits in the big picture of the organization)
• Staff roles	
• Space	• Skills
• Operation of organization	• Time
• Staff	• Routine tasks
• Organizational routines (schedule, etc.)	• Supplies/equipment
	• Occupational therapy routines

In addition to different types of fieldwork settings, the kinds of experiential learning experiences may vary for students from the typical block placement 1-week experience in a medical or community setting, to an experience that occurs once a week for a semester, the faculty-led experience, or a simulated learning experience. There are also role-emerging practice sites where supervision is provided by a licensed health care professional rather than an occupational therapy practitioner (AOTA, 2019). Table 8-14 illustrates how the student's learning experience may vary across Level I fieldwork sites and types.

Generally speaking, sites find that they are able to find ways to support the objectives of the academic program and provide suitable student learning experiences onsite. However, some challenges may occur. Some sites may have concerns regarding having Level I fieldwork students secondary to the student, restricted from touching the patient due to safety or hospital policy. However, there are many solutions to this challenge. Haynes (2011) identifies several strategies to address educator concerns with creating active participation opportunities for students in challenging settings in her research of FWed and student perceptions of participation in Level I fieldwork. One example Haynes (2011) uses for a site that will not allow a student to physically implement an intervention session is for the student to write a subjective, objective, assessment, and plan note to describe their observation. Table 8-15 illustrates several solutions to perceived barriers.

These are just a few examples. However, there are many ways to work around challenges and create effective student fieldwork experiences. Challenge yourself to be creative and think outside the box. Collaborate with the AFWC and problem solve potential solutions.

Box 8-3

QUESTIONS TO REFLECT ON THE FACILITY'S
ORGANIZATIONAL AND PHILOSOPHICAL ASPECTS

1. What is the mission/role and purpose of your site? (i.e., is your mission to provide respectful and excellent care to your patients, or if you are in a community setting, is your mission to provide purposeful activities and opportunities for socialization for adults with intellectual disabilities?)

2. What is the ultimate goal for the clients/consumers?

3. What is the client population, and how are they served?

4. What are the various staff positions, and what are their roles in the organization?

5. What is the role of the occupational therapist, and how does occupational therapy fit into the big picture of the organization (or clinic, facility, school, etc.)?

6. If there is not an occupational therapist at the facility, what is your role? What experiences do I have, and what processes/experiences does my site offer? (If there is not an occupational therapist onsite, it will be helpful to work with the AFWC to process different approaches to the occupational therapy process, or how the students might apply their learning in this setting.)

7. What prior experience, skills, and knowledge does the educator have in the occupational therapy field or other fields, and how might this support student learning? (What do I know, and how can I teach it? What is my role? What jobs/tasks do I perform? What skills could I perform?)

8. Does each discipline of the clinic operate individually, or do they come together for patient meetings to collaborate and set team goals?

9. Is the role of occupational therapy at your site consultative?

10. Is my setting a community setting where there are several staff who represent different disciplines (e.g., occupational therapist, recreational therapist, aids, teachers) and work as a team to support the clients and the program?

11. How do I measure progress or success of my consumers?

12. Does your organization philosophically support students in the setting?

13. Will having students in your facility affect consumers (in a positive or negative way)?

STEPS TO DEVELOPING A
LEVEL I FIELDWORK PLAN

Now that the FWed has reflected on connecting the academic program curriculum and sequence to their own situation and resources, the next stage is to develop a Level I fieldwork plan. There are three main steps to developing a fieldwork plan: (1) develop learning activities for course objectives, (2) develop a sequenced learning plan, and (3) create student orientation (Figure 8-3).

BOX 8-4

REFLECTION QUESTIONS ON FIELDWORK EDUCATOR'S PRACTICE/SETTING

1. What do you do at your site? (i.e., is your site an adult rehab site or an outpatient pediatric clinic?)

2. What does the occupational therapy process look like at my site? (i.e., do you evaluate and treat children, or do you work with volunteers and staff to help create programming that will support clients in their daily activities?)

3. Who do you serve (individuals/populations/etc.), and how do you serve them?

4. What is the role of occupational therapy/occupational therapy assistant at your site (or what could the role of occupational therapy/occupational therapy assistant be at your site)? Is the occupational therapist's role as a direct provider, a consultative role, or a collaborative role?

BOX 8-5

REFLECTION ON FACILITY'S RESOURCES, OPPORTUNITIES, AND CHALLENGES

1. Reflect on the space of the facility. How big is the space (or spaces)? How is the space used? How could the space be used?

2. Would your facility be able to accommodate a student or students in their space?

3. What are the hours of operation?

4. What are the regular routines that occur in the organization (i.e., breakfast is served, then a gross motor group, a creative group, and a wrap up group)?

5. What staff and/or volunteers are in the program? What are the roles of these individuals?

6. What staff are available to help support a student program? How could the staff support the student program?

Course Learning Objectives

When connecting the link between academia and fieldwork experience, the FWed starts by considering how academic course objectives and the fieldwork evaluation used by the academic program applies to the fieldwork site. The academic program develops objectives from a program perspective. These may be somewhat general or specific, depending on the curriculum. FWeds use these academic fieldwork objectives and translate them into application at their site. A sample of academic program learning objectives is provided in Appendix C. Figure 8-4 illustrates the process of translating academic fieldwork objectives and assessment items into the development of site-specific learning activities.

As discussed in the guidelines provided by AOTA for Level I fieldwork (AOTA Commission on Education, 1999), the Level I fieldwork site, through collaboration with the academic program faculty, should design learning activities to meet Level I objectives provided by the academic program. If providing Level I fieldwork for both technical and professional level occupational therapy students, the fieldwork site should have different learning activities for each level of education that clearly reflect role delineation. Learning activities are designed with these guidelines in mind, while also considering the expectations of the occupational therapy/occupational therapy assistant program as reflected in the items listed on the Level I evaluation. Table 8-16 illustrates the relationship between academic program learning objectives, Level I fieldwork evaluation items, and fieldwork learning activities.

When developing site-specific learning activities, it is helpful to think in the context of the format of the fieldwork and the student's learning opportunities. Think about the opportunities for a student who may be with you for a 1-week intensive fieldwork and what opportunities might be available for a student who participates in fieldwork 1 day a week for 10 weeks. The approach to developing a student's learning may look different, but the same objective may be used in both scenarios.

For example, if the student participates in a 1-week fieldwork at an outpatient pediatric clinic (block placement), they may be able to see a variety of patients but not be able to observe the occupational therapist perform an evaluation on a new child. In this scenario, the FWed may provide the opportunity for a student to perform a section of an assessment for a treatment activity with a child or have a student identify one assessment that might be appropriate to assess the child's current level of function and why they would choose this assessment.

On the other hand, if a student participates in a fieldwork experience that is 1 day a week for 10 weeks (dose model placement), they may be able to observe the occupational therapy practitioner perform an evaluation on a new patient. The student will also be able to observe a child's progress but may not see a large variety of children. To enhance the student's experience, the FWed might direct the student to observe intervention sessions provided by the speech therapist and/or physical therapist working with the client. The student may be able to observe an evaluation on a new patient administered by the supervising FWed or another occupational therapist onsite. Both approaches would meet the needs of the student. Table 8-17 illustrates some examples of learning activities that may be available in different settings.

Developing a Learning Plan: Sequencing Student Learning

The learning plan is the progression or series of experiences that provide students the opportunity to facilitate what they need to learn during their Level I fieldwork experience. In developing a learning plan, you will consider what experiences naturally occur throughout the day in your setting. This has been discussed earlier in this chapter. Think about how a student might learn in your setting and then consider the process or sequence that will assist the student in their learning.

Chapter 2 discussed several learning theories. Each curriculum identifies learning theories that influence instructional strategies throughout the program (ACOTE, 2018). Familiarity with the learning theories guiding the academic curriculum of partnering institutions can be helpful to the FWed when planning and sequencing student learning activities. Bloom's Taxonomy, which was one of the learning theories explored in Chapter 2, will be used to illustrate how learning activities might be sequenced following a learning theory.

Bloom's Taxonomy, which is a commonly used resource by educators, proposes levels of complexity to learning—from basic to more complex. The new version of Bloom's Taxonomy identifies six levels or stages of thinking: Remember, Understand, Apply, Analyze, Evaluate, and Create (Hoque, 2016; Table 8-18). The FWed can apply this theory to teaching their fieldwork students. For example, if a student is in semester two of their occupational therapy or occupational therapy assistant program, they may still be working on understanding and applying information they have learned in their classes. Individually, students may be at different stages of learning during any given semester. Therefore, in developing learning activities and a learning plan, it is important

TABLE 8-13
NATURALLY OCCURRING EXPERIENCES IN A COMMUNITY OUTPATIENT SETTING

Assessment and reassessment in the classroom: Students practiced interview- and observation-based assessment protocols	**Assessment and reassessment on Level I fieldwork:** Students interview/observe a new program participant to determine placement in a specific job or role in a supported employment program. The experience may be working alongside the food service group to see what habits and skills the participants have as well as how the group works together.
Treatment planning in the classroom: Students learn to write short- and long-term goals with a focus on occupational performance	**Treatment planning in the community outpatient setting:** Students attend a treatment team meeting where patient progress and plans are discussed and work with client to formulate goals that are reflective of the client's interests.
Therapy intervention in the classroom: Students practice leading peer groups following a structured seven-step format for group leadership	**Group therapy intervention in the outpatient setting:** Students participate in a grocery-shopping group or a social skills group, and assist the leader in activity setup, introducing the learning activity, providing directions and support and processing group learning.

> ### Box 8-6
> ## DESCRIPTION OF THE OCCUPATIONAL THERAPY PROCESS AND LEVEL I FIELDWORK IN BRAIN INJURY REHABILITATION
>
> **Role of occupational therapy:** The goal of occupational therapy in this setting is to collaborate with the patient on setting goals and facilitating rehabilitation. Occupational therapists provide services, modify environments, and recommend adaptive equipment to increase function, participation, and level of independence in activities of daily living. Occupational therapists evaluate and treat adolescents/adults with brain injuries. Occupational therapists treat the patient individually and in groups. Occupational therapists collaborate with the rehab team to identify what multidisciplinary groups would be beneficial for the patient.
>
> **Role within the rehabilitation team:** The occupational therapist is a member of the rehabilitation team, working alongside a physical therapist, speech therapist, nurse, physician, vocational rehabilitation specialist, recreational therapist, and social worker. The team may set team goals as well as individual discipline goals for the client. The occupational therapist may treat individually or in groups and co-treat with another discipline. The team works together to support the goals of the client and their family.
>
> **Evaluation process includes:** Patient interview, pain scale, assessment of upper extremity function/movement/sensation, assessment of cognition, assessment of vision, assessment of basic activities of daily living, and, if applicable, home management/community management skills.
>
> **Intervention may include:** Instruction of safe functional transfers, dressing, grooming, bathing, toileting, upper extremity movement/functioning, etc. The patient may participate in groups like exercise groups, grocery/meal planning groups, leisure groups, etc.
>
> **Other learning experiences may include:** Case management: researching community resources; patient and family education; team meetings; community outings; co-treatment; collaboration with other disciplines; collaboration with physicians and specialists.

to understand the curriculum sequence, as well as the level of experience and growth of each student. In setting up a fieldwork plan, the FWed needs to think about where the student is in terms of their learning process. Most Level I occupational therapy students are working within the first four stages of thinking based on of Bloom's Taxonomy. Table 8-19 illustrates how the FWed can create learning activities to develop the student's learning in a basic occupational therapy skill.

The learning plan is developed by taking the objectives and breaking them down into steps that are sequenced from basic to more complex. As you develop sequential learning activities for students within your setting, reflect on what skills are required to work as an occupational therapy practitioner in your setting. Then, think backward and reflect on the developmental steps to get to that point. What are some of the pieces that make up the big picture of an occupational therapy/occupational therapy assistant practitioner? For example, if an entry-level practitioner needs to evaluate and treat adults with brain injuries, then what common assessments do they need to perform? Stepping back farther (in terms of learning), what are the simplest/most basic assessments (or components of assessments) to administer and learn? Figure 8-5 illustrates how to break down the skills and knowledge of an entry-level practitioner into basic components.

This process of facilitating a student's learning helps the FWed to identify the basic components of their own practice. Similar to performing an activity analysis for an activity for a patient, the FWed performs an analysis of the progression of performing occupational therapy skills. For example, the educator reflects on the assessments used in their setting considering

TABLE 8-14

STUDENT LEARNING EXPERIENCES
ACROSS TYPES OF LEVEL I FIELDWORK

SETTING	STUDENT LEARNING EXPERIENCE
Outpatient pediatric setting: Block placements	Occupational therapist evaluates and treats pediatric clients for developmental delays and functional challenges. The occupational therapist/occupational therapy assistant works on facilitating increased participation and function with children using age appropriate activities/tasks and equipment. The clients may receive therapy for several years. Assessments may include the Peabody Developmental Motor Scale, Developmental Test of Visual Perception, Sensory Profile, Motor-Free Visual Perception Test, the Bruininks-Oseretsky Test of Motor Proficiency, etc. Treatment may include groups and individual treatment. Available learning experiences may include observation or participation in an occupational therapy assessment, working with swings, therapy balls, fine motor toys, gross motor toys, dressing, eating, sensory activities, etc.
Outpatient neuro rehabilitation day program: Block placement	Occupational therapist evaluates clients on self-care, home management, leisure, community reintegration, etc. The occupational therapist/occupational therapy assistant works on individual goals for the client but also establishes group goals in collaboration with the other disciplines. Occupational therapist/occupational therapy assistant works within the clinic as well as takes the client on outings (e.g., grocery store, library, gym). Occupational therapist meets weekly to discuss patient progress. Clients participate in grocery groups, exercise groups, etc. Assessments may include evaluation of upper extremity function/movement/sensation, self-care, home management, driving/community reintegration, work skills, cognition, vision, etc. The occupational therapy student is able to observe and participate in select elements of the occupational therapy process.
Day program for young adults with development delays: Dosing placement model over the course of a semester	Occupational therapist collaborates with staff and volunteers to develop program to facilitate participation and socialization of members. Occupational therapist/occupational therapy assistant's role is consultative and supportive. The occupational therapist helps to assess the program and its components to make sure it meets the needs of the client. The program may include a gross motor group (playing games, exercise, etc.), cooking group, and a cognitive group (participants play games or participate in activities that encourage participants to interact with one another and problem solve). The occupational therapist/occupational therapy assistant's role is to observe clients and collaborate on activities that will engage clients. They will also adapt activities to meet the individual's needs. The goal of the members is to participate in functional/purposeful activities and social interaction.

(continued)

TABLE 8-14 (CONTINUED)

STUDENT LEARNING EXPERIENCES
ACROSS TYPES OF LEVEL I FIELDWORK

SETTING	STUDENT LEARNING EXPERIENCE
Camp for adolescents with brain injuries: Role-emerging fieldwork setting	There may not be an occupational therapist/occupational therapy assistant on staff. The role of an occupational therapist/occupational therapy assistant student is to support the campers and help modify the activities so that the camper is successful and able to complete the task and feel good about it. The occupational therapist/occupational therapy assistant student may stay in the cabins and help the campers perform their daily self-tasks. They can adapt the task so that the camper may be more independent. The student has the opportunity to see what the camper is able to do from a self-care, leisure, and social perspective.
Simulated adult rehab setting	In this setting, trained actors play the role of the patient and caregivers. The occupational therapy process in this setting may include evaluation and treatment of a simulated patient. The student can perform an assessment or a more comprehensive evaluation on the patient. The student can write up their results/findings, set goals, and plan one to two treatment activities for the patient.
Online/virtual simulation activity	There are multiple online/video simulation activities that fulfill the criteria for Level I fieldwork experiences. These activities provide opportunities for students to observe a simulated patient and assessment or work through a written case study. Students apply their clinical reasoning in these scenarios. The student can assess the patient using their observations and information provided. They can recommend additional assessments, practice writing an evaluation summary, set goals, and develop treatment plans.

---

which assessments (or components) are simplest and which assessments are more complex. Box 8-7 illustrates an example of identifying the simple or more basic components of an occupational therapy evaluation.

In thinking about sequencing of student learning experiences, it is important to consider the breadth of activities that might occur related to each step of the occupational therapy process. For example, if you wished to offer your student learning experiences related to learning how to administer an evaluation, you would need to consider the types of evaluation experiences that you offer your clients but also the complexity of the evaluation and its purpose. If you were to sequence the complexity of the evaluation process, you might start with considering the population that you serve and the range of complexity of their conditions and have students start with a less complex client. You would also consider the steps of the evaluation. If using Bloom's Taxonomy to structure a learning sequence, you would consider what information students need to *know* before engaging in the assessment. This might include familiarity with a select portion of the assessment instrument but also familiarity with associated processes, such as how to complete a chart review, client application, or interview a teacher or caregiver about a student's performance prior to a more formal evaluation. How would you ensure that the student *understands* the information they have gathered before engaging in the evaluation process? For example, the student might discuss their knowledge and their plan for their portion of the assessment process with the FWed prior

	TABLE 8-15	
SOLUTION TO PERCEIVED BARRIERS TO FIELDWORK AT SITE		
SETTING	PERCEIVED BARRIERS	SOLUTIONS
Community site	No occupational therapist on staff: FWed and site feel unqualified to supervise a student.	• Student might research in advance potential roles for occupational therapy in similar settings (e.g., role of occupational therapist in supported employment, community mental health). • Student might complete a literature review on the population prior to the Level I placement and identify common needs and successful intervention approaches. • During the placement, the student can attend programming offered, interview the members (or individuals) and staff, and explore what processes and activities work well and which components of the site environment present challenges. • During the placement, student might attend programming with one to two select clients and apply informal interviewing and observation to identify client needs. The student might share their observations with site mentor and discuss alignment of observations with completed literature review. • Student might identify one to two appropriate occupational therapy goals and discuss with supervisor how they might be achieved in the context of the fieldwork setting. • Student could assess the environment and the participants within the environment and recommend potential modifications to support function.
Neonatal intensive care unit	FWed feels the patients they serve are too fragile for students.	• The FWed could share with a student the clinical reasoning process used when working with an infant, a staff member, or a parent. • The FWed could discuss assessments and positioning and have the student simulate an evaluation on a doll. • The FWed could give feedback on the scores and functions of the simulated patient and then have the student respond based on the feedback. • The student could practice positioning an infant using the doll.

(continued)

TABLE 8-15 (CONTINUED)
SOLUTION TO PERCEIVED BARRIERS TO FIELDWORK AT SITE

SETTING	PERCEIVED BARRIERS	SOLUTIONS
		• The student could observe the therapist complete an evaluation of a patient. • The student could write up what they observe and compare with the therapist's observations. • The student could look up research articles to support different treatment strategies in the neonatal intensive care unit and write up some basic education sheets to give to parents.
Telehealth	FWeds feel having multiple people on the screen may be confusing or distracting to the client. Another challenge may be the perception that the student is not getting *hands-on* experience with the client.	• FWed can introduce the students to the client (with the student on video) and then explain to the client that the student will hide their video so that they will not distract the client. • When the student is treating the client, they can turn the video on. • The FWed could practice performing a task with the student acting as a client. • The FWed might reverse roles and have the student treat the practitioner. • A follow-up idea might be to have the student practice "treating" the practitioner via a virtual platform.

to implementation. Or if the student were assisting with a wheelchair transfer, they might talk the FWed through the steps of transferring a patient from wheelchair to bed or bed to wheelchair prior to *applying* their knowledge and understanding to assistance of a transfer with a client. Next, you would consider what kinds of experiences you might provide for the student to *analyze* or *evaluate*? If completing an assessment, the student might *analyze* or determine the meaning of performance scores in relation to client-identified goals, or a student might observe a client session and document what the client is able to do, as well as their challenges/barriers. An occupational therapy/occupational therapy assistant student might observe a child as they practice writing during class, considering the child's posture/how the child is sitting/where the child's feet are, and identify the implications for client goals. Reflection about a past treatment session provides another means for the student to analyze what went well, challenges, and changes that might be made in future sessions (Boud et al., 2002; Hanson et al., 2011). *Evaluation* occurs when the student has the opportunity to evaluate two or more competing choices and make a decision. This might occur when a student collaborates with the Level I FWed to make a decision as to which assessment tool to use among two to three options.

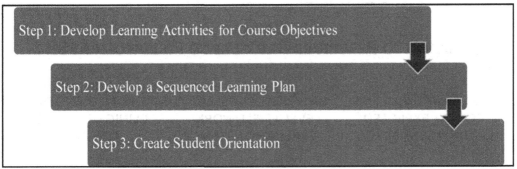

Figure 8-3. Steps to creating a Level I fieldwork plan.

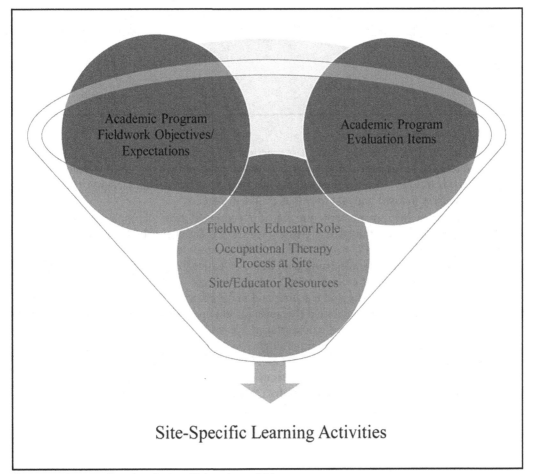

Figure 8-4. Process of creating site-specific learning activities.

An important element of sequencing student learning experiences is the ability to supportively challenge students by encouraging them to consider questions for themselves, try new ideas, and learn from the consequences. Scaffolding student learning involves the provision of intentional supports that can be reduced as students incrementally develop independence and mastery (Kaelin & Dancza, 2019; Schell & Schell, 2018). While engaging them in progressively more difficult activities, be sure to also provide adequate time for reflection, discussion, and emotional support

TABLE 8-16

SOLUTION TO PERCEIVED BARRIERS TO FIELDWORK AT SITE

UNIVERSITY/COLLEGE COURSE EXPECTED LEARNING OBJECTIVE	UNIVERSITY/COLLEGE LEVEL I FIELDWORK EVALUATION ITEM	POST–CONCUSSIVE DISORDER OUTPATIENT CLINIC LEARNING ACTIVITY
Student will: Describe to relevant stakeholders occupation and discuss how it relates to occupational therapy practice and its relationship to health and well-being.	Student will: Articulate specific occupational therapy role functions within the setting.	Student will: Demonstrate understanding and articulate the role of occupational therapy in telehealth practice to one caregiver/patient (or simulated patient) receiving services in the post–concussive disorder clinic.

(Dancza et al., 2021). Keep in mind the *best practices* to support clinical reasoning development that were discussed in Chapter 5, and how use of an occupation-focused model or frame of reference might be helpful to structure the student's learning. Your partnering academic program may also have resources to assist you and to enhance student success.

Learning plans help create structure and an organized plan of implementation for the fieldwork experience. Once this plan is created, it makes it easier for the FWed to host students because the process has already been created. It will also provide the structure to help support students learning. Developing a learning plan makes it easier for the educator to be purposeful in educating the student in the occupational therapy process. It allows the FWed to step back and reflect on their own practice and teaching and make changes to meet the needs of students. Many occupational therapy/occupational therapy assistant programs have similar expectations in fieldwork. Therefore, once the FWed has developed a learning plan in conjunction with one program, it can often be modified to apply to multiple academic programs. Keep in mind that when students undertake prolonged or consecutive Level I fieldwork experiences in the same facility, the learning activities should reflect a sequence from simple to more complex requirements (AOTA Commission on Education, 1999). See Appendix D for an example of a learning plan that demonstrates a sequence from simple to more complex requirements.

Student Orientation

The final step in developing a fieldwork learning plan is to design a student orientation. Although the orientation of the student comes before the remainder of the learning experiences, you are best able to design your orientation once you have developed your learning plan. The purpose of the student orientation is to introduce the student to expectations for professional behavior, site expectations, and the overall context and expectations for their learning experience (Hanson & Schumacher, 2014). To accomplish a comprehensive orientation for students, it is helpful to develop a student Level I fieldwork manual. Under the tab of education and fieldwork, the AOTA website provides an excellent resource to guide a FWed or site coordinator to develop a Level II fieldwork manual, and this information could be modified for the Level I experience. The recommended content for a Level II fieldwork manual is summarized in Table 8-20.

TABLE 8-17

SOLUTION TO PERCEIVED BARRIERS TO FIELDWORK AT SITE

UNIVERSITY/ COLLEGE COURSE EXPECTED LEARNING OBJECTIVE	UNIVERSITY/ COLLEGE LEVEL I FIELDWORK EVALUATION ITEMS	SITE-SPECIFIC LEARNING ACTIVITIES
Student will: Demonstrate reliable and safe work habits.	Student will: Adhere consistently to safety regulations and use sound judgment to ensure safety. Follow fieldwork setting's policies and procedures for client safety. Demonstrate awareness of hazardous situations and report safety issues to supervisor (AOTA, 2017a, p. 2).	Student will: *Acute Inpatient Rehab Setting* Identify one to two safety precautions related to treating an individual with a total hip replacement by the end of the fieldwork experience. Articulate how to set up the environment (patient room) to promote safety and optimal participation in therapy. *School System Setting* Demonstrate understanding of safety protocols for school by identifying a protocol to follow during one occupational therapy session (i.e., cleaning procedures) by the end of the fieldwork experience. *Supportive Employment Program for Adults With Brain Injuries (No Occupational Therapy)* Identify two environment safety concerns in one working unit by the end of the fieldwork experience (food prep unit, environmental services unit, etc.). *Upper Extremity/Hand Clinic* Identify two safety precautions to consider when applying heat to patient by the end of the fieldwork experience. Demonstrate understanding of safety risks when using hot pack by applying hot pack to one client, adhering to precautions, by end of the fieldwork experience.

For the Level I fieldwork manual, the learning objectives will be provided by the academic site, so if you are providing Level I fieldwork for multiple academic programs, you might have a separate tab for the learning objectives of each academic program. Instead of a sample weekly schedule or week-by-week schedule, the Level I orientation manual would identify site-specific learning activities for each learning objective, and a learning plan that sequences learning activities over the course of the Level I experience. Since some Level I experiences are 1-week block placements, the plan would represent learning activities over the week. For other Level I experiences, such as the

TABLE 8-18

STAGES OF THINKING BASED ON THE REVISED BLOOM'S TAXONOMY

Basic Thinking Skills					Complex Thinking Skills
REMEMBER	**UNDERSTAND**	**APPLY**	**ANALYZE**	**EVALUATE**	**CREATE**
Recall facts	Explain the meaning of the facts/information	Implement what was learned	Find/identify relationships	Critique	Use all the information learned and hypothesize and create something new

Adapted from Anderson, L. W. (Ed.), Krathwohl, D. R. (Ed.), Airasian, P. W., Cruikshank, K. A., Mayer, R. E., Pintrich, P. R., Raths, J., & Wittrock, M. C. (2001). *A taxonomy for learning, teaching, and assessing: A revision of Bloom's Taxonomy of Educational Objectives.* Longman.

TABLE 8-19
STAGES OF THINKING BASED ON THE REVISED BLOOM'S TAXONOMY

Basic Thinking Skills			Complex Thinking Skills
	REMEMBER	UNDERSTAND	APPLY
Activities	• Identify norms for upper extremity range of motion (ROM)/ movement	• Student observes assessment of upper extremity ROM/ movement • Discuss how measurements apply to function	• Student completes upper extremity ROM/movement assessment on patient • Have student reflect on their own performance • Have student observe same patient perform a daily task • Discuss what *functional ROM/movement* you observe • Discuss what might be challenging for the patient based on what you saw the patient do
Measurement	• Have student recall norms for upper extremity ROM/ movement	• Student writes up results with comparison to norms	• Student writes up results and assessment part of note (the O and A portion of a subjective, objective, assessment, and plan note)

	ANALYZE
Activities	• Student completes upper back dressing with patient • Have student reflect on their own performance and discuss what they might do differently in the future • Have student reflect on what was challenging for the patient during the activity and how that relates to their upper extremity function • Have student identify another activity that might support the patient in working on upper extremity skills
Measurement	• Have student explain to patient caregiver how assessment of upper extremity ROM/ movement applies to patient functioning • Have student identify, discuss, and provide rationale (explain why) for one treatment activity that might address the upper extremity function • Explain any modifications or adaptive equipment that might need to be provided

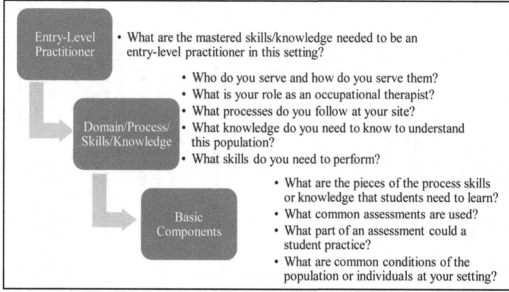

Figure 8-5. Developmental progression of skills and knowledge of entry-level practitioner.

dose placement model, the learning activities might occur over the semester or within a designated period of time. See Table 8-21 for an example of content in the Level I fieldwork manual.

Once the FWed has developed a student manual, a schedule can be created for the student for the first day/days at the site. The educator needs to review emergency and safety expectations, protocols, and information about the organization and the role of occupational therapy. The FWed will want to introduce the student to other employees who they will interact with over the course of their learning experience and to the space and resources they will use (Hanson & Schumacher, 2014). Student orientation sets the student up for success. It is like providing the directions for building a model. It helps the student begin to understand the structure and expectations for the experience.

SUMMARY

This chapter has provided the FWed with a roadmap for developing a Level I fieldwork learning plan that supports the learning objectives of the partnering occupational therapy/occupational therapy assistant educational programs. Through understanding the relationship between the ACOTE standards and the Level I fieldwork experiences, the novice FWed or AFWC are better able to situate the learning plan in the overall context of higher education. Throughout this chapter, emphasis has been placed on the understanding that Level I fieldwork is a course within the curriculum of an academic program. Thus, the academic program and its curriculum sequence must be tightly intertwined with the fieldwork learning experiences. Strategies have been provided for the FWed to analyze site resources and experiences to support and complement the academic program expectations and curriculum. A format for developing site-specific learning activities corresponding to the learning objectives of the Level I fieldwork course was offered and strategies for development of a learning plan were explored.

Having a broader understanding of Level I fieldwork, based on the ACOTE accreditation standards, the occupational therapy/occupational therapy assistant program curriculum and the occupational therapist's role in the site will help guide the FWed to create effective learning experiences for students. These experiences will not be stand-alone experiences, but opportunities

---

BOX 8-7

EXAMPLE OF RANGE OF COMPLEXITY OF EVALUATION PROCESS IN BRAIN INJURY REHAB

Range of Simple to Complex Components of Evaluation

Simple ➤➤➤	**Complex**
Component of patient interview (name, support system, roles, home environment)	Full interview
Assessment of reality orientation	Assessment of functional cognition
Complete unaffected upper extremity range of motion and movement	Range of motion/ strength
Complete one section of the motor-free visual perception test	Full oculomotor exam
Complete pain scale for verbal patient	Pain scale for nonverbal patient
Complete upper body dressing	Upper and lower body dressing
Simple functional transfers	Complex transfers (Max assist x 2, etc.)
Remove and place foot pedals on wheelchair	Complete wheelchair/ mobility assessment

---

for the students to apply what they are learning in a professional environment. Once the FWed develops Level I fieldwork learning plans, they will find that these learning plans are compatible with multiple occupational therapy/occupational therapy assistant academic curriculums. These learning plans will help the site and educators be more purposeful in creating Level I fieldwork experiences for their students.

Upon concluding this chapter, you are encouraged to reflect on the resources and opportunities available at your site and reach out to a local academic program to begin a partnership process. If you have already been offering Level I fieldwork, you are encouraged to review your learning plan in view of what you have learned in this chapter and make revisions to support student learning success. The following additional learning activities are provided to help you apply what you learned from this chapter to your own context.

TABLE 8-20

AOTA RECOMMENDED CONTENT FOR LEVEL II FIELDWORK MANUAL

1. Outline of orientation
2. Patient rights or patient confidentiality information
3. Guidelines for documentation
a. Sample forms (completed and blank)
b. Acceptable medical abbreviations
c. Evaluation procedure and form
d. Billing
4. Behavioral objectives and expectations (including communication with the FWed)
5. Sample weekly schedule
6. Week-by-week schedule of responsibilities (AOTA, 2021)

LEARNING ACTIVITIES

1. With a specific partnering academic program in mind, consider the impact of accreditation standards on the design of Level I fieldwork experiences by reviewing Tables 8-2 through 8-5 and Appendix A. Do you have questions or concerns about your implementation of any of the Level I fieldwork standards? What prompts provided will be helpful to you in following up with the AFWC of the academic program regarding your questions?

2. Consider Tables 8-6 through 8-8 with a specific partnering academic program Level I fieldwork request in mind. Using a format similar to that provided in the tables, identify the program and semester emphasis of the partnering academic program, and determine whether and how your fieldwork site could support the academic program curriculum and sequence.

3. Review the occupational therapy/occupational therapy assistant program mission statement and learning objectives provided in Box 8-1 and the samples provided in Tables 8-10 and 8-11. What learning experiences would best meet these learning objectives in your facility or fieldwork context? What new ideas do you have for designing learning experiences in your context to meet learning objectives?

4. Review the examples provided in Tables 8-16 and 8-17 showing the impact of the learning objective and Level I fieldwork assessment on the design of learning experiences. Identify a Level I fieldwork learning objective provided by your partnering academic program and the item on the Level I assessment tool that corresponds to the learning objective. What ideas does this provide about learning experiences that would be appropriate for meeting that learning objective?

TABLE 8-21

CONTENT FOR A LEVEL I FIELDWORK LEARNING MANUAL

Level I Fieldwork Learning Manual
1. Outline of orientation process
2. Safety and emergency procedures
3. Patient rights or patient confidentiality information
4. Guidelines for documentation and practice
a. Sample documentation forms (completed and blank)
b. Acceptable abbreviations
c. Evaluation procedure and form
d. Billing guidelines
5. Academic program learning plan
a. Academic program learning objectives
b. Summary of learning activities available for each learning objective
c. Sequenced learning plan for Level I fieldwork duration
6. Level I fieldwork forms (all forms pertinent to Level I fieldwork for each academic program)

5. Consider Boxes 8-2 through 8-5 and the examples provided in Table 8-14 and identify one to two learning activities that would be a fit for addressing the academic course learning objective and Level I fieldwork evaluation item:

Academic Course Learning Objective: Demonstrate reliable and safe work habits.

Level I Fieldwork Evaluation Item: Adheres consistently to safety regulations and uses sound judgment to ensure safety. Follows fieldwork setting's policies and procedures for client safety. Demonstrates awareness of hazardous situations, and reports safety issues to supervisor (AOTA, 2017, p. 2).

6. Review the sample student skills inquiry provided in Appendix B. In view of the context of your Level I fieldwork, how might a student skills assessment be helpful to you in structuring student learning experiences? What items would you include?

7. Review the occupational therapy/occupational therapy assistant program mission statement and learning objectives provided in Box 8-1 and the sample learning activities provided in Tables 8-10 and 8-11. Using one of the sample learning activities (or a learning activity specific to your Level I fieldwork context), break down the activity to describe a sequence of learning activities that would meet the learning objective. You may find the examples provided in Table 8-19 (using Bloom's Taxonomy) or Table 8-10 helpful to this process.

8. Consider Table 8-21 and the learning plan example found in Appendix D. What documents do you need to develop and/or assemble to make up your Level I fieldwork learning plan for a specific academic program?

REFERENCES

Accreditation Council for Occupational Therapy Education. (2018). *2018 Accreditation Council for Occupational Therapy Education standards and interpretive guide.* https://acoteonline.org/wp-content/uploads/2020/10/2018-ACOTE-Standards.pdf

American Occupational Therapy Association. (2006). Role competencies for a fieldwork educator. *American Journal of Occupational Therapy, 60*(6), 650–651. https://doi.org/10.5014ajot.60.6.650

American Occupational Therapy Association. (2009). *The occupational therapy model curriculum.* http://www.aota.org/Eduicate/EdRes/COE/Other-Education-Documents/OT-Model-Curriculum.aspx

American Occupational Therapy Association. (2017a). *Level I fieldwork competency evaluation for COTAs and OTRs.* https://www.aota.org/-/media/Corporate/Files/EducationCareers/Educators/Fieldwork/LevelI/Level-I-Fieldwork-Competency-Evaluation-for-ot-and-ota-students.pdf

American Occupational Therapy Association. (2017b). Philosophical base of occupational therapy. *American Journal of Occupational Therapy, 71*(Suppl. 2), 7112410045p1. https://doi.org/10.5014/ajot.716S06

American Occupational Therapy Association. (2019). *Fieldwork educator certificate program. Education module* [PowerPoint slides]. https://www.dropbox.com/home/Fieldwork%20Educators%20Certificate%20Workshop/2019%20Modules%20(FINAL)/3.%20Education?preview=3.+Education+Module+PowerPoint+new+logo.pptx

American Occupational Therapy Association. (2021). *AOTA recommended content for a student fieldwork manual.* https://www.aota.org/Education-Careers/Fieldwork/NewPrograms/Content.aspx

American Occupational Therapy Association, Commission on Education. (1999). *Guidelines for an occupational therapy fieldwork experience: Level I.* American Occupational Therapy Association.

Anderson, L. W. (Ed.), Krathwohl, D. R. (Ed.), Airasian, P. W., Cruikshank, K. A., Mayer, R. E., Pintrich, P. R., Raths, J., & Wittrock, M. C. (2001). *A taxonomy for learning, teaching, and assessing: A revision of Bloom's Taxonomy of Educational Objectives.* Longman.

Boud, D., Keogh, R., & Walker, D. (2002). Promoting reflection in learning: a model. In R. Edwards, A. Hanson, & P. Raggatt (Eds.), *Boundaries of adult learning.* Routledge.

Brenau University College of Health Sciences. (2020). *Brenau University School of Occupational Therapy Student Manual 2020-2021.* https://drive.google.com/file/d/1_kSGtwknRFYcg6z2tYviGJKVRuKt8v4V/view

Dancza, K., Copley, J. A., & Moran, M. (2021). PLUS Framework: Guidance for practice educators. *The Clinical Teacher, 18*(4), 431-438. https://doi.org/10.1111/tct.13393

Devoto, M. D. (2020). *OT 617: Level I fieldwork – Community based/mental health course syllabi: Fall 2020.* Brenau University. https://catalog.brenau.edu/preview_course_nopop.php?catoid=20&coid=34975

Hanson, D., Johnson, C., Sauerwald, C. & Stutz-Tanenbaum, P. (2016). Working "smarter" in the academic fieldwork coordinator role. In D. Costa (Ed.), *The essential guide to fieldwork education* (2nd ed.). AOTA.

Hanson, D., Larson, J. K. & Nielsen, S. (2011). Reflective writing in Level II fieldwork. *OT Practice.*

Hanson, D., & Schumacher, A. (2014). Preparing for Level I fieldwork students. *OT Practice.*

Haynes, C. J. (2011). Active participation in fieldwork Level I: Fieldwork educator and student perceptions. *Occupational Therapy In Health Care, 25*(4), 257-269. https://doi.org/10.3109/07380577.2011.595477

Hewitt, B. (2017). *Skills assessment Level I and II occupational therapy students* [Assessment]. Emory University Hospital, Emory University Orthopedic Spine Hospital and Emory University Hospital Midtown Rehabilitation Therapy Department Occupational Therapists.

Honey, A., & Penman, M. (2020). "You actually see what occupational therapists do in real life": Outcomes and critical features of first-year practice education placements. *British Journal of Occupational Therapy, 83*(10), 638-647. https://doi.org/10.1177/0308022620920535

Hooper, B., Krishnagiri, S., Price, P., Taff, S. D., & Bilics, A. (2018). Curriculum-level strategies that U.S. occupational therapy programs use to address occupation: A qualitative study. *American Journal of Occupational Therapy, 72*(1), 7201205040. https://doi.org/10.5014/ajot.2918.024190

Hoque, M. E. (2016). Three domains of learning: Cognitive, affective and psychomotor. *The Journal of EFL Education and Research, 2*(2), 45-52.

Kaelin, V. C., & Dancza, K. (2019). Perceptions of occupational therapy threshold concepts by students in role-emerging placements in schools: A qualitative investigation. *Australian Occupational Therapy Journal, 66*(6), 717-719. https://doi.org/10.1111/1440-1630.12610

Schell, B., & Schell, J. (2018). *Clinical Professional Reasoning in Occupational Therapy.* (2nd ed.). Walters Kluwer.

Stutz-Tanenbaum, P., Greene, D., Hanson, D. J., & Koski, J. (2017). Professional reward in the academic fieldwork coordinator role. *American Journal of Occupational Therapy, 71*(2), 7102230010. https://doi.org/10.5014/ajot.2017.022046

Stutz-Tanenbaum, P., Hanson, D., Koski, J. & Greene, D. (2015). Exploring the complexity of the academic fieldwork coordinator role. *Occupational Therapy in Health Care, 29*(2), 139-152. https://doi.org/10.3109/07380577.2015.1017897

APPENDIX A

Reflection Questions Regarding the 2018 ACOTE for the Level I Fieldwork Educator

	ACOTE STANDARD	FIELDWORK EDUCATOR/SITE REFLECTION QUESTIONS
C.1.1.	Ensure that the fieldwork program reflects the sequence and scope of content in the curriculum design, in collaboration with faculty, so that fieldwork experiences in traditional, nontraditional, and emerging settings strengthen the ties between didactic and fieldwork education.	1. Do I know what the academic institution's sequence and scope of content in the curriculum design is? (i.e., What courses do the students take throughout the occupational therapy program? What is the academic program's main threads?) 2. Does your site's mission and roles match up with the academic institute? 3. Is my site/program able to meet the academic institute's fieldwork objectives? 4. Can my site/program measure the student's progress with the fieldwork evaluation form the school/academic institute is using?
C.1.2.	Document the criteria and process for selecting fieldwork sites, to include maintaining memoranda of understanding, complying with all site requirements, maintaining site objectives and site data, and communicating this information to students prior to the start of the fieldwork experience.	1. Do I have a contract/memoranda of understanding with the academic institute? 2. What are my site requirements? 3. Have I filled out a site data form (contains information about my site)?
C.1.3.	Document that academic educators and FWeds agree on established fieldwork objectives prior to the start of the fieldwork experience and communicate with the student and FWed about progress and performance throughout the fieldwork experience. Ensure that fieldwork objectives for all experiences include a psychosocial objective.	1. Have I communicated and collaborated with the academic institute and AFWC regarding my/site's expectations and roles? 2. Have I collaborated with the AFWC on what my site-specific objectives are? 3. Am I communicating with my AFWC on my student's progress and performance throughout the fieldwork? 4. How am I incorporating psychosocial/mental health components in my practice?

	ACOTE STANDARD	FIELDWORK EDUCATOR/SITE REFLECTION QUESTIONS
C.1.4.	Ensure that the ratio of FWeds to students enables proper supervision and provides protection of consumers, opportunities for appropriate role modeling of occupational therapy practice, and the ability to provide frequent assessment of student progress in achieving stated fieldwork objectives.	1. What types of supervision is my facility/site able to provide? (1:1? Group based? 2:1? 1:2?) 2. What support and training am I providing the FWeds at my site?
C.1.5.	Ensure that fieldwork agreements are sufficient in scope and number to allow completion of graduation requirements in a timely manner, in accordance with the policy adopted by the program as required by standard A.4.7.	1. Do I have a signed agreement/contract with the academic institution?
C.1.6.	The program must have evidence of valid memoranda of understanding in effect and signed by both parties from the onset to conclusion of the Level I fieldwork and the Level II fieldwork if it involves an entity outside of the academic program. (Electronic memoranda of understanding and signatures are acceptable.) Responsibilities of the sponsoring institution(s) and each fieldwork site must be clearly documented in the memorandum of understanding.	1. Do I have a signed agreement/contract with the academic institution?
C.1.7.	At least one fieldwork experience (either Level I or Level II) must address practice in behavioral health, or psychological and social factors influencing engagement in occupation.	1. How do I address/take into consideration how behavioral health, psychological, and social factors affect a person's function? 2. What does this look like at my site? 3. What factors do I consider when treating patients? 4. How does this influence my practice? 5. How do I teach my student about these factors?

	ACOTE STANDARD	FIELDWORK EDUCATOR/SITE REFLECTION QUESTIONS
C.1.8.	Ensure that personnel who supervise Level I fieldwork are informed of the curriculum and fieldwork program design and affirm their ability to support the fieldwork experience. This must occur prior to the onset of the Level I fieldwork. Examples include, but are not limited to, currently licensed or otherwise regulated occupational therapists and occupational therapy assistants, psychologists, physician assistants, teachers, social workers, physicians, speech-language pathologists, nurses, and physical therapists.	1. Who are the individuals that would be supervising occupational therapy students at my site? What is their role in my organization? 2. Do my FWeds know and understand my partner academic institution's curriculum? 3. Do my FWeds understand the connection between the fieldwork experience and the academic institute's curriculum? 4. Are the FWeds able to support students at my site?
C.1.9.	Document that Level I fieldwork is provided to students and is not substituted for any part of the Level II fieldwork. Ensure that Level I fieldwork enriches didactic coursework through directed observation and participation in selected aspects of the occupational therapy process, and includes mechanisms for formal evaluation of student performance. The program must have clearly documented student learning objectives expected of the Level I fieldwork. Level I fieldwork may be met through one or more of the following instructional methods: • Simulated environments • Standardized patients • Faculty practice • Faculty-led site visits • Supervision by a FWed in a practice environment All Level I fieldwork must be comparable in rigor.	1. Am I documenting the correct experience (Level I or Level II)? 2. What does the occupational therapy process look like at my site? 3. Am I showing my student what the occupational therapy process looks like at my site? 4. Do I have an evaluation form to assess my student's performance (this is usually provided by the academic institute)? 5. Does the occupational therapy Level I fieldwork experience at my site fall under one of these instructional methods: • Simulated environments • Standardized patients • Faculty practice • Faculty-led site visits • Supervision by a FWed in a practice environment

Adapted from Accreditation Council for Occupational Therapy Education. (2018). *2018 Accreditation Council for Occupational Therapy Education standards and interpretive guide.* https://acoteonline.org/wp-content/uploads/2020/10/2018-ACOTE-Standards.pdf

APPENDIX B

Sample Skills Assessment/Inquiry

The following chart lists common skills used in our acute care practice. Please rate your level of comfort and exposure to the following skills that are currently associated with occupational therapy practice in acute care:

SKILL	LEARNED IN CLASS OR IN OTHER EXPERIENCES BUT PREFER A REVIEW	COMFORTABLE WITH PERFORMING	NOT TAUGHT IN CURRICULUM; NEVER PERFORMED
Basic patient interview			
1. Explain role of occupational therapy			
2. Orientation			
a. Name			
b. Date			
c. Location			
d. Situation			
3. Glasses/hearing aids			
4. Home environment			
a. House/apartment			
b. Number of steps (internal/ external)			
c. Rails (internal/ external)			
d. Outside surfaces to entrance/exit			
e. Assistive devices			
f. Durable medical equipment (raised toilet seat, tub bench/chair)			
g. Prior level of function			
h. Patient/family goal			
Upper extremity active ROM			
Upper extremity passive ROM			
Upper extremity manual muscle testing			
Sensation testing			
Proprioception testing			

SKILL	LEARNED IN CLASS OR IN OTHER EXPERIENCES BUT PREFER A REVIEW	COMFORTABLE WITH PERFORMING	NOT TAUGHT IN CURRICULUM; NEVER PERFORMED
Stereognosis testing			
Vision (acuity, tacking, saccades)			
Functional cognition			
Bed mobility			
a. Positioning			
b. Supine to sit			
c. Rolling, including log rolling			
Functional transfers			
a. Stand pivot			
b. Bed to chair			
c. Chair to chair			
d. Bed to bedside commode			
e. Toilet transfer			
f. Shower transfer			
g. Sliding board transfer			
Self-care assessment			
a. Bathing			
b. Dressing			
c. Grooming			
d. Toileting			
e. Feeding			

SKILL	LEARNED IN CLASS OR IN OTHER EXPERIENCES BUT PREFER A REVIEW	COMFORTABLE WITH PERFORMING	NOT TAUGHT IN CURRICULUM; NEVER PERFORMED
Instruction in adaptive equipment in lower body dressing			
a. Reacher			
b. Dressing stick			
c. Shoe horn			
d. Sock aid			
Vital signs			
a. Blood pressure			
b. Heart rate			
c. Respirations			

Adapted from Hewitt, B. (2017). *Skills assessment Level I and II occupational therapy students* [Assessment]. Emory University Hospital, Emory University Orthopedic Spine Hospital and Emory University Hospital Midtown Rehabilitation Therapy Department Occupational Therapists.

APPENDIX C
Sample of Level I Fieldwork Objectives

The University of Findlay
Occupational Therapy Program
Level I Fieldwork Objectives

OCTH 513 (MOT) & 534 (OTD) Level I Fieldwork A (Pediatric)
OCTH 514 (MOT) & 626 (OTD) Level I Fieldwork B (Adult)

Course objectives for these Level I rotations are the same.

The student will:

1. Use professional terminology and respectful communication when interacting with professionals and clients in the practice setting.

2. Demonstrate clear, concise, grammatically correct style in all written assignments.

3. Identify frame of references used in the assigned practice setting.

4. Describe the characteristics of a frame of reference that would make it appropriate for use with a particular client.

5. Identify the screening and/or assessment tools used in the practice setting.

6. Observe situational variables that impact accurate assessment results in the practice setting.

7. Review environmental modifications and assistive technology used in the practice setting and/or by a specific client.

8. Explain occupational therapy practice to a client or professional in the assigned practice setting.

9. Determine the process used when referring clients to specialists in the community.

10. Follow universal precautions and infection control if asked to participate in clients' treatment.

11. Critically analyze interactions between the occupational therapist, client, family members, and other professionals in the practice setting.

12. Determine the role of specialists in the practice setting.

13. Assess the therapist's therapeutic use of self and grading of occupations through observation during client treatment in the practice setting.

14. Examine the use of client/family education provided by the therapist in the practice setting.

15. Observe the teaching/learning techniques and strategies used by the occupational therapist when educating family members or other professionals.

16. Identify and describe the psychosocial factors that influence client's engagement in occupation.

17. Evaluate the collaborative role between occupational therapists and occupational therapy assistants, if applicable.

18. Assess relationship of stated goals, interventions and outcomes, through observation and questions asked in the practice setting.

19. Determine the procedures and documentation used for termination of treatment in the practice setting.

20. Review the documentation methods and procedures used in the practice setting.

OCTH 660 (MOT) and 702 (OTD) Level I Fieldwork C

Course Description: This Level I fieldwork course OCTH 660–Level I Fieldwork C provides students with an opportunity to observe and explore needs and services in a community setting. Students will identify the psychological and social factors influencing engagement in occupation for populations, groups, and individuals. The community site utilized in this fieldwork placement serves as the basis for other coursework related to community program development and preparation for grant writing. This course will be graded satisfactory/unsatisfactory.

Course Objectives

1. Educate community-based professionals about the role of occupational therapy and the possible benefits occupational therapy services would provide clients in their programs.

2. Identify the mission and philosophy of the community setting.

3. Describe the population and the population needs that are served in the setting.

4. Identify the psychological and social factors that influence the client's engagement in occupations.

5. Identify the environment and contexts in which programming occurs and how they positively and/or negatively impact the client's participation and engagement in programming.

6. Identify the client's areas of occupations being addressed in current programming.

7. Assess the roles and responsibilities of service providers in the community setting.

8. Assess the professional licensure and/or training required by the service providers.

9. Appraise current trends and policies that influence the provision of health and human service in the community setting.

10. Identify funding/reimbursement policies and sources.

11. Compare and contrast community service delivery models with traditional services (i.e. hospital, nursing facility).

12. Identify unmet needs and establish a plan of action to assist the site in investigating various methods to meet those needs.

APPENDIX D
Learning Plan for Addressing
Course Objectives Identified in Appendix C

COURSE OBJECTIVES FOR OTCH 513 AND 514	LEARNING PLAN
Objective 5 Identify the screening and/or assessment tools used in the practice setting.	a. Student is given a list of screening and assessment tools used within facility. b. Student reviews notes for three patients to identify how assessment tools were used to identify treatment goals. c. Student observes an assessment process and interacts with FWed in discussion of how assessment results will influence treatment goals and interventions. d. (Advanced) Student reviews assessment tool in advance of client assessment, participating in administration of selected elements of the assessment.
Objective 6 Observe situational variables that impact accurate assessment results in the practice setting.	a. Student reviews notes for three patients, identifying assessment tools used and how situational variables might have impacted accurate results. b. Student observes an assessment process by an occupational therapist or a different health professional and identifies situational variables that might have impacted assessment results. Student discusses observations with FWed. c. Student participates in selected aspects of assessment administration. Upon assessment completion, student writes reflection identifying situational variables that might have impacted accurate assessment results.

Objective 7	a. Student observes three different treatment interventions, identifying environmental modifications and assistive technology used.
Review environmental modifications and assistive technology used in the practice setting and/or by a specific client.	
	b. Student engages in discussion with three different occupational therapist practitioners as to environmental modifications and assistive technologies used in their practice.
	c. Student observes an intervention provided to a specific client involving assistive technology and notes effect of technology on occupational participation.
	d. Student assists in testing of assistive technology use to improve occupational performance of specific client.
	e. (Advanced) After observing client occupational performance, student investigates assistive technology or environmental modification that may benefit client and provides information to treating therapist.
COURSE OBJECTIVE FOR OTCH 660	**LEARNING PLAN FOR OTCH 660**
Objective 3	a. Student reviews program documents to identify common populations served in setting.
Describe the population and the population needs that are served in the setting.	
	b. Student informally interviews at least five treatment providers or their clients to identify their perspectives on services they are providing or obtaining in the setting.
	c. Student observes occupational therapy practitioner providing client interventions, and identifies population needs served. Student discusses perspectives with FWed.
	d. Student observes an intake process, identifying needs identified and services provided to address needs.
	e. Student reviews documentation records for several clients and identifies general population needs addressed. Student discusses with FWed their observations.

Objective 4 Identify the psychological and social factors that influence the client's engagement in occupations.	a. Student discusses with FWed the psychological and social factors that influence client's engagement in occupations. b. Student observes interventions provided, noting psychological and social factors that influence client's engagement. c. Student observes and then assists FWed in engaging clients in occupations. Following intervention, student discusses with FWed their observations as to factors influencing client engagement in intervention session. d. (Advanced) Student co-plans with FWed an intervention session, taking into account psychological and social factors influencing client engagement in occupations.
Objective 5 Identify the environment and contexts in which programming occurs and how they positively and/or negatively impact the client's participation and engagement in programming.	a. Student observes an individual and a group intervention session provided to the same client. Student identifies how the environment/context influenced client participation/engagement. b. Student identifies differences in client response to interventions provided in a secluded vs. an open physical environment and discusses observations with FWed. c. Individually or in pairs, students develop a list of questions and discuss with client or client caregiver the impact of the environment/context on the client's participation/engagement in programming. d. Student assists therapist in provision of intervention services to the same client or group of clients in two different environment/contexts, sharing observations with FWed as to the impact of environment/context on client engagement. e. (Advanced) Student co-plans with FWed for programming that will modify environment/context to positively impact client engagement. Student assists FWed in provision of programming and discuss results.

Unit III

Situational Topics in Level I Fieldwork Learning

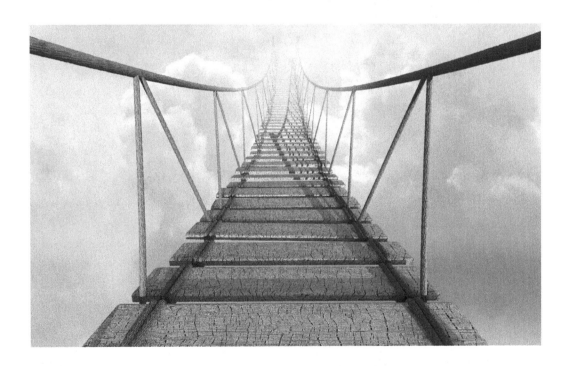

9

Taking Advantage of Emerging Learning Opportunities Onsite

Rebecca L. Simon, EdD, OTR/L, FAOTA

Level I fieldwork is a time for students to practice many of the skills they have learned in the classroom in the *real world*. While previous chapters have described how a fieldwork educator (FWed) can prepare in advance for student success, this chapter will look at the *in-the-moment* experiences that happen when students are in the field. As occupational therapists, we are skilled at improvisation and are able to take the changing and sometimes challenging environment and mold it as a meaningful, therapeutic moment for our clients. The examples provided in this chapter will further explore the same concept but focus on using available opportunities to extend the learning of students. It is the role of the FWed to both model for the student, as well as to let them experience the moment, react, and reflect afterward. These teachable moments are sometimes equally as valuable, if not more valuable, than preplanned student learning experiences.

This chapter will focus on attending to those serendipitous fieldwork moments which may have a significant impact on students, yet cannot be planned in advance. Just as we cannot predict the *a-ha* moments with our patients or clients, we often cannot predict those that occur with our students. Using an understanding of adult learning and examples from practice, this chapter aims to support aspects of the Intentional Fieldwork Education Model (IFWEM; Crawford & Hanner, 2019) while defining and providing specific examples of how one might look for and capitalize on the *here and now* moments.

Hanson, D., & DeIuliis, E. D. (Eds.).
Fieldwork Educator's Guide to Level I Fieldwork (pp. 269-289).
© 2023 Taylor and Francis Group.

LEARNING OBJECTIVES

By the end of reading this chapter and completing the learning activities, the reader should be able to:

1. Understand the importance of spontaneous interactions and how they can lead to new learning.

2. Apply techniques to engage students in the learning process as situations present themselves.

3. Provide direct feedback in a way that fosters student learning.

4. Evaluate appropriate methods of reflection that can be utilized to enhance learning.

SERENDIPITOUS INTERACTIONS

While many planned activities can occur on fieldwork (as described in Unit II of this book), it is the unplanned moments that happen during the day-to-day of life as a therapist that sometimes have a large impact on professional development, clinical reasoning, and setting-specific learning. In the academic setting, it is understood that students are not simply "recipients of facts" but assemblers of knowledge (Hooper, 2006, p. 21). This also applies to fieldwork and really means that a FWed cannot just tell a student what they need to know but must allow them to begin to put important pieces of information together as they occur. Students need the opportunity to experience things as they happen, as part of the unwritten agenda of fieldwork, and try to make sense of it all.

As therapists, we understand that serendipitous interactions can assist students in the process of piecing ideas, practice, and reality together to form a bigger picture, which lends to better understanding and their ability to grow as a therapist and professional. It is often after these *off the cuff* and unexpected experiences that students are able to realize their interaction style, confidence, or areas of growth. It is within these experiences that they develop more awareness about how they will react in unexpected situations and what their natural style of interaction may be. It is important to process this with them and assist each student in developing a detailed awareness of their professional self.

Aligned with a key cornerstone of the occupational therapy profession, fieldwork education should also be viewed through a person-centered lens. Students should be treated as individuals who have emerging abilities that can be brought forth through facilitated interaction, guidance, and reflection (Vygotsky, 1980). As seen in Figure 9-1, the IFWEM, also known as the Intentional Fieldwork Education Model (Crawford & Hanner, 2019) modernizes this approach and focuses on the importance of collaborative relationships, effective communication, and feedback. With foundations in intentional learning, this model addresses both the end product of learning, as well as the learning process itself (Blumschein, 2012).

Four primary elements are emphasized: (1) day-to-day interactions; (2) direct experience with clients; (3) feedback; and (4) reflection. With these elements in mind, FWeds should be prepared for the learning opportunities that spontaneously occur during **day-to-day interactions** and allow for immediate **feedback** (Johnson Coffelt & Gabriel, 2017) while supporting teachable moments through **reflection**.

With the IFWEM (Crawford & Hanner, 2019) in mind, Level I FWeds can utilize serendipitous interactions to promote growth and the development of clinical reasoning, professional behaviors, and competence with basic therapeutic skill required on Level I fieldwork. The guidance of the skilled therapist (and sometimes the client) enhances the learning experience and allows the students to not only apply what they learn in school to fieldwork but also to apply what is learned on fieldwork in school. Capitalizing on these spontaneous interactions between students, clients, and professionals, providing immediate educator feedback, and supporting self-reflection will be the focus of this chapter.

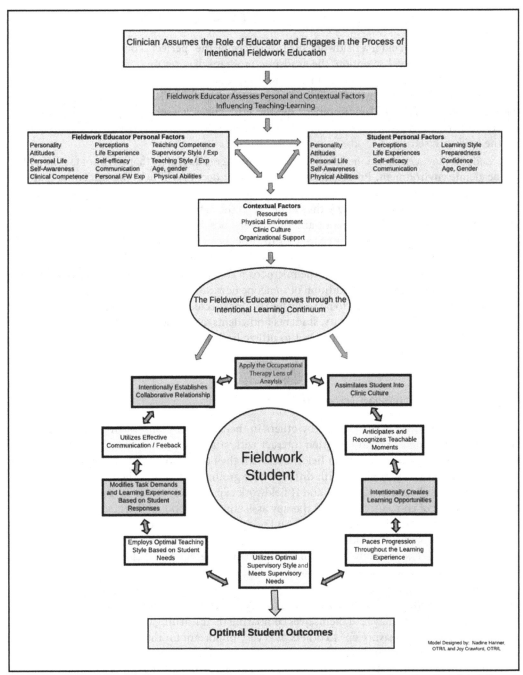

Figure 9-1. The Intentional Fieldwork Education Model. (Reproduced with permission from Crawford, E. J., & Hanner, N. [2019, February]. *The intentional fieldwork educator: Applying the intentional fieldwork education model [IFWEM].* University of St. Augustine for Health Sciences. https://soar.usa.edu/cgi/viewcontent.cgi?article=1010&context=ot.)

DAY-TO-DAY INTERACTIONS

Students can often enter a fieldwork site influenced by the "perfect" conditions of the academic institution. With good intention, the academic program may set up opportunities for positive interactions within contrived environments that lend to neat and clean case studies with obvious issues that can be resolved hypothetically. Once on Level I fieldwork, students may notice differences between the real world environment and the academic one, especially when interacting with others who may be unpredictable or just simply different from what they expected when preparing for the fieldwork setting.

Students may see practitioners, other students, or clients do things that were not taught within the academic environment. Processing the reaction that occurs will help the student prepare for the realities of a clinical or community environment. It is important to entertain open and honest discussion with the student to ensure they understand the nature of the interaction, the unpredictability of working with other humans, and the importance of being honest and humble, learning from each. FWeds should also be prepared for the unexpected interactions that may occur simply by introducing the new, yet temporary, individual (fieldwork student) into their setting.

As occupational therapists know, the microcosm of an organization has a culture of its own and jostling of the norm with an addition of someone new can create a bit of chaos. While this can be easily settled, the FWed needs to be ready for the unexpected interactions that can occur. These interactions can be between students, students and clients, and students and other professionals. As a FWed, it is important to be prepared to utilize both positive and negative interactions as a learning experience for all.

Student-to-Student Interactions

Students are typically surrounded by others in their own programs during the didactic portion of their programs and do not often interact with students with different perspectives from other programs until they go out on fieldwork. With the occupational therapy profession having multiple points of entry, students with different backgrounds often find themselves on fieldwork together. This can be a mix of Level I and II fieldwork experiences, as well as a mix of educational levels and points of entry (occupational therapy assistant, occupational therapy bachelor's, master of science in occupational therapy [MSOT], and occupational therapy doctorate [OTD]). This mix offers the perfect opportunity for students to learn from each other, receive feedback, and gather new perspectives. The spontaneous learning occurring together in a fieldwork situation can be very positive yet also can present some challenges.

From a positive perspective, students are exposed to or explore different ways of thinking about the same client or situation. Alternately, the introduction of sharing space and resources can be a challenge. Students may find themselves comparing their learning to other students onsite and wondering how they "measure up" to others. It is very important for the FWed to be acutely aware of the possible teachable moments that will arise from multiple students, as well as the challenge and conflict that may rear its head. If the FWed notices an exemplar behavior of a student, pointing this out to the other students may reinforce positive behaviors and set an example of expectations, *or* it may make the other students feel inadequate. The educator should be cautious not to overly praise one or two students while ignoring others, but there are times where these moments can and should be used as a demonstrable model. Most times this type of peer modeling interaction should be followed up by a group or individual discussion to reflect not only on what was done correctly, but why and how it may be replicated by all. If the educator can use these experiences as learning moments, all will depart fieldwork having learned quite a bit about the realities of practice and their role within a team in a very pragmatic way (Box 9-1).

Box 9-1

CASE EXAMPLE ONE

Milania, Georgia, Chloe, and Luis are Level I fieldwork students in an inpatient mental health hospital. They are from a variety of schools and a mix of academic levels. Thomas, their FWed, is on the floor with them running a group. He notices Georgia and Chloe have come to the group prepared and ready with all materials. He mentions this when they arrive, in front of the other students, and compliments them on their preparedness. Georgia and Chloe confidently begin the group, which requires a multistep art project.

During the group, Chloe notices that one of the clients, who speaks primarily Spanish, is struggling to understand one of the tasks. She sits next to the client and begins to help interpret English into Spanish. Milania sits quietly observing. Meanwhile Luis, who stated he was feeling lost initially, is walking around from person to person. While he is not engaging verbally, he is monitoring the task and assisting the clients in retrieving items and helping with materials as needed. Thomas compliments him verbally, in front of the group, for assisting. He once again thanks Georgia and Chloe at the end of the group for their preparedness and has the clients clap for them.

At the end of the group, Milania is feeling a bit self-conscious because she did not hear the praise Thomas gave to the other students. She recognizes that she needs to be as prepared as Georgia and Chloe when she runs the group with Thomas next week and knows that they will need to be more interactive based on what Thomas has said to the group. Luis feels confident that he has been helpful based on the praise from his educator but knows he and Milania need to work together to be as organized as Chloe and Georgia were. These feelings were all based on the observations of the FWed and other students. Of course, Georgia and Chloe exit the group feeling great and whisper that they hope Milania and Luis will be able to pull it together next week, especially since Milania "just sat there."

Interactions on fieldwork are sometimes obviously positive or negative, and the students may reach out to the FWed for assistance or guidance, allowing discourse and open communication. However, there are also times where the FWed must step in to assist the group in understanding the interaction, why it happened, and what can be learned. In this case, *debriefing* can be quite helpful to maximize student learning and process the interactions in a different, more positive way.

Debriefing is generally defined as communication after events of care that allows improvement of future performance through group reflection on the shared experience (Kessler et al., 2015). Debriefing is commonly used in medical practice as well as post-simulation for training in both physical and occupational therapy education (Shoemaker et al., 2011). Debriefing provides long-lasting results and can be composed of simple interactions between the FWed and student (Mackenzie, 2002), individually or as a group. In Case Example One (see Box 9-1), group debriefing guided by the FWed can provide clarity on interactions, learning preferences, and how each party participated vs. allowing the students to form their own conclusions, which may be erroneous and lead to division between them. It also encourages students to follow the example of open dialogue set by the FWed. This type of *debriefing as you go* is equally as important to student learning as providing the student with direct, private opportunities for debriefing and feedback on their actions for corrective purposes. For example, had the previously described debriefing session not happened, each student would potentially have left with a very different opinion of the student participants, and the clients may not have benefitted as much the next session (Box 9-2).

> **Box 9-2**
> ## ACADEMIC FIELDWORK EDUCATOR TIP
>
> While it is easier to predict group roles and interaction styles when you place students from your program together, it is important to prepare students to self-reflect and talk to other students about learning styles when they are with students from other programs. Awareness of leadership, group roles, and learning styles are helpful tools for both Level I and II fieldwork placements. Sending students with this information or including it in the student packet is quite helpful to FWeds for planning learning activities but also to prepare them for situations where they need to manage multiple students' interactions.

DIRECT EXPERIENCE WITH CLIENTS

While students have the intention of building rapport and developing a therapeutic relationship with clients without issue; in reality, they may experience something completely different. The client may refuse therapy, be argumentative, have different lifestyle choices, or be disagreeable in general. These experiences can be used as learning moments in which the student can grow and develop their therapeutic use of self and intentional relationship building with the client, even in a nonideal situation. Interpersonal events that occur naturally can be emotionally charged, producing strong feelings from all parties (Taylor, 2020a).

Challenging interactions can be as powerful as the rewarding interactions. Teaching students in these moments can lead to future growth by shaping the interaction in a positive way and learning from exploration of various aspects of communication with clients. For example, if a client demonstrates a behavior that is undesirable, and perhaps unexpected, the FWed can capitalize on this moment to model proper behaviors and ways to handle the situation. Since Level I fieldwork is generally short in duration, the student may not get the opportunity to see the client again in an opportune situation, so even the experience of observing the skilled occupational therapy practitioner handling a negative behavior may assist them in future interactions (Box 9-3).

When challenging interpersonal issues arise, **modeling** can provide the student with an example of exemplary behavior. While the previous example was resolved relatively easily, some interactions require more work and even more debriefing afterward. If clients do or say something hurtful or display cultural insensitivity, students will need help depersonalizing the event. It is important to create a safe space for the student to discuss the event (Whitgob et al., 2016). The FWed needs to help the student unpack the situation to understand that the nature of therapy is sometimes to work with those who think very differently from the way we do. It is important to make time, in those situations, to assist the student in understanding the nature of therapy; this is also another instance where debriefing may be beneficial to the student. Taylor (2020b) describes therapeutic modes as a source of interpersonal interaction. The modes include advocating, empathizing, collaborating, encouraging, instructing, and problem solving (Taylor, 2020b, p. 83). Each has its unique phrases and practical applications and can be selected based on the situation. Taylor (2020b) notes that therapists facing difficult client behavior typically use the therapeutic modes of instructing and problem solving. Each of these can be direct, active, and require a questioning approach. Helping students to understand why a FWed might be more directive when obstacles arise is important for the unpacking that must be done when these events happen. Reviewing the modes of interaction to find what the student relies on in challenging situations may make the student more comfortable. Students will often model the FWed, but if their style and mode of interaction is different, that needs to be discussed. It is an important step to gaining a deeper understanding of the student's interpersonal style to discuss and possibly role play various methods of interaction with challenging clients.

Box 9-3

Case Example Two

Jillian, a second year MSOT student, is walking into a client's room in a skilled nursing facility with her FWed, Sam. Sam has told Jillian that Mrs. Simonelli is a wonderful client who loves cooking and use of the kitchen has been a positive motivator for therapy.

Upon arriving in the room, Mrs. Simonelli sees Jillian and immediately comments on her hair (which is long, braided, and ombreé) and a visible piercing. Mrs. Simonelli tells Sam that she doesn't feel comfortable working with some "hippie" who clearly "smokes pot" and will not know a thing about being in the kitchen. Jillian retreats and begins to defend herself, but Sam steps in and smiles calmly at Mrs. Simonelli.

Sam gently inquires about her experiences with hippies, and why she thinks they can't cook. With a smile, Sam also tells the client that Jillian has a lovely pasta recipe, which they were hoping to share. Sam also asks Jillian to tell the client a little about her plan, what it will be working on, and why she decided to choose it as a "special" activity for Mrs. Simonelli since it was her grandmother's recipe which she has made several times. As Mrs. Simonelli smiles and relaxes a bit, Sam also tells the client that Jillian purchased the items for the session on her own even though she works while in school, and it was a challenge to collect all necessary materials.

Mrs. Simonelli seems surprised by this and states that she is impressed that Jillian has made it before, works, and goes to school. She says she likes to "joke" and tells Sam she will give the young "whippersnapper" a chance. Jillian feels more confident and tells Mrs. Simonelli how happy she is to work together. As she walks to the kitchen, Mrs. Simonelli tells Jillian how much her hair has changed over the years and mentions that she misses being able to braid her hair as she did when she was younger. She even jokes about asking her hairdresser to do her hair in the same colors Jillian has in hers so they can be twins. The student suggests that they work on some different independent hair grooming techniques for the next session since that might be meaningful to her. Sam thinks this is a great idea and lets Mrs. Simonelli know they will plan it.

As they enter the kitchen, the client stops to tell Jillian that she should consider removing her piercing. Jillian now has the confidence to answer and lets the Mrs. Simonelli know it has special meaning to her. With that said, Mrs. Simonelli begins unpacking the ingredients for the pasta. They continue with the session leaving the words, which were initially hurtful, in the past.

When things do not go as planned (e.g., client refuses, someone vomits, a colostomy bag explodes), the FWed's response to these interactions is valuable to the student. The ability to be flexible is contagious, and it is extremely important to be flexible in action and thinking as an occupational therapist in unpredictable situations. Hvenegaard (2011) asserts that students gain a more well-rounded education when they have opportunity to learn skills and gain insights through experiential learning in real time. While self-assessment, supervisory assessment, and structured preparation are important, spontaneous opportunities and interactions can provide direct learning toward the objectives on fieldwork. Anticipating these unexpected interactions and using them as learning moments lends to significant learning.

Box 9-4

CASE EXAMPLE THREE

Roger, an occupational therapy student, is placed in a Level I fieldwork experience with a Level II occupational therapy student as one of his FWeds. They are also working on an outpatient team with a physical therapist, a physical therapy student, and a physical therapist assistant student. With flu season, the caseload is down, and there are not as many patients present in the times when Roger is there.

In the downtime, Roger asks the physical therapist as many questions as he does the occupational therapy student who is supervising. Roger often eats lunch with the physical therapist and physical therapist assistant, as well as the occupational therapy student, and they discuss the events of the day and break down some of the differences between the professions and even the occupational therapy program philosophies between the two schools present onsite.

His FWed is a little worried about Roger's experience due to the low caseload and contacts the academic fieldwork coodinator (AFWC) at his school to determine how they might improve going forward.

The AFWC is surprised and tells him that Roger has many clinical examples to share in class and often talks about multiple aspects of clients he has seen. Upon engaging further, Roger tells the AFWC that it was the discussions he had at lunch that were most important. He felt that the safe space between students and the positive feedback he witnessed between the physical therapist and occupational therapist were uplifting and inspiring. Roger reports he would now like to return to a setting for Level II fieldwork that will allow him to have the same intercollegiate experiences, supervisory experiences, and as many interprofessional experiences as possible.

Interprofessional Interactions

One of the best features of fieldwork, either Level I or II, is interacting with other professionals and students from other professions. Interprofessional education and interprofessional collaboration in practice are considered essential to the growth and development of team-based and leadership skills for the occupational therapy practitioner. Interprofessional education is defined as "students from two or more professions learn about, from, and with each other to enable effective collaboration and improve health outcomes" (World Health Organization, 2010, p. 7), and interprofessional collaborative practice is "when multiple health workers from different professional backgrounds work together with patients, families, health care workers, and communities to deliver the highest quality of care" (World Health Organization, 2010, p. 7). Having the opportunity to experience each of these through interaction and observation on Level I fieldwork can create meaningful spontaneous learning opportunities. The FWed should be attuned to these interactions and acknowledge their importance as they occur, not only with the client but with each other.

In Case Example Three (Box 9-4), it is the discussion and debriefing between professions, and even between students, that has been most important. A FWed should attempt to be involved in these conversations as much as possible, but it is also the organic nature of intra- and interprofessional discussions that can sometimes be more of a learning moment than seeing clients. The conversations that take place on fieldwork help students to learn about other professions and see things from a different perspective. FWeds do not always have to make time for formal supervision to make a lasting impact.

BOX 9-5

CASE EXAMPLE FOUR

Marie has been an occupational therapy assistant in a school system for 5 years and is now enrolled in a bridge to MSOT program. She is on her adult rehabilitation Level I fieldwork experience and is working with a team of occupational, physical, and speech therapists. Marie has spent the morning observing her FWed, Joan, assess a client with a right cerebrovascular accident. In a staff meeting later that day, Joan mentions the client needs a swallow study and further cognitive assessment before returning home.

The speech-language pathologist in the room whispers loudly to the physical therapist that she is surprised the client isn't on her caseload. She says she cannot understand why the occupational therapist has not referred the client to her and wonders "what is up with that?" Marie is in awe because in the school system where she worked, the therapists worked as a team and referral (or lack thereof) was never an issue. Marie's FWed looks directly at the speech-language pathologist and explains that she should bring any concerns to her directly vs. speaking to a peer in the meeting.

The room becomes quiet and Joan gently, but firmly, explains that she is quite capable of completing the necessary cognitive assessment and that the swallow study is being required by the doctor as part of their return to home protocol. No issues were noted in the evaluation. Marie nods silently as she knows her FWed watched her client eat earlier, and they discussed that she did not think she needed further assessment. The speech-language pathologist looks sheepish and apologizes for not being more direct, stating she was just making a point and didn't mean for it to sound the way it did. The physical therapist then joked aloud to Marie that they are actually a really cohesive team, unless there was a "shoulder to fight for." Everyone laughed.

Later, Marie and Joan discuss the situation and unpack how conflict sometimes arises on a team, even when it isn't meant to be negative. Marie mentioned her experience in school systems was very different, but she appreciated how the tension in the room was cut by humor. Marie also mentioned that she liked how Joan handled the situation and made it about the client, not about the therapists. Joan also reminded Marie that tensions can sometimes be higher based on their current productivity expectations, so everyone is trying to work on increasing their own caseload. Joan also tells Marie that the professional disagreement did not hurt their personal relationship and that she and the speech-language pathologist will most likely get together and talk more at lunch tomorrow. Marie left with a different understanding of the team dynamic and was able to reflect on the dynamics with her classmates later that week.

In addition to their own personal interactions, students may also be able to observe the day-to-day camaraderie and team approach between professionals while onsite. Some students may expect competition between therapists, and students might be surprised to see how challenges can be worked through positively, as long as all parties understand each other's perspectives. This happens spontaneously in the work environment, and students should be encouraged to discuss and reflect on how the culture of the facility and shared team approach is important. It is a hidden aspect of fieldwork that is not always as obvious since we tend to provide client-focused learning. It is also important for students to mirror positive behavior as they, at times, may feel competitive with the other students onsite. If a FWed is attentive to the group dynamic, a positive outcome can be reached. If there is tension, it is better to address it in-the-moment and utilize it as a learning experience vs. waiting for the teachable moment to pass. The example in Box 9-5 illustrates how a tense situation between professionals can become a learning moment for the student and a positive experience for all involved.

Box 9-6

ACADEMIC FIELDWORK COORDINATOR TIP

Be sure your FWeds **and** students are aware of your expectations for interactive learning. Sometimes it is easy to fall into an observation only situation on Level I fieldwork. If they know your expectations initially, it is easier to begin dialogue to enhance experience. If Case Example One or Case Example Two had been observation only, the students would not have been able to modify their interactions and come out better prepared for a more independent Level II fieldwork experience.

The open conversation in Case Example Four (see Box 9-5), along with the observation, will allow Marie to frame the interaction differently than if she had just observed it without a response or further discussion. Marie's FWed set an example by being firm, but kind, and not allowing the conflict to take over the meeting. The educator also gave Marie a chance to unpack the situation and discuss the differences in settings and the reasons for some behaviors she may have seen. Instead of ignoring the situation, or "letting it slide," the educator took the time to demonstrate and reflect on professional interactions and what makes for positive conflict resolution.

Although most students have been (or will be) exposed to different professionals and disciplines within their educational programs within a contrived, positive environment, the reality of team dynamics in less than perfect conditions is important to see. Students need to be prepared to advocate for their role as an occupational therapy practitioner, as well as working toward becoming a strong, positive member of a team with other professionals. The interactions that occur spontaneously may bring stress or disagreement, but students need to see that it can be dealt with professionally. This important impromptu interaction can become a teachable moment and is, once again, a reminder that interactions are an unpredictable, yet important, part of our lives as occupational therapy practitioners.

PROVIDING DIRECT FEEDBACK

While FWeds are asked to provide written feedback to students on Level I fieldwork experiences via evaluation mechanisms, real-time, direct feedback is a valuable tool for teaching and learning. de Beer and Mårtensson (2015) found that students' clinical reasoning skills improved more when the feedback was accompanied by direct suggestions on how to improve, which can easily happen in the course of spontaneous events occurring during Level I fieldwork. Constructive feedback focused on specific skills assisted the students in respecting the viewpoint of the FWed and improved overall learning (de Beer & Mårtensson, 2015). Simply providing corrective feedback is not enough to elicit change. Students respond to timely, specific suggestions using real-time components and suggestions for change. For example, if a student is hesitant to touch a client during an activities of daily living interaction, the FWed must not only provide feedback of the importance of therapeutic touch after the session but must direct the student in-the-moment. The FWed can use a variety of direct feedback methods including a hand-over-hand guidance, a verbal prompt to touch the client, or even a direction on how to move the client's body if needed. The student must understand that they need to be in-the-moment with the FWed and client and not simply a passive observer during the session (Box 9-6).

While on Level I fieldwork, students are often called upon to improvise under the direction of someone with experience, knowledge, and skill. As they begin to understand the big picture, students must piece together moments in time to make meaningful use of the experiences and begin to transform their thinking.

TABLE 9-1
THE FIVE STEPS TO THE ONE-MINUTE PRECEPTOR

Ask a question that requires a firm answer (*"Why do you think Juan is losing his balance?"*)

Ask follow-up questions (*"Are there any medications that may be contributing to his unsteady gait?"*)

Teach a general rule (*"We usually like to look at the medication side effects to rule out any other causes."*)

Identify specific behaviors that the student did well (*"You did a nice job asking questions about his home environment and any obstacles to balance."*)

Correct mistakes (*"A quick chart review may have told you that he was placed on a pain medication that might have caused a temporary loss of balance vs. chronic condition."*)

Adapted from Neher, J. O., Gordon, K. C., Meyer, B., & Stevens, N. (1992). A five-step "microskills" model of clinical teaching. *Journal of the American Board of Family Practice, 5*(4), 419-424. https://doi.org/10.3122/jabfm.5.4.419.

Hooper (2006) challenges us to surpass the technical skills required for occupational therapy practice and assist the students to embrace the tensions and variability that often come with the role of occupational therapy practitioner. This is where the unexpected moments of fieldwork can be utilized to discover the learning content that enhances clinical reasoning, professional skills, and client-centered practice. Using the serendipitous moments to assist the flow of knowledge will empower students to engage in learning and build their professional and clinical skills. FWeds can use models of teaching that can guide students to learn from these experiences in a more organized way. While many exist, a popular model, the One-Minute Preceptor (Neher et al., 1992), can help to organize these feedback experiences.

The One-Minute Preceptor

While many teaching strategies might be applied within Level I fieldwork, a widely accepted strategy to provide feedback efficiently is the One-Minute Preceptor (Neher et al., 1992). Each step of this model is meant to bring awareness and understanding to the student about their actions and help the student to utilize the feedback to improve. When this method is used, students tend to provide high ratings to supervisors and often describe learning more than expected (Gatewood et al., 2020). Using concepts from the One-Minute Preceptor (Neher et al., 1992), students should be encouraged to be independent but receive appropriate follow-up after a clinical event. FWeds can use questioning to understand their perspective but still identify areas of improvement and give specific direction, if needed, to avoid future errors. See Table 9-1 for a scenario using the One-Minute Preceptor Approach.

Allowing the student to struggle a little before jumping in to provide support is one strategy that can be frustrating yet beneficial. FWeds have an ethical responsibility to their clients to keep them safe and progressing in therapy, but a moment of struggle for the student will not thwart that effort. Instead of jumping in to "save them," the FWed may choose to give space in-the-movement and let the student self-correct. Again, the One-Minute Preceptor supports reinforcing what was done well and making corrections, but in certain circumstances, the student's learning is better served if it is done after the student is allowed the freedom to perform a little trial and error, even if the One-Minute-Preceptor is used as a follow-up (Box 9-7).

BOX 9-7

CASE EXAMPLE FIVE

Sam, the occupational therapy assistant, is observing his student Joni (completing her final Level I fieldwork placement) working with a family in the home during an early intervention visit. She has been with Sam for several visits with this family, and he thinks she is ready for a direct intervention experience. She plans the treatment, they review it, and she is ready to go.

Joni is positioning the 6-month-old on her stomach over a ball to build strength while reaching for a toy held at eye level. The baby does not like this position and begins to resist by crying. Then screaming. The parents are watching the treatment session, and Joni is looking to Sam for help. Sam has to make the decision to hold off on saving Joni since the child is fine, but resistant to the position. Sam chooses to give Joni the space to continue to try to calm the child. She removes the ball and places the child in prone on a blanket. The child continues to cry, and once again, Joni looks at him for help. Sam tells the family that the resistance is due to her weakness and that even though this is not a preferred position, it is an important one.

Joni feels more confident about her choice to keep the baby in prone and continues to work on positioning the child, even with the resistance. The baby calms and reaches for preferred item, which Joni has now offered her. This in-the-movement experience of learning to adjust was important to Joni. She was able to realize that a small shift in her intervention made the difference, and the child could still work on what was needed. Her confidence is higher, and she feels ready to discuss what happened after the session is over.

Using the One-Minute Preceptor Model, after exiting the home, Sam **asks** her why she thinks the ball was an issue. He then asks her **follow-up questions** about what other methods could be used to grade the activity going forward. He also **teaches** Joni that it is helpful to explain what is happening to the family so they don't become concerned as the child is crying. He **identifies that she did a great job** persisting, adjusting, and bringing in a preferred toy. He also reviews how to **correct her mistake** by explaining why it is important to keep the family invested and knowledgeable about what is happening to their child.

While the feedback and correction were able to occur in detail after the session, Sam also gently guided her within the session without jumping in to position the child himself. In this way, Sam protected his client yet educated all present effortlessly and followed up in more detail after the fact.

Task-Level Feedback

While a slow, deliberate method of providing feedback is an effective strategy in many cases, there are times that the nature of the interaction requires immediate correction without following the steps identified in Table 9-1. For instance, if the student is required to plan an activity, and all goes well, the steps can be utilized easily. Yet, as we all know, the intervention plan may need to be adjusted quickly based on a myriad of reasons and may need to be immediately adjusted with direct intervention by the FWed if safety is a factor. This task-level feedback is specific to the issue at hand and should not contain higher processing since it is often not generalizable and specific to the error, or scenario, at hand (Brooks et al., 2019). When this happens, the FWed still needs to provide follow-up knowing that the student may feel vulnerable and inadequate. The FWed may need to walk the student through the error, unpack the reasoning behind it so it does not happen again, and also help the student to recognize that this error is not solely representative of their abilities.

Box 9-8

CASE EXAMPLE SIX

Maria, the occupational therapy student in her last week of Level I fieldwork, attempts to help the certified nurse assistant with a transfer. The patient is status-post a hip replacement. Maria is about to allow a movement that is restricted due to the postoperative precautions. Tonya, the FWed who was standing nearby, immediately tells her to "STOP" and runs over to assist in the transfer. During this event, there is no time for Tonya to slowly explain what Maria did correctly and incorrectly. The fact that the motion might hurt the client is more important than providing slow and kind feedback. The firm words may embarrass or cause Maria to feel stress, especially in front of the client, but it is what Tonya needed to do.

Mastery leads to self-esteem, and for some students, the need for intervention in-the-movement may leave them feeling deflated. FWeds can, through direct feedback with support, foster a growth mindset in which the error is viewed as a learning moment instead of a failure. The hope is that the student is able to accept the feedback without deflecting or becoming self-defensive (Forsythe & Johnson, 2017). To do this, FWeds simply need to provide follow-up to the correction using a variety of methods, rewarding improvement rather than results, and focusing on the reward instead of the risk (Briggs, 2019; Box 9-8).

In Case Example Six (see Box 9-8), the direct task-related feedback was essential and will assist the student in not making the same mistake twice. However, to further reinforce her learning and create generalization, it is appropriate to provide correction and ask the student to take responsibility for her learning, perhaps even producing evidence on proper techniques that could have been applied to the client. Following up with feedback and, if possible, giving the student another chance with the same, or similar, situation will reinforce this learning and provides a sense of mastery and self-esteem for Maria. The communication provided after the incident is also necessary in that it reinforces Tonya's desire to enhance learning instead of judging Maria based on one instance.

de Beer and Mårtensson (2015) note that students' clinical reasoning skills improve through corrective feedback *if accompanied by* suggestions on how to improve. Students, however, often note that they experience FWeds' written and face-to-face feedback as predominantly critical or negative (de Beer & Mårtensson, 2015). A common misconception from students is that the FWed only focuses on areas of improvement needed. Balance may be reached if FWeds are able to use multiple forms of feedback with a growth mindset approach, following up as necessary and reinforcing strengths, learning opportunities, and other positive observations that happen organically during the Level I fieldwork experience.

LEARNING THROUGH REFLECTION

Reflection is a tool that can be used in multiple ways and can take many forms. Occupational therapy practitioners use reflective practice when they explore the thoughts, assumptions, and gaps in knowledge they may have and learn to build on an experience for self-improvement. Occupational therapy practitioners value reflection and agree that its purpose is to learn from experience in order to become a successful, self-directed learner (Knightbridge, 2019). Helping students understand the importance of reflection on Level I fieldwork experiences will help them to recognize the value reflection may have for future practice experiences.

Self-Reflection

Self-reflection is a tool that is foundational to adult learning. It aids in the development of professional behaviors and lifelong learning (Iliff et al., 2019). Using the metacognitive skill of self-reflection is quite useful and assists students at all levels in developing an awareness of their skills. Dunn et al. (2019) found that metacognitive awareness does not differ significantly between first-year occupational therapy assistant, occupational therapy, and OTD students; therefore, self-reflection can be utilized early in the educational process for all levels of the profession. Iliff et al. (2019) found that use of reflection expands the thinking of Level II fieldwork occupational therapy students in many ways. The participants valued the use of reflection to enhance their feelings of competence and decision making. This self-awareness is a critical step in learning to learn and grow. Beginning this in the Level I fieldwork experience can prepare students to utilize a variety of skills later in their academic and professional experiences.

When working with individuals with generational differences, it is also helpful to become aware of their specific needs and learning style as a group, as well as individually. Resources such as those presented in DeIuliis and Saylor (2021) can be quite useful in discovering strategies to optimize professional relationships with Generations Y and Z. Exploring implicit biases bidirectionally is also an important step in understanding communication style, and how different it may need to be with each student supervised.

As self-reflection can assist the student to build upon prior knowledge and experience (American Occupational Therapy Association, 2018), the FWed should cherish the moments of unplanned, *on the spot* learning and help the students reflect immediately following the experience to assist them in identifying their strengths and needs (Box 9-9). This may help them better move forward from that point in time.

In Case Example Seven (see Box 9-9), Matthew is able to use a simple form of self-reflection that has a big impact on the clients and even the FWed. Just by offering the opportunity to think and plan a session independently on Level I fieldwork, the FWed encourages critical thinking and therapeutic use of self. The in-the-movement decision Jason made to ask Matthew why he chose the activity and subsequently not modify Matthew's activity was important and led to a deeper level of learning and excitement. Self-reflection does not always have to be about a negative client interaction or a critical *big* moment. Instead, it can be encouraged spontaneously by asking students to perform and plan tasks on Level I fieldwork and explain (or justify) their rationale. After the session, the student can be asked to further unpack the details of the session—what went well, what did not, and why. This is another simple self-reflection activity that can create growth and learning in a detailed way.

FWeds can set an example of their own reflective journey by documenting what works, what does not, and how they may plan to improve the next time. They may also model successful mentor and peer interactions as we expect from our students. If we expect our students to continually accept feedback, we should also elicit feedback from each student and reflect on the feedback at the end of each fieldwork experience.

Guided Reflection

While self-reflection is an important skill, sometimes the FWed must intervene and help the student to understand the event at a deeper level. Very often, this type of guided reflection is prompted by a *critical incident*, which can be a negative or uncomfortable situation, or even an immensely positive experience, which requires us to explore our actions and feelings (Alphonso, 2007). There are a variety of models of reflection that can be utilized during Level I fieldwork but

---

Box 9-9

CASE EXAMPLE SEVEN

Matthew is a Level I fieldwork student placed in an elementary school with Jason as his FWed. Matthew has planned an in-class handwriting session with a classroom of children he has observed before. When Jason looks at his treatment plan, he is surprised to see the "Handwriting Olympics" as Matthew's primary activity. This is not something they had discussed, and he thinks it might make the kids too revved up.

When Jason expresses this, he also asks Matthew to explain why he chose this particular activity. Matthew states that last time he was in the class, Tyler (one of the students) told him about his love for sports, and how the class really misses going out to recess in the winter. Matthew reflected on his own childhood and how much movement and sports played a part of fun for him and his friends. Matthew noticed that the therapists often have the students sit down to do pencil and paper task, and the kids look bored. He recalls the time he volunteered in a skilled nursing facility, and the clients enjoyed a game of balloon volleyball. He says that it just seemed like they all were able to work on their strength while having fun, and he hoped this activity would do the same thing for the kids.

Jason reminds Matthew to check in with the group vs. one perspective going forward but allows Matthew to use that as his final activity with the class. Matthew plans and executes a variety of games, art, and dancing activities that meet the needs of the group in many ways while having fun. At the end of the session, Jason asks how he feels it went. He tells Jason that Tyler told him it was his "best day ever" and that he thinks "handwriting is cool." He also tells Jason that it was the first time he really "felt like a therapist" and now has the confidence to know he can be a great practitioner, maybe even in pediatrics, which he didn't think he liked initially. The "Handwriting Olympics" was a huge success, and Jason plans to use it going forward in other classes long after Matthew exits.

---

not all are appropriate for use in reflecting in action in the course of spontaneous events. Boyd and Fales (1983) described the first part of completing a reflection as an inner sense of discomfort. FWeds need to be able to recognize when this may be happening to a student and bring it to light through discussion. Initially, reflection is not an automatic reaction but needs to be brought forward with conscious, guided effort (Nichola, 2016). While several models guide reflection, Gibbs (1988) is a tried and true basic, easy-to-follow, easy-to-learn model that can be used quickly during fieldwork experiences.

Gibbs (1988) describes six distinctive reflective stages that can be used to guide students once an event occurs (Figure 9-2). The FWed begins by asking for a description of what happened, any feelings that were involved from a personal level, what the student thought was good and bad about the situation, leading to an analysis, conclusion, and action plan for the future if the situation happened again.

For example, if the student on Level I fieldwork is leading a cooking group for clients with self-injurious behaviors and forgets to remove the knives, the FWed can immediately remove the knives but guide the student through the reflection afterward. Once the group is over, the FWed can ask, "So what do you think you forgot to do?" or "Why do you think I removed the knives?" vs. just telling the student their rationale. The cycle can continue as the student identifies the issue and why they may have forgotten or not realized the importance of the removal. They can continue to identify what went right about the group, so they realize that it was not all bad. Further exploration into safe management of spaces and thinking ahead can be discussed. The educator can provide a

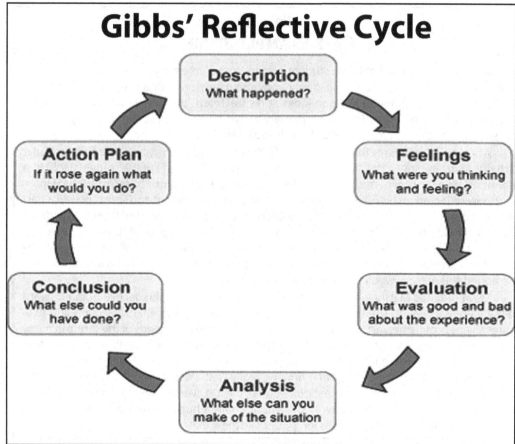

Figure 9-2. Gibbs' Reflective Cycle. (Reproduced with permission from Gibbs' model at https://www.crowe-associates.co.uk/coaching-tools/gibbs-reflective-cycle.)

scenario in which the student was alone and guide them in figuring out how the knives could have been managed and preparing for this not to happen again in the future. An overall emphasis on generalized safety can be discussed, and the student should be allowed to talk through how they plan to meet the client's needs in the future while maintaining a safe environment, as well as the critical importance of assessing space before intervention. Guiding the student through this model initially may lead them to begin to do it on their own and become more aware of their strengths and needs.

Another in-the-moment reflection tool is the Brookfield Model (Brookfield, 2000). It can be used for personal growth and development immediately following a critical incident. The student is encouraged to analyze the situation from multiple perspectives and reflect deeply on the experiences of others, as well as themselves. The student would be asked to take self-reflection into account along with how any colleagues may have perceived the incident, how the client may have perceived it, and also if any academic literature exists to support the response. This offers a way to discuss the situation in-the-movement but give the student "homework" to consider how the interaction fits into practice and any impact it may have had on those in the environment. Using the previous example, the student would be asked to appreciate how having knives in the group session may have impacted the client who was self-injurious, as well as the other clients in the group should something have happened. They would also analyze why safety is of utmost importance and the steps that would have to be taken should something negative have happened. Finally, they

---

BOX 9-10

CASE EXAMPLE EIGHT

Katie is a Level I fieldwork occupational therapy student who has been struggling with her fieldwork placement, arriving late, and often appearing distracted even after feedback was provided by her FWed and fieldwork coordinator. She is working with another occupational therapy student who is there from her school, although on different days of the week.

Katie is almost about to fail when her FWed calls out sick so she is assigned to work with the social worker, Margaret. They plan to work together for 2 days to finish her hours in the day program while the FWed is out. After meeting a client with schizophrenia that morning, Katie breaks down in tears. Margaret immediately pulls her aside and asks her what happened and how she felt about it. Katie tells Margaret that seeing the clients with mental health issues has been hitting close to home. She discloses that one of her family members has a significant mental illness and being onsite is troubling at times. She told the social worker she had felt uncomfortable about being there and just seemed like she was not helping anyone. She also felt that the other student was doing much better since she came back to class and told everyone that the FWed asked her to treat a client independently, something that Katie has not been allowed to do.

The safe space of the meeting and guided reflection by the social worker gave Katie the ability to talk about what she was feeling and open up a bit more about why she felt that way. Margaret suggests Katie consider what she feels might be helpful for the population given her personal experience and how she might reflect on this experience in order to make some positive change. They decide that a project for Katie would be to create a resource binder of community supports for individuals. Katie begins the project excitedly and is able to see the usefulness of her role in the setting and how she might make a difference.

When the FWed returns and asks the social worker how Katie did, Margaret tells her what a wonderful student Katie is and how helpful she was in creating the binder. Katie also goes back to school and speaks to her AFWC about the issues she may have working with the mental health population and wants to begin to consider options for Level II fieldwork based on her personal experiences and stress level among that population.

---

would be encouraged to consider not only the safety of the client but how the imagery of the knife may have an impact as related to trauma, for example, or to find examples of how cooking groups can be managed to support clients with psychosocial needs.

Guided reflection might also be a valuable tool to address student issues with professionalism or psychosocial issues that interfere with student-to-client interactions (Box 9-10).

In this case example illustrated in Box 9-10, the guided reflection done by the social worker was essential in-the-movement to learn why Katie had not been as invested. It also uncovered important information that Katie needs to know about herself to create a positive change. Had her FWed initially took the time to help Katie reflect on her behaviors during the initial portion of the placement, Katie (and the FWed) may have had a better experience. Her goals may have been clearer and her FWed may have been able to plan something meaningful for her. As noted in the example, guided reflection does not only have a powerful impact in-the-movement but can also affect future growth and impact planning for Level II fieldwork and future clinical practice.

Reflection can be a powerful tool when used properly. FWeds can both guide reflection and encourage more independent self-reflection through simple actions described in the previous sections, and many more creative ways that can just happen unexpectedly. Knowing the importance of exploring actions and feelings, in addition to teaching best practice methods of care, will help FWeds bring out the best in their students and help students learn to find their inner potential, no matter the setting. This process may be especially helpful for students with disabilities who may not have disclosed their disability prior to Level I placement. More information on the topic of working with students with disabilities during Level I fieldwork will be explored in Chapter 10.

Spontaneous Learning in Alternative Level I Fieldwork Settings

The Accreditation Council for Occupational Therapy Education (2018) added standard C.1.9 to the 2018 educational standards. This new standard allows for the use of different instructional modalities to satisfy Level I fieldwork, such as simulation, standardized patients, and faculty-led visits, which are discussed in Chapter 4 of this book. In each of these instructional methods, it is important to understand that the students may be entering the placement with a more academic mindset due to the nature of the experience. They may expect to be exposed to simulations that look like case studies where they have time to think, process, and receive feedback on *correct* answers. While simulated scenarios do need to be well planned and thoughtful, some of the experiences should mirror the nature of the unpredictable and spontaneous interactions of the traditional fieldwork site. Gormley and Fenwick (2016) discuss the need for medical professionals to receive training in situations of uncertainty and complex dynamics. Not unlike crisis management, students need to practice these skills in a safe space. The authors maintain that even familiar practice routines that feel comfortable for students can fall apart when complex system dynamics are introduced (Gormley & Fenwick, 2016). Therefore, if we do not simulate practice environments effectively, the student may not be prepared for the unexpected nature of therapist-client, therapist-therapist, and even student-student interactions that naturally occur in the faster paced real world setting.

While preparation is essential for simulated or standardized fieldwork placements, the in-the-moment experiences described in this chapter are quite valuable for these alternative settings as well. The combination of (1) flexible thinking during real-time interactions along with, (2) proper feedback, (3) debriefing, and (4) reflection will lead to a more introspective student who is not only ready for the unexpected but able to self-reflect enough to learn from it going forward.

Even individuals who cross the borders between academia and traditional/community placements (such as within a faculty-led Level I fieldwork practice) should be aware of the dichotomy and encourage true *in-the-moment* unexpected learning opportunities, which can lead to the developments described. Sometimes it is a challenge to let the academic side of ourselves go a bit and let the student struggle with an unexpected situation and learn naturally, but these opportunities can be much more effective than contrived opportunities.

Within the simulation or standardized patient fieldwork model, students should be encouraged to expect the unexpected, which can allow them to think quickly and flexibly. If their simulated client, who is being seen for a self-care session, suddenly loses balance and begins to fall, the student will have to respond to an unexpected outcome of what they thought might be a simple session. This can be quite effective and a way to provide immediate feedback on how to support the client and stop them from falling in a safe space of learning. In less immediate situations, formal debriefing is also an extremely effective tool. As a simulation is occurring, the action can stop and direct connections to the program's didactic curriculum can be made. This pause and reflection can allow students to more readily identify specific areas of the Level I fieldwork experience that relate to a learned experience in the classroom. For example, if the student is leading a simulated evaluation and begins to proceed with an assessment tool in a nonstandardized way, the action can be stopped, and the error can be discussed as related to what was learned in the classroom and why competency in assessment administration is important prior to providing service.

While video recordings of sessions often cannot be used in traditional placements due to client confidentiality, they can be an effective tool for self-reflection within a simulated environment, especially given both examples described earlier. The student may not have even realized they were making any errors or that they did not react quickly enough to prevent a fall. This method provides students with very specific visual and auditory feedback, which can allow them to self-reflect on their interactions, learn, and grow from the experience itself—even if it is not traditional.

SUMMARY

As demonstrated in the chapter, the road to being a skilled, creative, flexible occupational therapy practitioner begins with experiences on Level I fieldwork that build off the didactic learning experience. The opportunities afforded to students through spontaneous, **day-to-day interactions**, **feedback**, and guided or self-directed **reflection** allow students the freedom to learn and grow. The FWed needs to be astutely aware of all of the micro events happening as they are working on teaching practical skills. While not easy, it is very rewarding for all parties.

FWeds should remember to allow learning opportunities to develop naturally and be flexible in style and supervision to give the students room to grow with a safety net of protection as needed. As creative, skilled *improvisationalists*, occupational therapy practitioners have the abilities to effectively utilize the strategies described in this chapter. Doing so will serve to customize the learning experience for each student and make best use of opportunities for feedback and reflection, thereby promoting lifelong learning for both the student and the FWed.

LEARNING ACTIVITY

Please read the following case and answer the questions utilizing what you have learned about working through challenging interpersonal issues, providing feedback, and reflection:

> As an intervention session is occurring between Gigi, a certified occupational therapy assistant, and Herman, an occupational therapy assistant student, the supervising occupational therapist comes into the gym area to work with another client. Gigi is educating Herman on transfer strategies using a slide board. Upon seeing this, the registered occupational therapist comments that the client has been advanced to a stand pivot transfer.
>
> While the activity is in session, Gigi comments that this new information is helpful and shifts the client to a stand pivot transfer with Herman assisting. By doing this, Gigi models professional flexibility in moving the client from one position to the other, as well as acknowledging the change, which was not known before that moment. Later, Herman asks Gigi how she felt about being corrected in-the-movement unexpectedly.

Stop and Reflect

1. Based on what you have read in this chapter, if you were Gigi, what would YOU say in this case? Why? What examples given in the chapter support your decision?

2. How might you use this interaction as a learning moment for Gigi? For Herman?

3. What **feedback** would you provide, and how would you provide it based on what you have read in this chapter?

4. Would you utilize the One-Minute Preceptor in this case? Why or why not?

5. How might you encourage **reflection** after this event? Do you think it is best to use self-reflection or guided reflection in this case? Why?

6. Look back at Figure 9-2. How would **Gibbs' Reflective Cycle** be applied here? What questions would you ask? Why?

7. What if the certified occupational therapy assistant, Gigi, was supervising an OTD student in this scenario? Would it have been the same or different? (*Remember that MSOT and OTD students can have certified occupational therapy assistants as their Level I FWeds.*)

8. What if there was another student in the room? How might you address that? What challenges to **interpersonal interaction** does this present?

REFERENCES

Accreditation Council for Occupational Therapy Education. (2018). 2018 Accreditation Council for Occupational Therapy Education standards and interpretive guide. *American Journal of Occupational Therapy, 72*(Suppl. 2), 7212410005p1-7212410005p83. https://doi.org/10.5014/ajot.2018.72S217

Alphonso, C. D. (2007). Reflection on a critical incident. *Contemporary Nurse, 24*(1), 89-92. https://doi.org/10.5172/conu.2007.24.1.89

American Occupational Therapy Association. (2018). Philosophy of occupational therapy education. *American Journal of Occupational Therapy, 72*(Suppl. 2), 7212410070p1-7212410070p2. https://doi.org/10.5014/ajot.2018.72S201

Blumschein, P. (2012). Intentional learning. In N.M. Seel (Ed.), *Encyclopedia of the sciences of learning.* SpringerLink. https://doi.org/10.1007/978-1-4419-1428-6_37

Boyd, E. M., & Fales, A. W. (1983). Reflective learning: Key to learning from experience. *Journal of Humanistic Psychology, 23*(2), 99-117. https://doi.org/10.1177/0022167883232011

Briggs, E. (2019, July 16). *How to give feedback with a growth-mindset approach.* Your Brain at Work. https://neuroleadership.com/your-brain-at-work/feedback-strategies-growth-mindset/

Brookfield, S. D. (2000). The concept of critically reflective practice. In A. L. Wilson & E. R. Hayes (Eds.), *Handbook of adult and continuing education* (pp. 33-49). Jossey-Bass.

Brooks, C., Carroll, A., Gillies, R. M., & Hattie, J. (2019). A matrix of feedback for learning. *Australian Journal of Teacher Education, 44*(4). http://doi.org/10.14221/ajte.2018v44n4.2

Crawford, E. J., & Hanner, N. (2019, February). *The intentional fieldwork educator: Applying the intentional fieldwork education model (IFWEM).* University of St. Augustine for Health Sciences. https://soar.usa.edu/cgi/viewcontent.cgi?article=1010&context=ot

de Beer, M., & Mårtensson, L. (2015). Feedback on students' clinical reasoning skills during fieldwork education. *Australian Occupational Therapy Journal, 62*(4), 255-264. https://doi.org/10.1111/1440-1630.12208

DeIuliis, E. D., & Saylor, E. (2021). Bridging the gap: Three strategies to optimize professional relationships with generation Y and Z. *The Open Journal of Occupational Therapy, 9*(1), 1-13. https://doi.org/10.15453/2168-6408.1748

Dunn, L. S., Lewis-Kipkulei, P., & Bower, R. (2019). Metacognition of first year occupational therapy students: A comparison of entry-level degrees. *Journal of Occupational Therapy Education, 3*(4) 1-15. https://doi.org/10.26681/jote.2019.030401

Forsythe, A., & Johnson, S. (2017). Thanks, but no-thanks for the feedback. *Assessment & Evaluation in Higher Education, 42*(6), 850-859. https://doi.org/10.1080/02602938.2016.1202190

Gatewood, E., De Gagne, J. C., Kuo, A. C., & O'Sullivan, P. (2020). The one-minute preceptor: Evaluation of a clinical teaching tool training for nurse practitioner preceptors. *The Journal for Nurse Practitioners, 16*(6), 466-469.e1. https://doi.org/10.1016/j.nurpra.2020.03.016

Gibbs, G. (1988). *Learning by doing: A guide to teaching and learning methods.* FEU.

Gormley, G. J., & Fenwick, T. (2016). Learning to manage complexity through simulation: Students' challenges and possible strategies. *Perspectives on Medical Education, 5*(3), 138-146. https://doi.org/10.1007/s40037-016-0275-3

Hooper, B. (2006). Epistemological transformation in occupational therapy: Educational implications and challenges. *OTJR: Occupation, Participation & Health, 26*(1), 15-24. https://doi.org/10.1177/153944920602600103

Hvenegaard, G. T. (2011). Making the most of fieldwork learning experiences. *The Teaching Professor, 25*(4).

Iliff, S. L., Tool, G., Bowyer, P., Parham, D., Fletcher, T. S., & Freysteinson, W. M. (2019). Occupational therapy student conceptions of self-reflection in Level II fieldwork. *Journal of Occupational Therapy Education, 3*(1). https://doi.org/10.26681/jote.2019.030105

Johnson Coffelt, K., & Gabriel, L. S. (2017). Continuing competence trends of occupational therapy practitioners. *Open Journal of Occupational Therapy, 5*(1). https://doi.org/10.15453/2168-6408.1268

Kessler, D. O., Cheng, A., & Mullan, P. C. (2015). Debriefing in the emergency department after clinical events: A practical guide. *Annals of Emergency Medicine, 65*(6), 690-698. https://doi.org/10.1016/j.annemergmed.2014.10.019

Knightbridge, L. (2019). Reflection-in-practice: A survey of Australian occupational therapists. *Australian Occupational Therapy Journal, 66*(3), 337-346. https://doi.org/10.1111/1440-1630.12559

Mackenzie, L. (2002). Briefing and debriefing of student fieldwork experiences: Exploring concerns and reflecting on practice. *Australian Occupational Therapy Journal, 49*(2), 82-92. https://doi.org/10.1046/j.1440-1630.2002.00296.x

Neher, J. O., Gordon, K. C., Meyer, B., & Stevens, N. (1992). A five-step "microskills" model of clinical teaching. *Journal of the American Board of Family Practice, 5*(4), 419-424. https://doi.org/10.3122/jabfm.5.4.419

Nichola, B. (2016, May 2). *Guide to models of reflection—When and why should you use different ones.* Lifelong Learning with OT. https://lifelonglearningwithot.wordpress.com/2016/05/02/different-models-of-reflection-using-them-to-help-me-reflect/

Shoemaker, M. J., Beasley, J., Cooper, M., Perkins, R., Smith, J., & Swank, C. (2011). A method for providing high-volume interprofessional simulation encounters in physical and occupational therapy education programs. *Journal of Allied Health, 40*(1), 15E-21E.

Taylor, R. R. (2020a). Complexities within client-therapist relationships: Inevitable interpersonal events in therapy. In R. R. Taylor, *The intentional relationship: Occupational therapy and use of self* (2nd ed.). F. A. Davis

Taylor, R. R. (2020b). Knowing ourselves as therapists: Introducing therapeutic modes. In R. R. Taylor, *The intentional relationship: Occupational therapy and use of self* (2nd ed.). F. A. Davis

Vygotsky, L. S. (1980). *Mind in society: The development of higher psychological processes.* Harvard University Press.

Whitgob, E. E., Blankenburg, R. L., & Bogetz, A. L. (2016). The discriminatory patient and family: Strategies to address discrimination towards trainees. *Academic Medicine, 91*(11), S64-S69. https://doi.org/10.1097/ACM.0000000000001357

World Health Organization. (2010). *World Health Organization framework for action on interprofessional education and collaborative practice.* https://www.who.int/hrh/resources/framework_action/en/

Developing Supportive Fieldwork Accommodations for a Student With a Disability

Angela M. Lampe, OTD, OTR/L; Julia Shin, EdD, OTR/L; and Anna Domina, OTD, OTR/L

Occupational therapy practitioners are uniquely qualified to help students with disabilities adapt to academic, independent living, social, and mobility demands of postsecondary education settings (American Occupational Therapy Association [AOTA], n.d., 1998, 2013; Dirette, 2019; Kornblau, 1995). Transitioning to postsecondary education (Mamboleo et al., 2015) and then to fieldwork (Kornblau, 1995) can be challenging for students who may be unsure of how their disabilities will impact them or their future career. This chapter will provide an overview of inclusion and laws related to student disability in postsecondary education, discuss considerations for placement and reasonable accommodations, and provide practical suggestions for designing and evaluating Level I fieldwork experiences that set up occupational therapy and occupational therapy assistant students with disabilities for success. In addition, collaborative strategies for maximizing student learning while addressing unexpected situations related to disabilities will be discussed, and postplacement recommendations will explored.

Hanson, D., & DeIuliis, E. D. (Eds.).
Fieldwork Educator's Guide to Level I Fieldwork (pp. 291-316).
© 2023 Taylor and Francis Group.

Learning Objectives

By the end of reading this chapter and completing the learning activities, the reader should be able to:

1. Evaluate federal laws pertaining to postsecondary education that inform the process of disclosing a disability, setting up placement and reasonable accommodations, and guiding fieldwork students with disabilities.

2. Examine the steps, key players, and best practices to install supportive accommodations during Level I fieldwork.

3. Describe commonly requested reasonable accommodations and unexpected issues and events that can arise during Level I fieldwork.

4. Apply practical and collaborative strategies to promote positive learning experience and outcomes for students with disabilities during Level I fieldwork.

Key Words

- **Disability:** "A person who has a physical or mental impairment that substantially limits one or more major life activities, a person who has a history or record of such an impairment, or a person who is perceived by others as having such an impairment" (U.S. Department of Justice, 2020, para 2).

- **Family Educational Rights and Privacy Act (FERPA) (20 U.S.C. § 1232g; 34 CFR Part 99):** A federal law enacted in 1974 that protects the privacy of student education records.

- **Invisible, or hidden, disability:** A disability that is not immediately apparent to others, for example renal failure, diabetes, anxiety, depression, and chronic pain (Disabled World, 2020).

THEORETICAL OVERVIEW

The Americans with Disabilities Act (ADA) defines an individual with a disability as:

a person who has a physical or mental impairment that substantially limits one or more major life activities, a person who has a history or record of such an impairment, or a person who is perceived by others as having such an impairment. (U.S. Department of Justice, 2020, para 2)

Students entering postbaccalaureate degree programs with a disability have been on the rise in recent years (Jung et al., 2014; National Center for Education Statistics [NCES], 2019; Ozelie et al., 2019). Therefore, it is essential fieldwork educators (FWeds) are prepared to support a student with a disability in a clinical setting.

According to a report published by the NCES (2019), 19.4% of undergraduate and 11.9% of postbaccalaureate students in 2015 to 2016 reported having one or more of the following disabilities: blindness or a visual impairment not corrected by wearing glasses; hearing impairment; orthopedic or mobility impairment; speech or language impairment; learning, mental, emotional, or psychiatric condition (e.g., serious learning disability, depression, attention deficit disorder); or other health impairment or problem. Furthermore, there are some differences noted in the data with 13.3% of postbaccalaureate women compared to 9.9% of postbaccalaureate men reporting a disability (NCES, 2019). Postbaccalaureate students over the age of 24 were more likely to report a disability compared to their younger classmates, as well as postbaccalaureate students who had served in the military (NCES, 2019).

In a national survey of occupational therapy practitioners, Ozelie and colleagues (2019) found 47 of 292 respondents (16.9%) reported either a visible or invisible disability. Of these 47 respondents, only slightly more than half chose to disclose their disability during their postsecondary education experience. When occupational therapy students did disclose a disability, anxiety, depression, and migraine headaches were most reported (Ozelie et al., 2019). Given the growth of occupational therapy education programs by 58% between 2007 and 2017 and occupational therapy assistant education programs' growth of 73% in the same time period, there are more students entering experiential learning rotations (Stagliano & Harvison, 2018). Accommodating the growing number of students for experiential learning is a challenge for clinical settings and practitioners (Stagliano & Harvison, 2018). FWeds must be ready to address the growing number of students and the potential increase in the number of students requesting accommodations for visible and invisible disabilities during fieldwork experiences.

The challenge of the growth in occupational therapy and occupational therapy assistant students may become compounded because many of the students are coming from a generation with self-reported high levels of stress and other mental health concerns (American Psychological Association [APA], 2018b). As pertains to mental and invisible disabilities, FWeds and academics should be aware of a recent survey that indicates Gen Z (individuals born after 1997) reported a poorer mental health status than any other generation (APA, 2018b). More specifically, 35% of Gen Z women and 18% of Gen Z men reported their mental health as fair or poor (APA, 2018b). Twenty-three percent of adult Gen Z'ers reported they have been diagnosed with depression, and 18% reported a diagnosis of an anxiety disorder (APA, 2018b). Mental health issues, including anxiety and depression, are real concerns for Gen Z who may feel sad and nervous and show lack of interest, motivation, or energy in an academic or clinical setting (APA, 2018b). Everyone involved in higher education must recognize and effectively respond to the concern of student mental health issues (Kiuhara & Huefner, 2008).

FEDERAL LAWS PERTAINING TO POSTSECONDARY EDUCATION AND STUDENTS WITH DISABILITIES

Occupational therapy practitioners, particularly those working in school-based practice settings, are likely intimately familiar with federal laws, such as the Education of All Handicapped Children Act of 1975 (P.L. 94-142, 89 Stat 773) and the Individuals with Disabilities Education Act (P.L. 108–446, 118 Stat 2647). These two federal laws mandate occupational therapy services to students with disabilities in elementary, middle, and secondary school settings. Fewer practitioners may be aware that two federal laws, Section 504 of the Rehabilitation Act of 1973 and the ADA of 1990 (Title II of the ADA for public postsecondary schools and Title III for private postsecondary schools) provide protections for students with disabilities related to equal access to educational opportunities, including opportunities in postsecondary educational settings (U.S. Department of Education [USDE], 2011). Nearly all school districts and postsecondary schools in the United States must abide by one or both laws. The ADA of 1990 was amended in 2008, commonly known as the Amendments Act of 2008, to specify:

> that reasonable modifications in policies, practices, or procedures shall be required, unless an entity can demonstrate that making such modifications in policies, practices, or procedures, including academic requirements in postsecondary education, would fundamentally alter the nature of the goods, services, facilities, privileges, advantages, or accommodations involved. (U.S. Equal Opportunities Employment Commission, 2008, Sec. 6[a][1][f])

Under the Rehabilitation Act of 1973 and the ADA of 1990, public and private postsecondary institutions may not discriminate against and are required to provide accommodations to a student who has a documented disability (APA, 2018a). Postsecondary institutions must ensure the academic and extracurricular activities, including fieldwork, are accessible to a student with a disability. Flexibility and finding ways to accommodate, rather than exclude, students with disabilities is a must (Kornblau, 1995). Accommodations for a student with a disability in postsecondary institutions may range from architectural accommodations to providing aids, such as interpreters, large-print material, and ensuring material presented in an online format is accessible. Specific to Level I fieldwork, accommodations may include a variety of changes to the work and/or environment to support a student with a visible physical disability. For a student with an invisible disability, accommodations may be needed to support such things as communication and information exchange, fatigue, ergonomic, and/or psychosocial needs of the student.

As previously cited, accommodations and aids must be provided unless it is determined they would fundamentally alter the program or result in undue financial or administrative burdens (APA, 2018a; U.S. Equal Opportunities Employment Commission, 2008). As long as it does not fundamentally alter the nature of the program, modifying policies and procedures, such as allowing a student a short break throughout the clinical day, or giving a student additional time for chart review and/or documentation, are ways fieldwork settings may accommodate a student with a disability.

> The determination of what is a fundamental alteration, however, is one which requires specific steps and a reasoned, determinative process on the part of the campus community, and necessitates that colleges and universities question their notions of what is truly fundamental and provide for alternate methods of achieving the results intended by the educational program. (APA, 2018a)

For example, should a fieldwork setting allow double time for documentation to a student with a disability, it does not need to lower or substantially modify the process or quality of documentation produced by the student. Lowering or modifying the standard would be an example of fundamentally altering the nature of the program and is not required under the Rehabilitation Act nor the ADA (USDE, 2011).

Disclosing a Disability

Although protections exist, it is the responsibility of the student in postsecondary institutions to request accommodations (Aquino & Bittinger, 2019; Kiuhara & Huefner, 2008; USDE, 2011). As differentiated in Table 10-1, in postsecondary education settings, the responsibility of disclosing a disability shifts to the student, and this shift is significant. A student may elect to request accommodations for the academic component of a program but not disclose their disability for the clinical experience. Academic fieldwork coordinators (AFWCs) and faculty should positively support, and even empower, a student with a disability to disclose and request a needed accommodation (AOTA, 2003; Mamboleo et al., 2015). Students who have a positive experience disclosing and requesting an accommodation, as well as positive perceptions of instructors, are more willing to disclose a disability (Mamboleo et al., 2015). "From a self-advocacy standpoint, if students fail to take the initiative to seek accommodations, which may inevitably require disclosure of disability, they may miss opportunities for a more supportive environment for their college success" (Mamboleo et al., 2015, p. 9). To avoid potential problems that may arise in fieldwork, Kornblau (1995) stressed students must be willing to share their need for accommodation in a timely and suitable manner with those who need to support the student. And when a student does disclose, flexibility and open communication between all involved are important factors in creating a positive fieldwork experience (Kornblau, 1995).

TABLE 10-1

PRIMARY DIFFERENCES BETWEEN SECTION 504 AND THE ADA AND IMPLICATIONS FOR FIELDWORK EDUCATORS

SECONDARY INSTITUTIONS (HIGH SCHOOLS)	POSTSECONDARY INSTITUTIONS	IMPLICATIONS FOR FIELDWORK EDUCATORS
Under Section 504, secondary school districts must provide a free appropriate public education including regular or special education instruction, related services, and aids to all students with a disability in the school district's jurisdiction (USDE, 2011).	Postsecondary institutions are not required to provide free appropriate public education but must provide necessary academic adjustments to ensure they do not discriminate based on disability. Cannot deny admission to any student with a disability who meets the school's admission requirements (USDE, 2011).	Given the growth of occupational therapy and occupational therapy assistant programs (Harvison, 2018) and high level of stress of Gen Z'ers (APA, 2018b), FWeds should be prepared to supervise students with documented disabilities.
Required to identify an individual with a disability's educational needs and provide education in a regular classroom, education in regular classroom with supplemental services, or special education including related aids and services designed to meet the individual's needs (USDE, 2011).	A student with a disability attending postsecondary institutions is not required to report their disability. Postsecondary institutions are only required to provide academic adjustments to students who disclose their disability (USDE, 2011).	FWeds should be prepared to supervise students who chose to disclose a disability and be mindful some students may enter the fieldwork experience without disclosing their disability.
Required to identify students with disabilities and assess the needs of those students (USDE, 2011).	Not required to identify students with disabilities, nor are they required to assess the needs of students with disabilities, unless the student voluntarily discloses the disability to the institution (USDE, 2011).	FWeds should be prepared to work with the AFWC to determine the needs of a student who discloses a disability as pertains to Level I fieldwork.

(continued)

TABLE 10-1 (CONTINUED)

PRIMARY DIFFERENCES BETWEEN SECTION 504 AND THE ADA AND IMPLICATIONS FOR FIELDWORK EDUCATORS

SECONDARY INSTITUTIONS	POSTSECONDARY INSTITUTIONS	IMPLICATIONS FOR FIELDWORK EDUCATORS
Parental permission is required prior to the initial evaluation of a student with a disability. Evaluation and placement decisions are shared with parents who have the right to appeal any decision through an impartial hearing (USDE, 2020).	Will work with students who request an academic adjustment but will not invite parents to be involved in the process (USDE, 2011).	FWeds should be mindful parents of postsecondary education students are not a part of the accommodation process.
Required to develop an individualized education plan for a student with a disability (USDE, 2011).	An individualized education plan is not developed for a student who discloses a disability (USDE, 2011).	Appropriate accommodations do need to be communicated formally with the Level I site through a documented process from the AFWC.

Accommodations may be requested by the student at any point, and the student can deny accommodations based on their preference and perception of service functionality (Aquino & Bittinger, 2019). When a student opts to request an accommodation either for academic and/or clinical experiences, the student must present documentation by a physician, psychologist, or other professional who is familiar with the student and their disability (Barnard-Brak et al., 2010). The documentation provided should validate the disability, as well as recommend appropriate accommodations. Under FERPA, institutions must have written consent from the student before disclosing any information about the student (USDE, 2018). More specific information about requesting accommodations is discussed later in this chapter.

The possibility of being labeled, as well as shame, may prevent students from reporting a disability (Coduti et al., 2016; Demery et al., 2012). Collins and Mowbray (2005) offer a variety of reasons that students with psychiatric disabilities in postsecondary educational settings identify as barriers to accessing university-provided disability services (Figure 10-1). Collins and Mowbray (2005) also reported the most frequent issues reported by students with psychiatric disabilities in higher education settings are accommodations, coping with school, and attendance issues. Students with psychiatric disabilities also report issues with anxiety, low self-esteem, social skills/ personal skills, and memory/concentration issues (Collins & Mowbray, 2005) that may interfere with successful completion of fieldwork experiences. Over half of faculty, staff, and administrators question or have a need for general information, such as how to work with a student who has a psychiatric disability (Collins & Mowbray, 2005). Faculty, staff, and administrators also question if a student with a psychiatric disability will pose behavior problems in the classroom, attendance problems, and if the student can handle the course load (Collins & Mowbray, 2005). These latter questions and problems may certainly also be questions of AFWCs; will the behavior pose a problem in the clinic, attendance problems, and can the student handle the caseload and provide safe interventions?

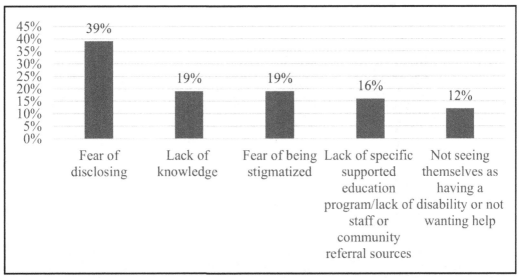

Figure 10-1. Top five barriers to accessing disability services reported by higher education students with psychiatric disabilities. (Adapted from Collins, M. E., & Mowbray, C. T. [2005]. Higher education and psychiatric disabilities: National survey of campus disability services. *American Journal of Orthopsychiatry, 75*[2], 304-315. https://doi.org/10.1037/0002-9432.75.2.304)

Ozelie and colleagues (2019) surveyed occupational therapy practitioners to determine accommodations they used/did not use while they were entry-level students. Over half of the practitioners did not disclose their disability during their entry-level program (Ozelie et al., 2019). A variety of reasons for not disclosing a disability were cited amongst occupational therapy practitioners (Figure 10-2; Ozelie et al., 2019). Yet, 22 of the 47 respondents in Ozelie's and colleagues' study (2019) reported their disability was a challenge for them while completing fieldwork rotations. The challenges experienced during fieldwork rotations ranged from mental exhaustion (the most frequently identified challenge) to communication (written and verbal with their supervisor or patients), to distractibility, physical exhaustion, and time management (Ozelie et al., 2019). Of the respondents who did not disclose their disability, Ozelie et al. (2019) reported that more breaks during the day and an altered daily schedule would have been helpful fieldwork accommodations.

In summary, choosing to disclose a disability is a complicated decision for a postsecondary education student. The literature indicates there are many factors a student considers when deciding to disclose a disability. To make an informed decision, the student must be aware of the laws and resources available to support them. A student must feel supported by AFWCs, faculty, and FWeds when/if they choose to disclose a disability. Given the barriers cited by students for not disclosing, AFWCs and faculty must be mindful of the ramifications perceived by students disclosing a disability. It is important for AFWCs and faculty to be knowledgeable about the laws enacted to support students with disabilities in postsecondary education. AFWCs and faculty must also be knowledgeable about the literature that discusses disabilities and accommodations in postsecondary education and encourage students to make informed decisions regarding their academic and fieldwork success. FWeds must be prepared to support a student who requests accommodation for their Level I fieldwork experience. This support may require changes in clinical practice routines by the FWed and should always include close communication and teamwork with the student and AFWC, so the student has a positive and successful experience.

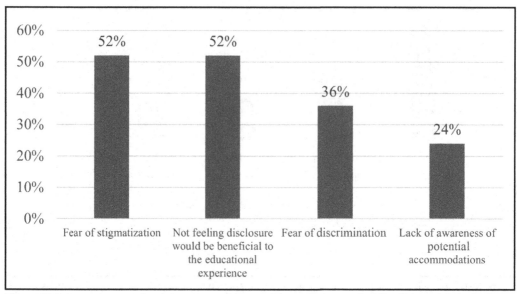

Figure 10-2. Reasons occupational therapy practitioners did not disclose a disability (Adapted from Ozelie, R., Delehoy, M., Jones, S., Sykstus, E., & Weil, V. [2019]. Accommodation use by individuals with disabilities in occupational therapy fieldwork. *Journal of Occupational Therapy Education, 3*[4]. https://doi.org/10.26681/jote.2019.030407)

LEVEL I FIELDWORK PURPOSE AND ACCREDITATION STANDARDS

For both occupational therapy and occupational therapy assistant students, "the goal of Level I fieldwork is to introduce students to fieldwork, apply knowledge to practice, and develop understanding of the needs of clients" (Accreditation Council for Occupational Therapy Education, 2018, p. 41). Prior to the start of Level I fieldwork, occupational therapy programs must inform Level I fieldwork supervisors about the curriculum, fieldwork program design, and ascertain agreement on standard fieldwork objectives in order to satisfy the educational program accreditation requirements. In the case of a student with a disability requesting accommodations, these standard fieldwork objectives continue to guide the experience and the determination of reasonable accommodations. For example, a standard fieldwork objective for a Level I fieldwork site may be to access and synthesize information from the medical chart to complete a chart review. A student with a documented accommodation may receive extra time to access the chart and synthesize the information as this does not fundamentally alter the practice skill the student is demonstrating. In contrast to Level II fieldwork, Level I fieldwork accreditation standards permit instruction to occur in a variety of ways ranging from simulated environments, to faculty-led site visits, and instructions to using standardized patients (Accreditation Council for Occupational Therapy Education, 2018). The flexibility offered by the accreditation standards for Level I fieldwork may be advantageous to accommodating students with disabilities.

Value of Experiential Learning

The National Collaborative on Workforce and Disability for Youth is a proponent of community-based work experiences, such as internships, apprenticeships, and other on-the-job training opportunities, such as Level I fieldwork experiences, which give students with disabilities the opportunity to learn specific job skills and work experiences (USDE, 2017). Occupational therapy and occupational therapy assistant students benefit greatly from Level I fieldwork experiential opportunities. The most meaningful Level I fieldwork experiences for students are those experiences that involve active participation (Haynes, 2011; Heine & Bennett, 2003; Kautzmann, 1987). Haynes (2011) suggests that Level I fieldwork should be designed with a "*just-right* challenge" (p. 265), so students can practice, assess, and confirm their academic knowledge in clinical situations to prepare the student to transition to Level II fieldwork experiences and ultimately clinical practice. Designing the just-right challenge for a student with a disability takes collaboration between academic faculty, the FWed, and the student.

ACCOMMODATION PROCESS PRIOR TO LEVEL I FIELDWORK

As discussed previously, the process of accommodations starts early in a student's educational career once they have disclosed a disability. It is important to acknowledge that in health sciences programs, accommodations must be considered for both didactic learning and clinical components such as fieldwork (Ozelie et al., 2019). Accommodations frequently requested by students for a Level I fieldwork may include extended time for testing, documenting in a private or distraction-free space, extended time for documentation, need for breaks during the day, accommodations for lighting or vision, or an altered schedule (Ozelie et al., 2019). In order for the student to determine the appropriate and reasonable accommodations that may assist with progression in the program, it is essential they work closely with a representative from the educational institution for the office of student disability services, as well as a faculty member of the occupational therapy program, which for Level I fieldwork experiences would include the AFWC. The team should take into consideration the technical standards available from the university for the program of study as a guide at this stage in the development of reasonable accommodations. Technical standards provide an overview of the nonacademic requirements that an occupational therapy student should understand as essential to completing the program (Kezar et al., 2019) and should be available at all education institutions for a program such as occupational therapy. It is important to note that technical standards vary greatly among academic institutions and are different from essential functions, which are the requirements that an occupational therapist or occupational therapy assistant must perform as their job duties at a place of employment (Kezar et al., 2019). Kezar and colleagues (2019) also noted that technical standards may not be compliant with ADA standards and may require updating or revision at many educational institutions. Still, the technical standards partnered with the standard objectives for a fieldwork experience may help guide all parties in determining reasonable and appropriate accommodations that meet the expectations of student learning.

Key players to consider when determining accommodations for a fieldwork placement include the following:

- Student
- Representative from student services for individuals with a disability from the academic institution
- AFWC
- Student advisor

These key players each bring different knowledge, skills, and experience to the table to best address the student need. The student is the first key player as they must disclose to begin the process. The student is also the individual that has the most intimate knowledge of how an accommodation may or may not work to meet their individual needs on fieldwork. The student disability services office is the next key player that ensures documentation is in place for the student accommodation, as well as provides essential understanding of the legal implications. The AFWC is also

> ## Box 10-1
> ## Vignette on Disclosure
>
> Jenny, the occupational therapy student, discloses to Mary, the AFWC, that she has a disability on file with the office for students with a disability at the school and is seeking advice on the accommodation process for fieldwork. Mary asks Jenny if she could provide a copy of her current academic accommodations so they can begin to discuss what may be reasonable to consider for the fieldwork setting. Jenny sends a copy of her academic accommodations, which includes extended time for testing and testing in a separate and quiet space. Mary then asks Jenny to think about scenarios from her shadowing or other experiences in a clinical setting that she anticipates she may need accommodations for. Mary also accesses a copy of the technical standards for the program and the Level I fieldwork standard objectives. Jenny is able to easily identify that documentation is her main concern. Mary asks Jenny to consider if she would need additional time for chart review, evaluation report, intervention planning, or other site-specific assignments. Mary also asks her to consider the environmental factors that may impact her fieldwork performance, such as lighting, screen time, or the noise level in the clinic. Once they have agreed on the general accommodation needs, Mary explains the process for accommodation requests in fieldwork to ensure Jenny's understanding.

a key player as this faculty member is the one that will have direct communication to the Level I fieldwork site regarding the accommodation request. The fieldwork site must have an affiliation agreement in place with the educational institution in order to accept students, and through this agreement, works with the AFWC on student placements, fieldwork objectives, student education, and accommodations as needed. The final key player in some situations may be the student advisor. Students may be assigned an advisor during their time in the program to assist with academic advancement and to provide support when concerns arise. This individual may be a positive support for a student who is seeking accommodation on fieldwork and can be a member of this team should the student request it.

The following case example (Box 10-1) will help illustrate the integration of these recommended steps for the Level I fieldwork process for accommodation. Meet Jenny, who is an occupational therapy student preparing for her first Level I fieldwork experience and currently has academic accommodations in place at the university. Jenny has scheduled her first appointment with the AFWC, Mary, to learn about the process to request for accommodations during fieldwork.

Once initial accommodations have been identified and agreed upon, it is time to work with the Level I fieldwork site to ensure the site understands the accommodation request process. This leads to the next step that occurs prior to the start of the Level I fieldwork, which is to create an accommodation request letter for the fieldwork site. An example accommodation request letter is available in Appendix A. It is advisable that the student placement process occur first based on the processes of the educational institution. Once the student has been placed and confirmed for a Level I fieldwork, it is then time for the student to review and approve the final accommodation request sent to the site by the educational program. The fieldwork site should be provided adequate time to review the accommodation request and provided a means to set up a meeting or ask clarification questions if necessary. It is important that a fieldwork site is aware that they are considered, by way of the affiliation agreement with the academic institution, an extension of the occupational therapy program. This means the student is eligible for accommodation within the fieldwork setting same as they are in the postsecondary educational setting. The accommodation request letter provides the fieldwork site with notice of the expected action to provide the student with an accessible education. Once the accommodations are reviewed, and if they are considered reasonable for the fieldwork site, it is best practice to collect a signed copy of the accommodation request letter should any concerns in meeting the accommodations arise during the fieldwork experience.

The question that often arises at this point in the process, from the academic institution and the fieldwork site, is how to determine if an accommodation is reasonable within the fieldwork setting. Looking at the legal and ethical mandates of the ADA, it is possible to consider scenarios that may go past the point of a reasonable accommodation. Any requested accommodation that "fundamentally alters the nature of the goods, services, facilities, privileges, or advantages" offered by the school would be considered an inappropriate request (U.S. Equal Opportunities Employment Commission, 2008, Sec. 6[a][1][f]; Weis et al., 2016). This may be harder to decipher in a clinical setting vs. an academic setting. For example, a student who requires testing in a quiet space during their didactic coursework can easily be accommodated in a testing center provided by the school. This is not fundamentally altering any processes or the nature of the services a school would already provide. However, in a clinical setting, a similar accommodation of documenting in a quiet and private space could present a concern. A fieldwork site may have a policy for Health Insurance Portability and Accountability Act protections that therapists can only document at their assigned computer in the therapy office. This is likely not a quiet space, but another approved documentation area may not be available. In this case, the reasonable accommodation may be noise cancelling headphones if the student is expected to participate in documentation. A recent study in nursing education (Horkey, 2019, p. 209) suggests that clinical accommodations have been poorly studied with literature providing only "hypothesized recommendations," which increases the challenge in making determinations around reasonable accommodation in a clinical setting.

The individual that can best speak to how an accommodation will or will not work in the fieldwork setting is the student themselves. When questions are raised about reasonable or appropriate accommodations by the fieldwork site, it is prudent that the AFWC or the office of disability services representative from the educational institution gathers details of why the accommodation could not be met, and what alternatives the fieldwork site may be able to offer the student to engage in the placement. Once this information is gathered, a meeting with the fieldwork site representatives, the AFWC, and the student may be necessary to reach final agreement on what are reasonable and appropriate accommodations for the setting. Box 10-2 provides an example of a meeting that may occur in a case where there are concerns with reasonable accommodations. This case highlights the conversation between Mary (the AFWC) and Brian (the FWed).

While this case example presents a scenario where the student, fieldwork site, and university were able to agree to the accommodations, it is possible in these early stages prior to fieldwork that a student and a fieldwork site may also agree that it is not a match and decide to terminate the placement. As a result, the fieldwork placement process and request for accommodations must start again for the student. Due to the additional steps that are involved in ensuring accommodations are in place, it is important the AFWC is planning ahead for placement, allowing ample time for any students who disclose a disability to go through the accommodation request process prior to starting the Level I fieldwork experience. It is also essential that students disclose the need for accommodation in a timely manner to the AFWC to facilitate the accommodations request process on their behalf. Key steps to setting up student accommodations from the perspective of the student, AFWC, and Level I fieldwork site is outlined in Table 10-2 in greater detail.

Preparation for students with a disability does not only include the process to request accommodations but also should include preparation of strategies for success on the Level I fieldwork. As mentioned earlier and shared in Figure 10-2, top reasons occupational therapy practitioners did not disclose a disability during their entry-level program were (1) fear of disclosing and (2) not feeling like disclosing a disability would be beneficial for their educational experience (Ozelie et al., 2019). To support students in disclosure, it may be ideal to introduce all students to their specific learning and communication styles to help them identify strategies in advance that can support their learning (Table 10-3). For students with a disability, this is also an opportune time to think through how to maximize learning in the fieldwork environment, considering their

Box 10-2

Vignette on a Discussion About Reasonable Accommodations

Brian, an occupational therapist at a hand clinic, is expecting a Level I fieldwork student to arrive in 4 weeks. Brian has mentored multiple Level I fieldwork students from the same program over the years. Brian feels ready and excited to meet his new Level I fieldwork student. A week later, Brian receives an email from Mary, the AFWC, with a letter of accommodations attached. The letter explained that his student, Jenny, has a documented disability, which allows her to access reasonable accommodations during the week of fieldwork. The letter states that Jenny may experience intermittent episodes of headache and double vision during the day, which can be aggravated by prolonged screen time, florescent lights, and fatigue. Jenny's accommodations include access to a quiet, dimmed space when requested, time and a half for chart review and documentation on computer, and access to printouts of electronic files as needed. Brian has never worked with a student who has accommodations before. Reading the letter of accommodations, he is not certain if he can provide all the necessary support to assist Jenny during her week of fieldwork. Brian works across multiple hand therapy stations that are directly under fluorescent lights. Brian decides to reach out to Mary for questions and clarifications. Mary responds to Brian's request for a video conference meeting within one business day.

Mary: "Hello Brian, thank you for meeting with me. I am glad we could find a time to discuss the accommodations in more detail."

Brian: "Hi Mary, thank you for meeting with me to answer my questions. I just wanted to be as prepared as I can to make sure Jenny can be fully supported during her fieldwork. First, can you tell me how Jenny is performing in her classes given her disability?"

Mary: "Brian, I cannot share student performance from coursework with you as this is protected under FERPA. I am happy to talk about accommodations with you though for her experience at your facility."

Brian: "You are right, thank you for the reminder! I just wanted to gauge how her disability is impacting her day-to-day performance."

Mary: "Well, I understand from your email you have some concerns regarding the accommodation for dimmed lighting in the clinic, can you elaborate on this more?"

Brian: "Yes, that is exactly my concern. My clinic uses fluorescent lighting, which turns on automatically when someone enters the clinic. I am unable to turn these lights off, especially over my workstation. I am afraid that this will make Jenny feel uncomfortable during the day."

Mary: "I can understand your concern, and from speaking with Jenny, she is able to take breaks from the space as needed instead of having the lights adjusted."

(continued)

accommodations in congruence with their learning and communication styles. The first step is to have students complete a learning style and/or communication style inventory to learn more about themselves.

Once this is information is gathered, students should consider what strategies may best align with specific styles of learning or communication. For example, a student who learns well from reading written notes may also do well with written feedback from their FWed vs. only verbal feedback. This is a skill that may be directly linked to a Level I fieldwork objective. An example

---

Box 10-2 (continued)

Vignette on a Discussion About Reasonable Accommodations

Brian: "Okay, so you are telling me that I do not need to turn off these lights as long as she can take breaks, correct?"

Mary: "Correct, and we can put other strategies into place if you feel they may be of assistance, such as opening shades over windows to allow for more daylight, allowing Jenny to wear sunglasses indoors, and accessing and sitting in her car for a break so that you do not have to change the lighting."

Brian: "These possible strategies and solutions can definitely work. Thank you for your suggestions!"

Mary: "If you are comfortable with these solutions, I can provide you an updated copy of the accommodation request letter for you to sign and return, and I will then provide Jenny a copy."

At the end of this meeting, Brian feels comfortable and confident in his ability to provide the necessary support for Jenny. Mary is assured that Brian has a clear and tangible plan to support Jenny's success throughout the week of fieldwork.

---

standard objective may read: "*Student is able to receive and integrate feedback received in a professional and time effective manner.*" In this case, one strategy for Level I fieldwork students may be to carry a notepad so the student can record the feedback they are receiving verbally, allowing them to review it again later. However, a student with an accommodation may need to consider how they would best be able to access this information if they do better with written feedback but also need additional time for written work. A reasonable strategy in this case may be to have the FWed provide a copy of their written feedback from the day to the student to ensure they have access to the information to meet the Level I fieldwork objective. Putting thoughtful consideration into preparation for Level I fieldwork experiences for all students, and especially those students with a disability, can help to alleviate some of the stress or anxiety students may feel at this stage in their education.

LEVEL I FIELDWORK WITH ACCOMMODATIONS

The student, FWed, and AFWC should feel comfortable and clear in their expectations with implementing the plan of accommodations during the fieldwork experience. If there are any uncertainties and reservations pertaining to what, when, and how the accommodations will take place from any one of the stakeholders, additional group discussions are highly encouraged as facilitated by the AFWC prior to fieldwork. For academic programs considering Level I fieldwork that includes simulated environments, faculty-led site visits, and standardized patients, the same level of clarity in expectations should be provided for all stakeholders involved as related to the plan of accommodations. Within such contexts, the stakeholders can include additional individuals who can support the successful implementation of the accommodations, including the faculty who is arranging and directing the experience, representatives from the site who can assist with environmental modifications, and the simulated lab manager. The list of relevant resources, including key personnel, laws and resources, and feedback and communication tools, to support a successful Level I fieldwork with accommodations is outlined in Table 10-4.

TABLE 10-2

KEY STEPS TO SETTING UP STUDENT ACCOMMODATIONS FROM THE STUDENT, AFWC, AND LEVEL I FIELDWORK SITE PERSPECTIVES PRIOR TO FIELDWORK

STUDENTS

1. Ensure paperwork is filed with the office of services for students with a disability at the academic institution.

2. Disclose your need for accommodations to the AFWC at your academic institution in preparation for fieldwork.

3. Work with your AFWC to develop/approve the accommodation request letter.

4. Review feedback provided from Level I fieldwork site about accommodations requested.

5. In some instances, you may need to meet with AFWC and Level I fieldwork site in advance to discuss accommodation requests.

6. Once Level I fieldwork site agrees to accommodation request, keep a copy in your files of the signed letter along with your other necessary paperwork for Level I fieldwork provided by your academic institution.

AFWCS

1. Upon student disclosure of need for formal accommodations for Level I fieldwork experience, set up meeting with student.

2. Place student according to regular placement processes at the school for the Level I fieldwork experience if not already done.

3. Draft accommodation request letter for student review taking into consideration standard fieldwork objectives and technical standards.

4. Work with student to develop final version of accommodation request letter well in advance of Level I fieldwork experience dates.

5. Send request for accommodation letter approximately 1 to 2 months prior to the start of the Level I fieldwork experience.

6. Follow-up with Level I fieldwork experience site regularly until response received.

7. Assist student in reviewing any feedback from Level I fieldwork site in regard to concerns or questions about accommodations.

8. Facilitate meeting with Level I fieldwork site and student if further discussion is warranted on accommodations request.

9. If accommodations request is signed and approved by student and Level I fieldwork site, keep this on file for reference during the fieldwork experience.

10. If the accommodations request is not approved by one or both parties, start placement and accommodation process over with the student.

11. In the event there are concerns regarding a cancellation of a Level I fieldwork placement for a student over an accommodation request, seek legal counsel or advisement at the academic institution.

(continued)

TABLE 10-2 (CONTINUED)

KEY STEPS TO SETTING UP STUDENT ACCOMMODATIONS FROM THE STUDENT, AFWC, AND LEVEL I FIELDWORK SITE PERSPECTIVES PRIOR TO FIELDWORK

LEVEL I FIELDWORK SITES

1. Develop a review process for Level I fieldwork accommodation requests if it does not already exist at the clinical or community site.

   a. Consider technical standards from the school or essential functions available from the employer (these should be available through your Human Resources [HR] department or rehab manager).

   b. Ensure standard learning objectives for Level I fieldwork are available or request a copy from the academic institution.

   c. Connect with legal department, HR, or rehab director if needed to determine if accommodations are reasonable.

2. Review the accommodation request letter and ensure accommodations can be met as outlined.

3. If in agreement with accommodation request letter, sign and return to the AFWC to indicate ability to accept and provide the accommodations.

4. If there are concerns in ability to meet the accommodations requested, reach out to the AFWC with details of what can and cannot be met, and what alternatives may be available.

5. Participate in meeting with AFWC and student to discuss accommodation requests, and what is reasonable and appropriate as determined by the clinical setting. It is appropriate to ask the student to describe how they envision the accommodation being implemented in the clinical setting. It is not reasonable to request additional information about the student disability that was not disclosed or other information protected under FERPA. In situations where the site may be unsure of how to proceed, it may be appropriate to seek assistance from HR or legal counsel at the fieldwork site.

6. Request necessary and agreed upon adjustments and new letter to be sent for review.

7. If in agreement with accommodation request letter at this stage, sign and return the letter to the AFWC.

8. Prepare as needed for accommodations to be in place when student arrives on day one to the Level I fieldwork site.

9. In the event where the accommodations request is seen as unreasonable and a meeting with the student and AFWC does not resolve the concern, it is recommended to seek legal counsel or advisement at the Level I fieldwork site to determine next steps or if a cancellation of placement is appropriate.

TABLE 10-3

EXAMPLES OF TOOLS THAT MAY ASSIST IN DETERMINING LEARNING AND COMMUNICATION STYLES

TOOL	ABOUT	WEBSITE
The VARK (Visual, Aural, Read/Write, Kinesthetic) Questionnaire	Provides a tool to identify learning preferences which may help to better understand others and maximize learning experiences.	https://vark-learn.com/the-vark-questionnaire/
Myers-Briggs Personality Type Indicator	Provides insight into personality preferences, which can help with understanding motivation and intent.	https://www.myersbriggs.org/my-mbti-personality-type/mbti-basics/
Personal SWOT (Strengths, Weaknesses, Opportunities, Threats) Analysis	A review of strengths and weaknesses and planning for how to address this in daily life to achieve success.	https://www.mindtools.com/pages/article/newTMC_05_1.htm

Reviewing the Plan of Accommodations and Assessing Efficacy at the Start of Fieldwork

At the beginning of fieldwork, the student and FWed are encouraged to review the plan of accommodations. While prefieldwork preparations will largely assist with visualizing what these accommodations can look like, it is important to remember that they can continue to remain abstract and unclear for the student. Depending on the level of fieldwork and prior level of experience, requesting for and receiving accommodations may be an entirely novel experience for the student. In other words, although the student may appear to be knowledgeable and agreeable to the plan established, they may not fully understand the needs, challenges, and arrangements to be encountered in a new fieldwork environment. Therefore, the FWed should not assume that the plan is final, as the student must feel comfortable and confident with the accommodations discussed prior. As the first day at fieldwork unfolds, which can include orientation, a tour of the facility, skilled observation, set-up and tear-down of the sessions, assistance with treatment sessions, documentation, etc., the student and FWed may identify additional opportunities and develop further strategies for success. The student and FWed can also discuss about the fieldwork objectives, learning activities, and evaluation forms to ensure that the generated plan will sufficiently support meeting such requirements (Hirneth & Mackenzie, 2004). It is important to remember that the execution of the plan of accommodations is an open-ended process throughout the week of fieldwork. Similarly, the student completing Level I fieldwork using alternate methods should be given an ample amount of opportunities to ask questions, provide feedback, and brainstorm additional strategies for success, especially at the beginning of the scheduled experiences. Box 10-3 provides an example of how this process might unfold.

Following such recommendations, Brian (the FWed) invites Jenny (the student) to reflect on her first day of fieldwork.

TABLE 10-4

EXAMPLES OF COMMON LEVEL I FIELDWORK ACCOMMODATION REQUESTS BASED ON LEVEL I FIELDWORK COMPETENCY EVALUATION FOR OT AND OTA STUDENTS

SECTION FROM COMPETENCY EVALUATION	COMMON ACCOMMODATION REQUESTS
Fundamentals for practice	• Patient lifting restrictions • Additional individual with student to read monitors for student with visual impairment
Foundations of occupational therapy	• Additional time for tasks that require use of computer • Additional time for tasks that require gathering of materials such as research articles
Professional behaviors	• Double time or time and a half for assignment completion • Double time or time and a half for documentation • Permission to use notepad or clipboard to assist with organization and memory aids • Short breaks allowed during the day due to a student condition • Ability to eat and drink throughout the day due to student condition • Access to a private space for removal from sensory stimulation for short periods of time during day • Access to area and breaks for pumping for student who is nursing • Late arrival or early departure allowed with notice due to medical condition and need for medical care • Provided printed materials for frequently used medical terminology or materials student is expected to reference frequently
Screening and evaluation	• Double time or time and a half for chart review • Double time or time and a half for documentation • Provide printed template of evaluation if completed in electronic medical record
Intervention	• Additional time for tasks that require gathering of materials or setup • Patient lifting restrictions • Additional time for tasks that require gathering of materials such as research articles for intervention planning • Additional time for assignments such as intervention planning • Double time or time and a half for chart review • Double time or time and a half for documentation

---

Box 10-3

VIGNETTE ON ASSESSING EFFICACY
OF THE ACCOMMODATION PLAN

On the first day of fieldwork, Jenny arrives 30 minutes late. Brian gently reminds Jenny that her day will start at 8 a.m. and end around 5 p.m. After the tour of the facility, orientation, and meet and greet with clinicians and staff members at this clinic, Brian and Jenny sit down for a review of the accommodations. Brian and Jenny reflect on the daily schedule, expected demands, and clinic environments to develop additional strategies and modifications.

Brian: "Alright Jenny, that was the end of your first day. The rest of the week will look and feel much like how today went. Is there anything that you want to share with me, as far as the clinic schedule, space, lighting, policies, and/or expectations?"

Jenny: "I enjoyed my first day of fieldwork very much! I think it worked well for me to sit in the staff lounge with lights turned off during lunchtime. It helps me to rest my eyes there. I liked that we were able to work in natural lighting in the afternoon today. I think these strategies were helpful in managing my symptoms."

Brian: "I am glad this space can work for you to take your break during the day. Please feel free to ask me if you need to step away and access this space for the rest of the week. Is there anything else that you want to tell me as far as meeting your accommodation needs?"

Jenny: "I think the setup and the plan we have are working well since I did not have any headaches today. I am excited for the rest of the week!"

Developing a Plan for Continuous Communication, Modification, and Evaluation

Throughout the fieldwork experience, the student and FWed are recommended to set aside reserved time for continuous monitoring, feedback, and modifications. Typically, the student and FWed can use a combination of informal and formal methods of check-in during the fieldwork. The FWed may casually ask for verbal feedback at the beginning of the day, during lunch, or at the end of the day. In addition, the FWed may schedule for a structured time at mid-experience to review how the student is perceiving and using their accommodations. The student may feel more inclined to tolerate and endure through the fieldwork rather than advocating for additional changes to the existing plan due to many factors including fear of being misjudged, efforts to maintain rapport, and lack of confidence and experience (Aquino & Bittinger, 2019; Mamboleo et al., 2015; Ozelie et al., 2019). Therefore, it is important for the FWed to provide a welcoming and supportive environment and ample, intentional opportunities for the student to express their perspectives and needs throughout the fieldwork. When completing Level I fieldwork along with peers with faculty-directed activities and simulated labs, such discussions can occur in a private, reserved space for protection of confidentiality.

Ideally, the plan of accommodations should support the student to participate, engage, and complete all required activities and meet objectives established for fieldwork or scheduled learning experiences. If additional strategies and modifications are identified throughout the experience, as pertinent to the accommodations documented in the letter, they can be applied to better support the student's participation and success. All stakeholders are recommended to engage in continuous evaluation of what is working well, and what can be done differently to accommodate for the student's unique needs throughout the fieldwork, especially in preparation for fieldwork performance evaluation or learning assessment, as appropriate. While both informal and formal checkpoints are recommended to evaluate the student's progress with meeting the learning objectives, formal discussion involving the review of Level I fieldwork learning objectives and evaluation of performance and learning is strongly recommended at mid-experience in preparation for end of fieldwork.

Preparing for Performance Evaluation, Reflection, and Feedback at the End of Fieldwork

Entering the latter half of fieldwork experience, the student and FWed should prepare to provide constructive evaluation and feedback related to the fieldwork experience. With the plan for continuous communication, modification, and evaluation installed throughout the experience, there should be no surprises related to (1) whether or not the plan of accommodations were thoroughly implemented and provided and (2) whether or not the student achieved the required learning objectives with reasonable accommodations. The student and FWed can begin to review and complete the evaluation forms and assessments required as part of the experience. The student is strongly encouraged to self-evaluate their performance by filling out the forms on their own, which can allow opportunities for understanding standards and criteria for a passing fieldwork performance, self-reflection, and advocacy. The FWed can review all evaluation and assessment items and estimate the outcome of the student's fieldwork performance. The student and FWed can engage in additional discussions to ensure all questions are answered related to fieldwork performance and evaluation prior to last day, which facilitates mutual understanding and agreement on the outcome of the Level I fieldwork experience. If the student and FWed have questions related to the proper provision of the accommodations and evaluation of student fieldwork performance, they must be communicated early and regularly, in which case, the AFWC may be involved.

Troubleshooting and Managing Unexpected Events During a Level I Fieldwork With Accommodations

With participation of all stakeholders involved with proactive planning, open communication, and continuous monitoring, the student and the FWed can significantly reduce the likelihood of encountering problems and conflicts during a Level I fieldwork. However, a number of unexpected events can occur, as expected in any fieldwork experience with and without a plan of accommodations:

- The student and the FWed may realize that the plan of accommodations cannot be adequately supported due to nonmodifiable environmental, organizational, and contextual factors (i.e., the student experiencing shortness of breath with the kind of personal protective equipment applied at site, which must be donned at all times due to the organization's infectious disease control policy).

- The student and the FWed may under- or overuse the accommodations to the point they significantly interfere with the student's fieldwork performance (i.e., the student potentially abusing the policy by taking excessive breaks and avoiding assigned tasks and responsibilities).

- The student and the FWed may disagree on ratings/comments on the evaluation of fieldwork performance (i.e., the FWed assigning a *Below Standards* rating for the student to indicate opportunities for improvement with daily notes when the student is allowed additional time for documentation).

As a general rule of thumb, it is important to approach and handle each event on an individual basis due to the specificity and the uniqueness of the context involving the student, plan of accommodations, and prior expectations and agreements established. The student's and the FWed's prior knowledge and experience can assist but may not always lead to the best solution possible, especially when the situation involves nonmodifiable factors, misinterpretation and miscommunication, or conflicts of interest.

When encountering issues that cannot be resolved from a collaborative review of the plan, problem solving, and transparent and regular communication, the student and the FWed are recommended to immediately reach out to the AFWC. The AFWC can serve as an advocate for the student, as well as an accountable support for the FWed to positively navigate the situation. The AFWC will complete a thorough evaluation of the event, both from the student's and the FWed's perspectives. To assist with the initial investigation, the student and the FWed are encouraged to document all meetings, discussions, and strategies implemented and provide the information to the AFWC. The AFWC may schedule individual and/or group meetings to obtain all necessary information. Then, the AFWC may, in consultation with the office of student disability as needed, recommend creative strategies and modifications as allowed within the limits of the plan of accommodations; provide education, counseling, or professional conduct citation as appropriate; and propose termination of fieldwork and replacement to a new site or arrangement of a different fieldwork experience, as necessary. The student and the FWed can count on the expertise, experience, and recommendations of the AFWC to mitigate the unexpected events encountered on a Level I fieldwork. An example drawn from the previous case illustrates the nature of continuing accommodation adjustment.

In the Box 10-4 case example, Brian (FWed), Jenny (fieldwork student), and Mary (AFWC), engage in an transparent and collaborative process to develop solutions to challenges encountered during the week of fieldwork (Box 10-4).

LEVEL I FIELDWORK EVALUATION WITH ACCOMMODATIONS

As illustrated in the case example in Box 10-4, evaluation of student performance on fieldwork experiences can be challenging due to the variability in practice settings and expectations. The first step to ensure clear evaluation of a student on fieldwork is to have agreement between the academic program and the fieldwork site prior to the start of the experience on the standard fieldwork objectives. These objectives should clearly lay out the expectations for a student on a rotation in the practice setting and should be based on skills that are evaluated on the final evaluation of fieldwork. For Level I fieldwork experiences, students are generally evaluated using the *Level I Fieldwork Competency Evaluation for OT and OTA Students* (AOTA, 2017; Table 10-4). Students are graded based on a rating scale that assess the student's ability to perform the necessary skill or activity from a rating of unacceptable to outstanding. When evaluating a student with a disability, the same evaluation and rating scale is used, but students are allowed to use their agreed-upon accommodations to meet the items listed on the evaluation.

For example, one item on the Level I competency evaluation assesses the students time management skills during the fieldwork experience and states, "consider student's ability to be prompt, arriving and completing assignments on time" (AOTA, 2017, p. 3). A student with a disability who has an accommodation to allow for time-and-a-half for a chart review should not be graded at a lower rating on this item if they were able to complete the assigned activity at the expected level within the additional time they are allowed per the agreed-upon accommodation. This means the student who meets the expectation with the accommodation in place would still receive a *Meets Standards*, *Exceeds Standards*, or *Outstanding* depending on the quality of the outcome for this

Box 10-4

Vignette on Level I Fieldwork Evaluation With Accommodations

On the second day of fieldwork, Brian notes that Jenny arrives 10 minutes late to the first scheduled appointment. Brian also notices that Jenny frequently appears distracted, checking on her phone in her pocket several times during client interactions. During the first break, Brian invites Jenny for an open discussion. Brian clearly sets expectations that showing up on time and actively engaging with clients are required to successfully pass the fieldwork. Brian also asks if Jenny is experiencing any difficulties and if the current plan of accommodations is adequately supporting her needs. Jenny verbalizes her understanding of expectations and indicates that all of her needs are sufficiently being addressed. For the rest of the week, Jenny presents with additional challenges in her professional behavior, which are noted and documented by Brian. Brian communicates these challenges with Mary at the occupational therapy program mid-week. Mary recommends that Brian continue documenting all meetings, feedback, and accommodations provided.

On the last day of fieldwork, Brian and Jenny review the student performance evaluation. Jenny is surprised to see multiple *Below Standards* ratings on the Level I Fieldwork Competency Evaluation. Brian and Jenny reach out to Mary for a meeting to discuss about the discrepancies noted by Jenny on her fieldwork performance. At this meeting, Brian provides his observation and documentation of all events that took place during the week of fieldwork. Jenny also provides her perspectives on why she deserves higher ratings, given her medical needs and accommodations. Mary reminds Jenny of the expectation to adhere to the highest level of professionalism during fieldwork, regardless of medical needs and accommodations, which is an important part of clinical education. Mary and Brian invite Jenny to reflect on her promptness and level of engagement with clients throughout the week. Jenny admits that in her initial understanding, running a few minutes late and passively observing the client was permissible given her low stamina. After further in-depth reflection, Jenny agrees the *Below Standards* ratings that Brian initially gave are fair. Mary and Brian invite Jenny to think about how her performance during this week can inform her next Level I fieldwork.

Upon her return to the academic program for continuing coursework, Mary requests a short meeting with Jenny to review her experience on her first Level I fieldwork. During the meeting, they discuss if the accommodations that were in place provided Jenny the opportunity to access the Level I fieldwork experience as she had expected. Mary explains this is an opportunity to consider if there are any changes to accommodations that may be needed for future experiences. Jenny provides feedback about the experience and that she felt it was very successful. Mary and Jenny agree to use the same accommodations for the second Level I fieldwork experience.

specific item on the assessment. Examples of common Level I fieldwork accommodations based on the Level I Fieldwork Competency Evaluation sections are provided in Table 10-4 to assist in framing this further.

Students with accommodations are expected to meet the same fieldwork learning objectives and assessment items as students without accommodations. Level I fieldwork sites and academic programs should not decrease the rigor of the expectations but rather find reasonable accommodations to allow the student to perform at their highest level within the fieldwork setting.

SUMMARY

This chapter provides an overview of relevant laws pertaining to students with disabilities in postsecondary education, discusses considerations for placement and accommodations for a student with a disability, and offers practical advice for the student, AFWC, and Level I fieldwork site for developing supportive accommodations for students with disabilities. A toolbox for success in accommodating students on Level I fieldwork is provided in Table 10-5 to assist the AFWC and FWed in meeting these expectations. As occupational therapy students transition from the didactic component of their curriculum to experiential learning, they may find the complexity and ambiguity of clinical practice challenging. The challenges of clinical practice may be compounded for a student with a disability. Under the law, students in higher education have the option of disclosing their disability at any time in their educational trajectory including in preparation and during fieldwork. Faculty, AFWCs, and FWeds must be knowledgeable of laws pertaining to students with disabilities, as well as the related literature so they can support students with disabilities in their successful completion of Level I fieldwork.

LEARNING ACTIVITIES

1. For students considering disclosing a disability for Level I fieldwork: What advantage(s) does disclosing your disability have, and how will disclosing support your success on Level I fieldwork? Can you think of any disadvantages to disclosing a disability for your Level I fieldwork experience?

2. For AFWC and academic departments: Do our students routinely disclose a disability to support them on Level I fieldwork? Why or why not? How can my department and I better support our students with disabilities during the request for accommodation and Level I fieldwork experience?

3. For clinical fieldwork coordinators and sites: Reflect upon how you might accommodate a student with a disability in your practice setting. What reasonable accommodations from Table 10-4 could your practice setting accommodate? Are there any accommodations that would not work in your practice setting? Explain.

TABLE 10-5

EXAMPLES OF TOOLS THAT MAY ASSIST IN DETERMINING LEARNING AND COMMUNICATION STYLES

Key Personnel	1. AFWC 2. FWed 3. Student 4. Faculty or instructor of record involved 5. Site's student program coordinator 6. Site's director of rehabilitation/manager 7. Simulated lab manager

Pertinent Laws and Resources	1. To learn more about the FERP specific to postsecondary education settings, refer to the following resources:
	
	   ◦ https://studentprivacy.ed.gov/audience/school-officials-post-secondary
	
	   ◦ https://www.hsmcoalition.org/
	
	   ◦ https://www.aota.org/Practice/Manage/Multicultural/Cultural-Competency-Tool-Kit/NOTPD.aspx
	
	2. If you are interested in learning more about disability rights and laws, check out this website: https://www.ada.gov/cguide.htm. This website has a comprehensive list and information on several disability laws including the ADA, the Rehabilitation Act, the Individuals with Disabilities Education Act, and more.
	
	3. Most college and university campuses have a support department or office serving students with disabilities, and this may be a good resource for faculty, students, and AFWC.

Communication and Feedback Tools	1. Key Personnel Summary and Contact Form 2. Fieldwork Experience Assessment Tool 3. The VARK Questionnaire 4. Dominant Communication Style Quiz 5. Myers-Briggs Personality Type Assessment 6. Personal SWOT Analysis 7. One-Week Calendar/Scheduler
Forms and Paperwork	1. AOTA Level I Fieldwork Competency Evaluation for OT and OTA Students https://www.aota.org/-/media/Corporate/Files/EducationCareers/Educators/Fieldwork/Level1/Level-I-Fieldwork-Competency-Evaluation-for-ot-and-ota-students.pdf

REFERENCES

Accreditation Council for Occupational Therapy Education. (2018). *2018 accreditation council for occupational therapy education standards and interpretive guide.* https://www.aota.org/-/media/Corporate/Files/EducationCareers/Accredit/Policies/ACOTE%20Manual%20Complete.pdf

American Occupational Therapy Association. (n.d.). *Practitioners with disabilities.* https://www.aota.org/Education-Careers/Considering-OT-Career/Diversity/Disabilities.aspx

American Occupational Therapy Association. (1998). Occupational therapy for individuals with learning disabilities (statement). *American Journal of Occupational Therapy, 52*(10), 874-880. https://doi.org/10.5014/ajot.52.10.874

American Occupational Therapy Association. (2003). Role competencies for academic fieldwork coordinator. *American Journal of Occupational Therapy, 58*(6), 653-654. https://doi.org/10.5014/ajot.58.6.653

American Occupational Therapy Association. (2013). *Students with disabilities in postsecondary education settings: How occupational therapy can help.* https://www.aota.org/-/media/Corporate/Files/AboutOT/Professionals/WhatIsOT/CY/Fact-Sheets/Postsecondary-Education.pdf

American Occupational Therapy Association. (2017). *Level I fieldwork competency evaluation for OT and OTA students.* https://www.aota.org/-/media/Corporate/Files/EducationCareers/Educators/Fieldwork/LevelI/Level-I-Fieldwork-Competency-Evaluation-for-ot-and-ota-students.pdf

American Psychological Association. (2018a). *DART toolkit II: Legal issues–ADA basics.* https://www.apa.org/pi/disability/dart/legal/ada-basics

American Psychological Association. (2018b). *Stress in America: Generation Z.* https://www.apa.org/news/press/releases/stress/2018/stress-gen-z.pdf

Americans With Disabilities Act Amendments, Pub. L. No. 110-325 § 3406 (2008).

Aquino, K. C., & Bittinger, J. D. (2019). The self-(un)identification of disability in higher education. *Journal of Postsecondary Education and Disability, 32*(1), 5-19.

Barnar-Brak, L., Lechtenberger, D., & Lan, W. Y. (2010). Accommodation strategies of college students with disabilities. *The Qualitative Report, 15*(2), 411-429. https://doi.org/10.46743/2160-3715/2010.1158

Coduti, W. A., Hayes, J. A., Locke, B. D., & Youn, S. J. (2016). Mental health and professional help-seeking among college students with disabilities. *Rehabilitation Psychology, 61*(3), 288-296. https://doi.org/10.1037/rep0000101

Collins, M. E., & Mowbray, C. T. (2005). Higher education and psychiatric disabilities: National survey of campus disability services. *American Journal of Orthopsychiatry, 75*(2), 304-315. https://doi.org/10.1037/0002-9432.75.2.304

Demery, R., Thirlaway, K., & Mercer, J. (2012). The experiences of university students with a mood disorder. *Disability & Society, 27*(4), 519-533. https://doi.org/10.1080/09687599.2012.662827

Dirette, D. P. (2019). Disability services for students in postsecondary education: Opportunities for occupational therapy. *The Open Journal of Occupational Therapy, 7*(2). https://doi.org/10.15453/2168-6408.1609

Disabled World. (2020). *Invisible disabilities: List and general information.* https://www.disabled-world.com/disability/types/invisible/

Education of All Handicapped Children Act, Pub. L. No. 94-142 § 3500 (1975).

Haynes, C. J. (2011). Active participation in fieldwork Level I: Fieldwork educator and student perceptions. *Occupational Therapy in Health Care, 25*(4), 257-269. https://doi.org/10.3109/07380577.2011.595477

Heine, D., & Bennett, N. (2003). Student perceptions of Level I fieldwork supervision. *Occupational Therapy in Health Care, 17*(2), 89-97. http://doi.org/10.1080/J003v17n02_06

Hirneth, M., & Mackenzie, L. (2004). The practice education of occupational therapy students with disabilities: Practice educators' perspectives. *British Journal of Occupational Therapy, 67*(9), 396-403. https://doi.org/10.1177/030802260406700904

Horkey, E. (2019). Reasonable academic accommodation implementation in clinical nursing education: A scoping review. *National Education Perspectives, 40*(4), 205-209. http://doi.org/10.1097/01.NEP.0000000000000469

Individuals With Disabilities Education Act, 20 U.S.C. § 1400 (2004).

Jung, B., Baptiste, S., Dhillon, S. Kravchenko, T., Stewart, D., & Vanderkaay, S. (2014). The experience of student occupational therapists with disabilities in Canadian universities. *International Journal of Higher Education, 3*(1), 146-154. https://doi.org/10.5430/ijhe.v3n1p146

Kautzmann, L. N. (1987). Perceptions of the purpose of Level I fieldwork. *American Journal of Occupational Therapy, 41*(9), 595-600. https://doi.org/10.5014/ajot.41.9.595

Kezar, L. B., Kirschner, K. L., Clinchot, D. M., Laird-Metke, E., Zazove, P., & Curry, R. H. (2019). Leading practices and future directions for technical standards in medical education. *Academic Medicine, 94*(2), 520-527. https://doi.org/10.1097/ACM.0000000000002517

Kiuhara, S. A., & Huefner, D. S. (2008). Students with psychiatric disabilities in higher education settings: The Americans with Disabilities Act and beyond. *Journal of Disability Policy Studies, 19*(2), 103-113. https://doi.org/10.1177/1044207308315277

Kornblau, B. L. (1995). Fieldwork education and students with disabilities: Enter the Americans with disabilities act. *American Journal of Occupational Therapy, 49*(2), 139-145. https://doi.org/10.5014/ajot.49.2.139

Mamboleo, G., Meyer, L., Georgieva, Z., Curtis, R., Dong, S., & Stender, L. M. (2015). Students with disabilities' self-report on perceptions toward disclosing disability and faculty's willingness to provide accommodations. *Rehabilitation Counselors and Educators Journal, 8*(2), 8–19.

Ozelie, R., Delehoy, M., Jones, S., Sykstus, E., & Weil, V. (2019). Accommodation use by individuals with disabilities in occupational therapy fieldwork. *Journal of Occupational Therapy Education, 3*(4). https://doi.org/10.26681/jote.2019.030407

Stagliano, H., & Harvison, N. (2018). *Current trends in accreditation and higher education* [PowerPoint slides]. https://www.aota.org/~/media/Corporate/Files/EducationCareers/2018-conference-presentations/2018-Trends-in-Accreditation-Higher-Education.pdf

U.S. Department of Education. (2011). *Students with disabilities preparing for postsecondary education: Know your rights and responsibilities.* https://www2.ed.gov/about/offices/list/ocr/transition.html#note

U.S. Department of Education. (2017). *A transition guide to postsecondary education and employment for students and youth with disabilities.* https://www2.ed.gov/about/offices/list/osers/transition/products/postsecondary-transition-guide-2017.pdf

U.S. Department of Education. (2018). *Family educational rights and privacy act (FERPA).* https://www2.ed.gov/policy/gen/guid/fpco/ferpa/index.html

U.S. Department of Education. (2020). *Protecting students with disabilities.* https://www2.ed.gov/about/offices/list/ocr/504faq.html#:~:text=Section%20504%20prohibits%20discrimination%20on,by%20state%20and%20local%20governments

U.S. Department of Education, National Center for Education Statistics. (2019). *Digest of education statistics, 2018* (54th ed.). https://nces.ed.gov/pubs2020/2020009.pdf

U.S. Department of Justice. (2020). *A guide to disability rights laws.* https://www.ada.gov/cguide.htm

U.S. Equal Opportunities Employment Commission. (2008). *ADA Amendment Act of 2008.* https://www.eeoc.gov/statutes/ada-amendments-act-2008

Weis, R., Dean, E. L., & Osborne, K. J. (2016). Accommodation decision making for postsecondary students with learning disabilities: Individually tailored or one size fits all? *Journal of Learning Disabilities, 49*(5), 484-498. https://doi.org/10.1177/0022219414559648

APPENDIX A

Sample Accommodation Request Letter (From Educational Institution to Level I Fieldwork Site)

XXX Occupational Therapy Program Letterhead
Accommodation Request

DATE: September 1, 2023
TO: XXX Fieldwork Coordinator
               XXX General Hospital
FROM: XXX Academic Fieldwork Coordinator
RE: Student Full Name

The information in this memo is confidential and shall not be released to another party without the student's consent. The student has signed a release of information form to allow communication of this information to you.

Dear Clinical Coordinator,

Thank you very much for agreeing to accept our student from [school name] educational institution occupational therapy program for the upcoming Level I fieldwork placement. [student name], in accordance with Section 504 of the Rehabilitation Act of 1973, the Americans with Disabilities Act of 1990, and the ADA Amendments Act of 2008, has a documented disability that allows access to academic accommodations. The documentation of the disability is current and on file in the Office of Disability Accommodations. The student would like to request the following accommodations while at your facility in order to be proactive regarding possible needs during this fieldwork experience:

1. **Please allow student to complete documentation in a quiet, distraction-free space as much as possible.**

2. **Please allow extended time for documentation, if required, by allowing student to arrive early or stay late to meet same day or other time-sensitive documentation expectations.**

If you would like to schedule a time to speak about any of these requests over the phone or through video conference with [student name] and myself, please feel free to reach out.

Thank you for taking the time to review this request. If the accommodations are acceptable, please sign and return this form indicating that you will provide these accommodations to the best of your ability, given any facility/resident constraints. Please return by [insert date].

_____   _____
Name   Date

Psychosocial Factors
Impacting Level I Fieldwork

Joscelyn Varland, OTD, OTR/L, CLT

As occupational therapy practitioners, we are trained to think holistically. We are taught to evaluate and treat the whole person. We are skilled in understanding how "pieces of the whole" influence and affect one another. Occupational therapy practitioners evaluate and treat people physically, emotionally, mentally, and spiritually. We modify and grade our treatment approaches and style of therapeutic rapport based upon many variables, including the psychosocial needs of the client.

Fieldwork is at the cornerstone of occupational therapy education. Psychosocial factors will impact the performance of the student. Some psychosocial factors can support learning and increase student self-efficacy, while other factors can present as a barrier to learning and hide the ability of student. Additionally, these supports and challenges can impact student perceptions of their educational experience and performance.

Fieldwork educators (FWeds) should approach fieldwork education with the same mentality of holism and person-centered approaches that are used with clients. As do clients, each student has a distinctive lived experience, and each student presents with unique strengths and a set of challenges. In the role of FWed, we may also evaluate the physical, emotional, mental, and spiritual needs of our students. This can mean grading the teaching approach and style.

Hanson, D., & DeIuliis, E. D. (Eds.).
Fieldwork Educator's Guide to Level I Fieldwork (pp. 317-335).
© 2023 Taylor and Francis Group.

Based upon the known data on college-aged students, especially in rigorous academic programs such as occupational therapy, psychosocial factors can impact student learning (Beiter et al., 2015). FWeds should be well equipped to support their fieldwork student holistically. Experiential learning experiences, such as fieldwork, can create a significant emotional response for occupational therapy students. Awareness and understanding of these factors can help the student and the educator have a better experience. This chapter will provide a framework for the FWed to identify and discuss the common psychosocial stressors associated with fieldwork. The FWed will also be provided strategies to help students navigate these stressors and support learning during Level I fieldwork.

LEARNING OBJECTIVES

By the end of reading this chapter and completing the learning activities, the reader should be able to:

1. Identify the influence of psychosocial factors on student fieldwork performance.
2. Describe various psychosocial factors that impact student performance.
3. Compare and contrast strategies FWeds might use to support students' learning experience.
4. Identify strategies that students may implement to manage psychosocial factors.
5. Recognize the impact of addressing psychosocial factors on student confidence and performance.

THE CONNECTION OF PSYCHOSOCIAL FACTORS TO OCCUPATIONAL THERAPY AND LEVEL I FIELDWORK

Psychosocial is defined as "pertaining to intrapersonal, interpersonal, and social experiences and interactions that influence occupational behavior and development" (American Occupational Therapy Association [AOTA], 2004, p. 1). For occupational therapy practitioners, the impact of social factors on our clients is well recognized and prioritized when developing an effective plan of care. The interactional relationship of person, environment, and occupation illustrates the impact of what and who is around us. These interactions help to define who we are and how we approach life. Moreover, occupational therapists are trained to have additional knowledge and skills to work in mental health settings. When providing these services, occupational therapists evaluate the psychosocial factors affecting engagement occupation (AOTA, 2004). As a FWed, the consideration for the psychosocial factors impacting student performance is just as important.

The evaluation of psychosocial factors is embedded in all fieldwork experiences. Educational programs must "ensure that fieldwork objectives for all experiences include a psychosocial objective" and "at least one fieldwork experience (either Level I or Level II) must address practice in behavioral health, or psychological and social factors influencing engagement in occupation" (Accreditation Council for Occupational Therapy Education, 2018, pp. 39-40). Although curriculums vary by institutions, the purpose of Level I fieldwork is to improve clinical thinking and professional reasoning (Nielsen et al., 2017). Students are given the opportunity to work with clients to assist them in better understanding what they have learned in the classroom. The skills of clinical thinking and professional reasoning are often challenging for students to learn, as is the transition from student to entry-level practitioner. Students can feel as though they have less control over

---

BOX 11-1

HOW DO PROGRAMS PREPARE STUDENTS FOR THE TRANSITION FROM CLASSROOM TO EXPERIENTIAL LEARNING?

- Case scenarios
- Problem-based learning
- Clinical videos
- Lab experiences
- Simulated environments

---

their environment and may be negatively impacted by the perceived pressure of fieldwork. Level I fieldwork may be the first opportunity for students to demonstrate the skills learned through coursework. In addition, students are expected to integrate verbal and nonverbal communication, written communication, professional responsibilities, work behaviors, and management skills. Due to the expanded expectations for students while on fieldwork compared to the classroom, they often experience increased stress as a result (Hackenberg & Toth-Cohen, 2018). This stress will inevitably impact the fieldwork experience.

However, when the psychosocial factors are addressed, the educator can focus on the growth of clinical skills (Rezaee et al., 2014). Psychosocial factors can improve student interactions and outcomes or hinder learning and performance. There are many strategies and considerations that will support the student who is anxious, the student who lacks confidence in their abilities, and the student having difficulty with the transition from classroom to clinic. As we think about psychosocial factors, we can think about them as stress related to environmental transition, developmental/life stressors, diagnosed mental health concerns, emotional intelligence, and confidence.

TRANSITION STRESS

As part of the academic preparation, students are taught the content required to be successful in a clinical experience. Also, students have the opportunity to demonstrate practical skills through use of labs, role play, simulation, etc. (Box 11-1). Still, the experience of transitioning from classroom to a practice setting can be challenging. Students perceive a stark contrast in the demonstration of skills within the classroom vs. demonstration of skills in a clinical setting. Students are learning to provide care and are concerned about the opinion of their educator. Though clients rarely present in a "textbook" manner, students are expected to draw from the information and theory taught in the classroom in their work with clients. To successfully transition from the classroom to a clinical setting, the student must demonstrate many forms of knowledge within a new setting (Karp, 2020). When entering this new environment with increased expectations, students can experience an array of emotions, such as anxiety, concern, pressure, and nervousness. In this transition, heightened alertness and action are used as a protective response. Yet, if this behavior is used long-term, it can become maladaptive.

Due to these increased expectations and perceived differences, students can experience uncertainty and tend to focus internally on their own ability and the perceptions of those around them (Tran & Hendrickson, 2015). For successful learning, the student needs to shift from a focus on self to the clinical assessment of the client. Without this shift of focus, the ability of the student to fully demonstrate their skills can be impeded. Although the level of rigor and the amount of content to be learned are determined within the curriculum, considerations can be made in the delivery of information and the structure of the learning environment to support students and their psychosocial needs. Box 11-1 summarizes some of the approaches that may be used within the academic setting to prepare students for the realities of practice as experienced in Level I fieldwork.

In addition, the fieldwork site may also assist the student by recognition of the transition stressors, modeling expectations, explicit discussion of soft skills expected, and guided discovery to help student develop problem-solving skills needed for practice (DeIuliis & Saylor, 2021). Through identification of differences in student learning between academic and practice settings, there is opportunity to normalize the stress or anxiety experienced by the student. This may be introduced in an orientation session to Level I fieldwork and may be reinforced through brief check-ins and short debriefings of various learning experiences. It is important that the FWed does not assume the student is aware of expectations regarding professional behavior in the practice setting, whether simulated or actual, but explicitly discusses expectations related to professional communications (including cell phone use), stress management, and overall clinical protocol (DeIuliis & Saylor, 2021). Knowing when and how to take initiative for learning is often stressful for students (Mattila, 2019). Use of a guided discovery approach, such as the Cognitive Orientation to Daily Occupational Performance Approach, can be helpful (Houldin et al., 2018). Four steps are emphasized: Goal-Plan-Do-Check. In other words, the learning process includes identification of a goal, a plan to accomplish the goal, carrying out actions outlined in the plan, and then a check on the progress of the actions in accomplishing the plan. It provides a process for guiding students in creating a plan and finding strategies that work for them. In doing so, it is important that students are not provided answers, but supported in taking initiative for their own performance success (DeIuliis & Saylor, 2021).

DEVELOPMENTAL/LIFE STRESSORS

While stress is an unavoidable part of life, it is very widespread among university students and becoming a larger mental health concern (Beiter et al., 2015). "Stress is the feeling of being overwhelmed or unable to cope with mental or emotional pressure" (Mental Health Foundation, 2021). Stress is the body's reaction to pressure, and a variety of situations or life experiences can trigger stress. Stress is often triggered when we encounter something new or unexpected that threatens our sense of control over a situation. Individuals manage stress differently, and the ability to cope can be influenced by genetics, past experiences, temperament, and social and economic circumstances.

Common sources of stress for students include school, work, finances, relationships, and day-to-day inconveniences. Students report the greatest concerns are academic performance, pressure to succeed, postgraduation plans, and financial concerns (Beiter et al., 2015). Research indicates college students experienced adverse health concerns related to stress; these concerns included increased anxiety, depression, and other factors that negatively affect physical, mental, and social health (Almhdawi et al., 2018; American College Health Association, 2019). Individuals who experience extended periods of cognitive demands, such as occupational therapy students, can experience stress exhaustion, which presents as mental fatigue in high-level tasks, along with decreased ability to sustain attention. Difficulty with sustained attention and mental fatigue impact the student's ability to learn. These health concerns paired with limited coping skills can have a significant impact of student learning and performance (Krabbe et al., 2017). An illustration of the impact of developmental life stressors on Level I fieldwork is provided in Box 11-2.

In addition to having multiple causes, stress can manifest itself in a variety of different ways. There may be psychological signs, such as difficulty concentrating, worrying, anxiety, and trouble remembering, or physical signs can present, such as changes in weight, frequent colds, or infections (Wegmann et al., 2020). Within health care programs, students report school and fieldwork are the time when they experience their highest levels of stress (Almhdawi et al., 2018). As a result, many students enrolled in professional programs experience adverse health issues related

---

Box 11-2

SCENARIO

Sandra is scheduled to begin her first Level I fieldwork next week. She wants to do well but is very nervous. She is anxious about her living situation. Her placement is out of state, and she is unfamiliar with the city. She has found a place to stay for the duration of her fieldwork, but she is unsure how she will afford it while she is not able to work. Her educator has sent her a list of topics to review prior to starting. However, Sandra is anxious, stressed, and upset about her circumstances and has not been able to concentrate. She was not able to sleep the night before she started. Sandra knows she is unprepared and is afraid of starting her experience off on the wrong foot.

Box 11-3

SCENARIO

Sara is in her first year of occupational therapy school. Her father, who lives 2,000 miles away, has recently been diagnosed with cancer. The cancer metastasized and spread quickly. Sara returned home and was able to spend summer break with her father before he passed. Upon the return in fall, Sara was presenting with flat affect, turning in assignments late, and not doing as well as before. For her Level I, Sara was placed in a home health setting. On the first day, the educator and Sara went to a client's home. This client was recently diagnosed with cancer. Upon hearing this, Sara was triggered on her recent death of her father. Sara could not stop crying and told her FWed she was going to go home.

---

to stress (American College Health Association, 2019). The impact of stress can directly influence student performance during Level I fieldwork. For students, coursework is challenging, but the demonstration of skills within the clinical role adds additional pressure. When students are adversely impacted by stress, so is their learning. The impact of life stressors on student learning is illustrated in Box 11-3. Specific strategies for addressing these types of psychosocial stressors are provided later in this chapter.

DIAGNOSED MENTAL HEALTH CONCERNS

While the stigma around mental health problems is lessening, the impact of mental health disorders can worsen if not addressed. Mental illnesses affect concentration, energy, positivity, and cognitive ability. Students report that stress has an impact on academic performance and presents with an increase in hopelessness, depression, anxiety, and feelings of being overwhelmed (Wegmann et al., 2020). According to the American College Health Association (2019), more than 60% of college students said they had experienced "overwhelming anxiety." Anxiety disorders are the most widespread psychiatric problems among college students, with nearly 11.9% of college students experiencing an anxiety disorder. Research indicates that anxiety has a damaging effect on cognitive processes, such as attention (Hashempour & Mehrad, 2014; Robinson et al., 2013). Anxiety makes the learner uneasy, affects working memory, makes cognitive processes less effective, can lead to avoidance, and decreases emotional intelligence. Another prevalent mental health concern among college students is depression, with incidence rates in college students of 7% to 9% (Pedrelli et al., 2015), while Beiter et al. (2015) found a higher average for allied health profession students with 62% reported being depressed. Depression contributes to lower grade point averages

---

Box 11-4

"I Am Concerned About the Mental Health of My Student. What Can I Do?"

- Identify and differentiate mental health concerns from anxiety related to transitional or developmental/life stressors
- Reach out to the AFWC
- Talk to the student: Ask the student about their mental health
- Determine if the student is able to continue
- Inquire if the academic institution has a counseling center available to the student
- Refer the student to a professional

---

and may lead to the student dropping out of school. Although anxiety and depression are the most common, they are not the only mental health disorder with prevalence in college students. Students may present with mood, eating, addiction, and attention disorders. Likewise, most mental health conditions can lower quality of life, as academics, relationships, and physical health are all affected. In the long-term, these issues can hinder career, overall health, and future plans.

Most mental health disorders have their peak onset during early adulthood. Among traditional students, the significant issues related with attending college may worsen current mental health conditions or trigger an onset. Similarly, nontraditional students, who may have to meet the demands of their several roles (parent, caregiver, employee, etc.), may have an exacerbation of symptoms or a deterioration of lifestyle.

Fieldwork presents an opportunity for students to demonstrate what they know, and it also presents an opportunity for the pressure and stress to impact the overall health and wellness of a student. If the student is suspected of suffering from a mental health disorder that directly impacts the student's ability to be successful while on fieldwork, the FWed should communicate their concerns. Talk with the student and/or reach out to the academic fieldwork coordinator (AFWC). Help the student to recognize the importance and normalcy of seeking professional help for mental health concerns. This is not an issue the FWed should address alone, and it is important that the educator avoid the role of "therapist" with the student. Many universities have resources to address the needs of the student. A summary of strategies for addressing specific mental health needs of students is provided in Box 11-4.

EMOTIONAL INTELLIGENCE

Emotional intelligence is a psychosocial factor that has potential to positively impact student learning during a Level I fieldwork experience. A student with strong emotional intelligence can demonstrate strong interprofessional skills and communication, making the experience beneficial for both the student and the FWed. Emotional intelligence is the insight and understanding of one's own emotions, which means the student has the ability to be aware of, manage, and communicate their emotions. Students who have strong emotional intelligence can handle interpersonal relationships respectfully and with empathy. Understanding emotions directly links with the requirement for students to work well with their educator, to collaborate with clients and other professionals, and to engage in client-centered care (Brown et al., 2016). Moreover, research suggests that intuition and instinct have an affective element. For example, students must be aware of their emotions to access intuition and to trust their emotions enough to make use of their emotions when making decisions or solving a problem.

Research shows the use of emotional intelligence has a direct effect on clinical reasoning (Chaffey et al., 2012). For example, therapists with more years of experience report feeling more comfortable using their intuition in clinical reasoning than those with less experience. Completion of a self-appraisal, such as the Emotional Intelligence Self-Assessment Tool (Sterrett, 2000), can help students to better understand the impact of emotional intelligence on direct patient care. Emotional intelligence is a skill to be developed. Students can use information from appraisals and feedback from others to develop in the areas of low ability. See Box 11-5 for a summary of characteristics associated with strong emotional intelligence.

CONFIDENCE AND STUDENT EFFICACY

The foundation of knowledge and the skills alone are not enough for student success, there must be the ability to perform. Moreover, the student must believe in themselves before they are able to effectively demonstrate what is expected (Artino, 2012). Students with confidence have the capacity to manage clinical situations and provide care using safe, appropriate, and effective approaches with less stress and fear (Abdelkader et al., 2021). The student who refrains from questions, appears disinterested, or unprepared may be experiencing insecurity and lack of confidence. These behaviors will negatively impact the ability of the students to grow and learn from fieldwork experiences and will limit the ability of the FWed to be an effective mentor if not addressed.

Self-efficacy and confidence can be used interchangeably to define a student's perceived competence and are necessary for students to be competent in their role as therapists. For this reason, it is important to consider these concepts when discussing fieldwork (Andonian, 2017). Students recognize Level I fieldwork as an opportunity to cultivate confidence, which is a frequent goal of fieldwork. Still, most students question their confidence prior to fieldwork and report a lack of confidence as a barrier to being successful in fieldwork (Derdall et al., 2002; Mackenzie, 2002).

FWeds play a significant role in the self-efficacy of a student (Mackenzie, 2002). While it is up to the FWed to determine the best approach to teaching clinical skills while on fieldwork, *the provision of a structured experience* can help the student to feel more confident in their own ability. Students prefer structure from their preceptor. This concept is grounded by students knowing what is expected, having encouragement, and being involved in patient care, schedule development, and decision making where appropriate (Grenier, 2015). When the educator fosters the student's sense of self-efficacy, the student is better able to receive feedback and actively participate in fieldwork (Andonian, 2017).

> **Box 11-6**
> ## Structured Experience to Support Confidence
>
> - Provide students with a list of assessments and diagnosis to review prior to the fieldwork experience
> - Provide demonstration of skills (modeling)
> - Encourage participation in experiences (active learning)
> - Offer observation of other professionals or team members
> - Simulate experiences where possible
> - Provide direct supervision
> - Create a daily plan

Although fieldwork can be completed in a variety of settings and have different durations, placements should be long enough to *encourage students to develop professional relationships* and feel at ease in the environment; this can be more easily accomplished when providing the student with information about what to expect prior to fieldwork (Grenier, 2015; Mulholland & Derdall, 2007). The opportunity to develop familiarity and recognize the consistency of the setting will help the student to better understand the environment and the expectation for that setting. When the student and the FWed both understand the expectations of a fieldwork placement, it leads to a supportive, collaborative, and valuable learning experience (Ingwersen et al., 2017). An example of strategies that can assist in supporting student self-confidence is provided in Box 11-6. Students are seeking affirmation that the skills they have learned are effective in the field and as part of their transition into a clinician.

HOW CAN LEVEL I FIELDWORK EDUCATORS HELP?

There are many strategies that can support the student with their existing skills and ease the psychosocial factors that may be inhibiting learning. Students report a reduction of stress when having a more interactional relationship with the educator (Sarkar et al., 2020). Students prefer clear direction and expectations from their educator. Broad strategies that will be helpful in addressing psychosocial issues across all areas will be provided first, followed by a discussion of specific strategies that might be used to help students transition from the academic to practice environment, bolster a student's emotional intelligence, help students manage stressors, and increase student confidence.

Self-Assessment

Once the student and the educator understand the requirements for the fieldwork, it is important to begin the process of self-assessment. There are many tools to act as a guide for self-reflection for both the student and the educator. For this section, we will focus on self-assessment of fieldwork education, professional skills, and learning styles.

The AOTA offers FWed competency tools for self-reflection, such as Fieldwork Experience Assessment Tool for Educator and for Student (FEAT; AOTA, 2001) and Self-Assessment Tool for FWed (SAFECOM; AOTA, 1997). These tools allow educators and students to identify strengths and areas for growth. The areas identified for growth provide the opportunity to develop a plan for the enhancement of skills in the areas of practice, education, supervision, etc. FWeds may choose to have students complete a self-appraisal of their individual strengths and areas of need when preparing for fieldwork using the FEAT. The student can set measurable goals to address any areas of need and develop self-assurance with their individual strengths. Self-reflection creates opportunity to increase awareness of the skills that they already possess and leads to a feeling of competence (Iliff et al., 2019).

Professional skills are an important part of the successful transition from student to clinician and cover a wide variety of skills. Each student demonstrates strengths and areas of need in the development of professionalism. However, professional skills are learnable. Students should use feedback received from educators and peers in assessing individual ability, but students can also use self-assessment to identify the areas of professionalism that can support or hinder experiential learning. The Genos Emotional Intelligence Inventory (Genos EI; Gignac, 2008) and the Communication Styles: A Self-Assessment Exercise (Case, 1981) are two ways students can assess the professionalism in a clinical setting. Similarly, if needed, students can explore areas of problem solving, critical thinking, interpersonal, and leadership skills through self-assessment.

Understanding learning preferences and what methods of teaching are preferred can help a student to feel more self-assured in their ability to be successful with experiential learning. Although there is formal testing of learning styles, such as The VARK Learning Style Model (Fleming, 1995) and Kolb Learning Inventory (Kolb, 1976), just as valuable are the acts of reflecting, observing, and communicating with students about how they process their learning. Equally important as the educator knowing the learning style of the student is the educator knowing their own learning style. Exploring the learning styles and needs of the student may help create an opportunity to discuss concerns and areas of challenge upfront. When given the opportunity, the student can identify preferred learning styles and communicate needs to the educator. An opportunity for open acceptance of evaluation, communication, and critique clinical competence will be created. Students can develop an understanding of their strengths and challenges in a professional role and identify opportunities to improve. Table 11-1 provides a summary of helpful self-assessment tools.

Communication

Communication among students and their preceptors is a crucial part to experience a successful and positive placement. Students prefer to collaborate with a FWed who represents themselves as a facilitator or mentor for direct guidance rather than a general supervisor, meaning students want direct supervision and feedback. Lack of communication can lead to misinterpretations of the students' behavior, motivation, or ability to demonstrate clinical skills (Rezaee et al., 2014; Robertson et al., 2011). Communication related to expectations, objectives, providing feedback, and debriefing will provide the student with clarity and the opportunity to be successful.

If expectations are unclear, it is difficult for those involved to prepare (Rezaee et al., 2014). Communication begins by learning about the student prior to the placement. For example, you might request information about the student's past work and/or fieldwork experiences, as well as their professional interests and strengths. If you are asking students to complete any type of self-assessment prior to the Level I fieldwork, you may ask them to share the results before the start of the placement. A discussion with the student prior to fieldwork can facilitate increased self-awareness and allow the student to set goals for the experience. See Box 11-7 for strategies to facilitate communication prior to the Level I fieldwork experience.

Conveying information, such as diagnosis and assessments to review, schedule, dress code, parking, prerequisites, and learning expectations, can help the student feel more prepared and consequently help to calm nerves. For students, clarity of expectations and assignments can lessen

TABLE 11-1
SUMMARY OF SELF-ASSESSMENT TOOLS

FIELDWORK SELF-ASSESSMENT	PROFESSIONAL SKILLS INVENTORY	LEARNING STYLE ASSESSMENTS
FEAT This tool is used for self-appraisal of the educator or student to identify individual strengths and areas of need when preparing for fieldwork (AOTA, 2001).	*Genos EI* The Genos EI measures how often respondents report emotionally intelligent behavior in the workplace according to seven constructs (Gignac, 2008).	*The VARK Learning Style Model* Evaluates learning styles which represents our preference to receive information from the world around us (Fleming, 1995).
SAFECOM This tool is designed for the FWed at all Levels of experience (AOTA,1997).	*Communication Styles: A Self-Assessment Exercise* This self-assessment is a tool to identify communication style and strategies for adjusting to other communication styles (Case, 1981).	*Kolb Learning Inventory* The way we think about information is through the process of either concrete experience or abstract conceptualization thereby creating the continuum of learning (Kolb, 1976).

BOX 11-7
METHODS TO FACILITATE
COMMUNICATION PRIOR TO LEVEL I FIELDWORK

1. Request information about the student prior to placement (past experiences, professional interests, strengths).
2. Discuss individual student goals for fieldwork.
3. Ask student to discuss anticipated strengths and challenges related to fieldwork. Provide direct supervision.

---

unnecessary stress, therefore decreasing associated anxiety. Similarly, awareness of the fieldwork objectives will help the student to understand the expectations for their performance and allow the student to prepare accordingly. FWeds can promote student confidence in their ability to successfully master learning objectives. When completing a fieldwork, students are evaluated upon conclusion, and many times, the objectives are discussed during the final meeting to ensure the outcomes were met. Sharing the objectives and evaluation forms with the student at the beginning of the experience, as opposed to waiting until the end, is helpful. The discussion of learning objectives provides clear expectations and allows the educator and the student to review which skills the student will be expected to demonstrate. For a Level I experience, the AFWC will be a great resource in helping all to understand the objectives. The learning objectives of each fieldwork

> **Box 11-8**
>
> ## STRUCTURING COMMUNICATION THROUGHOUT FIELDWORK
>
> **Prior to Fieldwork:** Send the student a list of expectations; materials and assessments to review, prerequisites, dress code, where to park, expectations for lunch, etc.
>
> **First Day of Fieldwork:** Discuss objectives for fieldwork, discuss with student how feedback will be provided, provide measurable expectations, discuss how student will be evaluated.
>
> **During Fieldwork:** Provide updates as to student's strengths and challenges, provide outline of daily plan, provide measurable expectations for progress (i.e., number of treatment sessions or evaluations, independent demonstrations of assessments).
>
> **End of Fieldwork:** Review overall performance and provide an evaluation that is consistent with the feedback that has been presented throughout. There should not be any "new" feedback presented.

experience will be unique and align with the educational program curriculum and the sequence of the content that has been taught. These objectives should be collaborative and meet the requirements of the academic program while emphasizing the needs and expectations that are specific to the fieldwork experience.

The use of objectives can also help to create a daily plan. Many Level II fieldwork experiences have a weekly schedule to assist with progression of the fieldwork. A Level I fieldwork is less time intensive than a Level II experience, but a clear progression can still be valuable to the student and educator alike. A shared plan gives the student direction in how to prepare for each day. Plans can be general or specific depending upon the fieldwork. See Box 11-8 for a summary of strategies that may be used to clearly communicate and process learning expectations.

The next area of communication that is vital to a strong learning experience is *feedback*. Communicating expectations, providing positive feedback, and constructive criticism are part of the conversations that will strengthen student learning. Even if a student may experience angst and concern, this should not be a deterrent to provide feedback. It is important to keep in mind that students typically are more likely to report having a negative experience if there is a lack of communication. Effective communication should address the successes, as well as the areas for improvement (DeIuliis & Saylor, 2021). The acknowledgment of the positives with the challenges increases acceptance and learning of the student, especially for students from Generations Y and Z. Moreover, the receipt of constructive critique is a professional skill needed for a success in the professional working environment. Feedback can be provided in verbal or written format but is most productive when feedback is presented in a timely manner. One benefit of timely feedback is the opportunity for the student to have affirmation and reinforcement of positive behaviors or adjust accordingly. See Box 11-9 to consider factors that have influenced your own experiences with receiving feedback.

Feedback can be taken a step further with *debriefing*. Debriefing is described as a collaborative, thoughtful, two-way conversation. Debriefing sessions have been shown to increase student competence. When a debriefing component is incorporated into fieldwork, students can process their experiences and confidently incorporate them in future practice. Successful debriefing

---

Box 11-9

REFLECTION ON PERSONAL EXPERIENCES WITH RECEIVING FEEDBACK

Think about a time when you perceived the feedback you received was positive.
- What do you remember about the presentation of the feedback?
- Was the feedback expected?

Have you experienced an approach to feedback that encouraged you to be receptive?

Box 11-10

COMPARE AND CONTRAST FEEDBACK VERSUS DEBRIEFING

FEEDBACK	DEBRIEFING
• Compares learner performance with benchmark standards • Performance is satisfactory or unsatisfactory • FWed assesses performance	• Students consider the approaches, reactions, and outcomes • Performance/actions are considered within a range of appropriate on a continuum of skill • FWed and student assess performance

---

motivates the student and helps them to correct their performance. Debriefing is the time where learners evaluate their performance, recognize gaps in ability, consider areas for progress, and strengthen knowledge and skills. This allows clinical application with better outcomes (Voyer & Hatala, 2015). See Box 11-10 for a comparison of feedback and debriefing.

Emphasizing Learning Opportunities

The composition of Level I fieldwork is varied and provides a variety of learning environments and demonstration of skills. In order for Level I fieldwork to provide an optimal learning experience, the opportunity to improve advocacy skills, prove competence, and demonstrate teamwork are all important from the student's perspective. There are many ways to optimize learning during Level I fieldwork, such as observation, simulated experience, active engagement, reflection, and guided questions.

According to research, a positive Level I experience is one which the student can observe best practice with competent role models and actively participate (Koenig et al., 2003; Nielsen et al., 2017). Students benefit from observing demonstrations from faculty and educators. Seeing best practice in action will increase awareness. This increased awareness will support student confidence and decrease stress. Naidoo and Van Wyk (2016) revealed that students who observed treatment sessions and completed practice labs prior to Level I fieldwork displayed improvement in their learning, competence, and self-assurance. Allowing the student to see the educator interact with clients and deliver intervention will increase insight and self-confidence during fieldwork.

Simulated learning in occupational therapy academic programs has an impact on a student's educational experience to prepare for fieldwork. Simulation allows the participant to engage in learning in a low-risk environment and supports clinical reasoning, problem-solving, and

---

Box 11-11

SAMPLE GUIDED QUESTIONS

- What did you see?
- What is your rationale for choosing this activity?
- How did the client factors influence this treatment?
- What would you do differently if you were to approach the same problem again?
- How could you better support the client?

---

decision-making skills (Bethea et al., 2014). Students became more aware of their own behavior and are able to develop empathy and sensitivity using simulation. Simulation also helps students become more aware of the patient as a person (Bethea et al., 2014; Giles et al., 2014; Øgård-Repål et al., 2018). This approach can be utilized while on fieldwork through use of role play and simulated trials. Use of role play and practice in the administering of assessments and techniques will decrease fear and stress and prepare the student for demonstrating skill when working with a client.

Active participation is another way in which students can grow in their skill. There is often a misconception that Level I fieldwork is passive, hands-off, or similar to a shadowing experience. This is not accurate. Students must be offered ample opportunity to grow and develop skills. The more opportunity that is provided, the more comfortable the student can be in their ability. Through repetition, the student's skill is performed, practiced, and progressively becomes easier. As the student develops their ability, they will not need to think consciously about the activity. This allows the student to focus mental capacities to learning new skills and concepts. The hands-on experiences of fieldwork allow students the opportunity to manipulate materials and equipment and learn about the scope of practice via real world experiences. Allowing the student to be an active participant during fieldwork contributes to overall sense of ability and accomplishment as the student can demonstrate clinical skills, professional behaviors, and clinical reasoning (Haynes, 2011).

The creation of reflection and guided questions can support both the role of the educator and the role of the student. Reflection and guided questions allow the student to think more deeply about what they have seen and process the implications. Questions from Level I FWeds can enhance learning and support student perceptions about their own ability. Predeveloped questions allow the educator to organize the flow of information and the components of the experience the educator would like to emphasize. Guided questions allow the student to reflect more deeply about what they have experienced; these questions can also be taken home at the end of the day to allow time for reflection and review of materials. A sample of guided questions is provided in Box 11-11.

WHAT CAN A STUDENT DO TO MANAGE THE IMPACT OF PSYCHOSOCIAL FACTORS?

There are many strategies that can help to calm the student and ease anxiety. Students may ask FWeds for advice on how to manage the stress and anxiety they experience on fieldwork. Students can benefit from practical solutions and setting goals. When addressing this question, the FWed can start with some general strategies and recommendations to help students navigate psychosocial factors on Level I fieldwork, by discussing self-care, development of coping strategies, improving emotional intelligence, and improving confidence.

TABLE 11-2
STRATEGIES FOR MANAGING ANXIETY

MANAGING AN ANXIOUS BODY	MANAGING AN ANXIOUS MIND	MANAGING ANXIOUS BEHAVIOR
• Limit caffeine and alcohol • Well-balanced diet • Get enough sleep • Practice mindfulness • Utilize deep breathing exercises • Make time for exercise	• Stop catastrophizing • Debunk unreasonable thoughts • Avoid activities that increase anxiety • Stop anxious thoughts • Do the most difficult tasks first • Positive self-talk	• Organize and plan for your day—do not allow too much free time • Seek life balance and activities you enjoy during evenings • Have fun • Set goals and implement a plan

Adapted from Wehrenberg, M. (2008). *Ten best-ever anxiety management techniques.* WW Norton & Company, Inc.

Occupational therapy students have busy schedules and multiple demands; as a result, students can fail to recognize the importance of self-care. Practicing self-care can decrease anxious feelings and improve the student's ability to engage and learn. Following a sleep schedule, healthy diet, exercise, and social engagement are all vital to emotional health and wellness.

One approach that allows students to cope with stress and anxiety and have better learning outcomes is mindful meditation. Mindfulness is the exercise of intentionally focusing your mind on the present. This practice helps shift preoccupations toward an appreciation of a moment or physical and emotional sensations. Mindfulness allows students to have greater awareness of their physiological and physical state. Similarly, gratitude-based training has been found to have a positive impact. Individuals with mental well-being experience better client interactions and clinical awareness (Mattila et al., 2020). Table 11-2 provides a summary of strategies for self-care that holistically address the student's body, mind, and behavior.

The abilities that make up emotional intelligence can be learned at any time. The key skills for building emotional intelligence and improving the ability to manage emotions and connect with others are self-management and self-awareness. Self-management is the ability to handle emotions while receiving feedback or manage a difficult situation in a healthy way, such as taking initiative, following through on commitments, and adapting to changing circumstances. With self-awareness, students can recognize their own emotions and how they affect thoughts and actions. This awareness can assist in better understanding strengths and weaknesses. The skills of emotional intelligence can enable students to override stress and improve confidence.

Not everyone is born with an innate sense of self-confidence. Sometimes it can be difficult to build confidence, either because of past experiences or because of low self-esteem, but confidence can be learned and practiced. Therefore, it is important that students develop a growth mindset in regard to emotional intelligence (DeIuliis & Saylor, 2021) and incorporate opportunity to practice skills that will foster self-confidence. As the student becomes more comfortable with the skill, confidence and self-efficacy will improve. Also, students should focus on accomplishments thus far and set measurable goals for what they would like to accomplish. Setting goals allows the students to see small achievements that can build confidence.

HELPING STUDENTS NAVIGATE SPECIFIC PSYCHOSOCIAL FACTORS ON LEVEL I FIELDWORK

After having reviewed general strategies that are helpful for students in managing psychosocial stressors of Level I fieldwork, next we will discuss specific strategies that may be helpful in further assisting students to transition from the academic to practice setting and in managing mental health. In the transition to Level I fieldwork, students are expected to assume a new role. The process of learning and demonstrating knowledge in a classroom is different than synthesizing and applying knowledge with a client. The demonstration of new skill can leave the student feeling unsure about their own ability. Additionally, transitioning to a new environment for a fieldwork and with a new educator can leave the student unsure about what to expect.

For example, Sandra (see Box 11-2) is scheduled to begin her first Level I fieldwork and is anxious. She is concerned about a variety of factors directly and indirectly related to her fieldwork. She will show up to her first day unprepared and exhausted. To a FWed, she may present quiet and disinterested. The educator may be left wondering if this student is ready for fieldwork and if she has the skills to be successful as she progresses toward a Level II experience. This becomes a challenging situation for both the FWed and the student. However, there are specific strategies that can help the student transition to a new setting and help the FWed feel prepared to navigate these behaviors and create a strong learning environment; strategies for addressing the earlier scenario are illustrated in Box 11-12.

In the scenario from Box 11-12, general stress and nervousness about fieldwork can be anticipated in advance and predictably addressed by the educator, but there are those circumstances that the educator will not anticipate. There may not always be an anticipatory response available when handling mental health issues. This is the case with Sara (see Box 11-3). Most often, the student would not have divulged the loss of her father to a new FWed. Also, it is not likely that either the student or the FWed would anticipate a home health setting to trigger a psychosocial response. Even when signs of mental health distress become evident to the educator, it is often the case that a triggering event, such as the student leaving the session crying, would be the first indication for the FWed that a mental health issue is evident.

These circumstances are best navigated with the same compassion and empathy we have for our clients. Although there is not a "correct" way to respond, there are considerations for how to proceed. Determine what is happening with the student and the severity of the issue. Remember the student is an adult learner and is responsible for their education, so be sure to start with the student when shaping the outcome. Do not be afraid to ask questions, such as asking the student, "What happened?" When the student is composed enough to share, provide a listening ear. In Sara's case, the educator can ask how much time she needs, or if she is seeking professional help. Ascertain if the student is addressing their own needs or are already seeking support. A conversation should occur as to whether the student can or should continue the fieldwork. The student may not have shared this information with the AFWC yet, but the coordinator should be contacted if the mental health of student is impacting the progression of the fieldwork. If this is the case, the student may need to explore accommodations as examined in Chapter 10. Discuss with the student any plans to reach out to the school and queries that will be posed. There will be support available for the student and for the educator as is discussed in subsequent chapters of this book.

Box 11-12

Sandra's Fieldwork Experience

When provided the student's contact information, Tia, the educator, reached out to Sandra and requested a Zoom meeting. During the meeting, Tia asked Sandra about her previous experiences and her familiarity with the outpatient setting of her fieldwork. Sandra reported she had not spent time in an outpatient clinic but could complete some observation hours before her placement. They also discussed Sandra's strengths and challenges related to communication and learning. Tia discovered that Sandra prefers to see a demonstration first before being asked to complete a task herself. She also learned Sandra likes verbal feedback throughout the day but also likes an overall review of what went well, and what could be done different. Tia offered a list of assessment tools, diagnosis, a skills checklist, and site expectations to review before the placement. They reviewed the checklist and expectations together so Sandra would know which skills she would be required to demonstrate during her 1 week. Tia also let Sandra know she would be sent specifics about parking and schedule a week before she came. On Monday, Tia and Sandra met at the entrance to the building as planned. Tia let Sandra know they had a busy day scheduled, but they would have time to sit down and answer questions after sessions were complete. Sandra accompanied Tia for all her treatment sessions, and Tia would explain what she was doing during the sessions or immediately following. At the end of the day, they met to discuss, and Tia answered Sandra's questions. Tia let Sandra know the schedule for day two and that Sandra will have time to complete chart review and assist with the afternoon treatments. She also asked Sandra to create a written elevator speech explaining occupational therapy to a client. Tia has a new client on Wednesday, and if appropriate, she will have Sandra assist with the evaluation. Sandra showed up prepared Tuesday morning. She was able to present ideas for the afternoon session and practice her speech with her educator and get feedback. Sandra did well with her client interactions, and Tia was able to see her confidence grow. The end of day two, when meeting, Tia was able to ask Sandra what she thought went well, and what were the challenges of the day. Together they discussed the day and considered alternative approaches and outcomes. The meeting ended with a schedule for the rest of the week, as well as a list of guided questions for Sandra to spend time reflecting and preparing for the next day. Tia was able to create a structure that supported Sandra and facilitated communication. The outcome was a successful fieldwork that deepened the student's understanding and learning.

SUMMARY

Experiential learning experiences, such as fieldwork, will often create a significant emotional response for occupational therapy students. As occupational therapy practitioners, we consider a holistic approach. We evaluate and treat the whole person, addressing the psychological, emotional, mental, and spiritual factors. We modify and grade our approaches and style of therapeutic rapport based upon many variables, including the needs of the person. As FWeds, we can approach the role of Level I FWed with this same mindset of a person-centered and holistic approach.

Each student has a unique lived experience, intrinsic sense of motivation, and distinctive set of strengths and challenges. These challenges and experiences impact the way the student will perceive and respond to their fieldwork experience. FWeds should be prepared to support their fieldwork student utilizing a framework to identify and discuss the psychosocial stressors associated with experiential leaning. The FWed can also use strategies to better prepare students to navigate and manage these stressors during Level I fieldwork.

LEARNING ACTIVITIES

1. Reflect upon how psychosocial influences may impact your ability to supervise a Level I fieldwork experience.

   a. What behavior may be noted in a student who is experiencing anxiety related to their fieldwork experience? How can you best address the student's anxiety?

   b. How can you structure the experience to decrease student stress and support learning?

   c. How may a student with a mental health crisis present? How would your response differ?

2. Alicia is your occupational therapy student who you will be supervising for 2 weeks in a block Level I fieldwork placement. She is at the end of the first week and is very quiet and tends to stand off to the side during sessions. During each session, you explain your rationale and treatment; following each session you check in to see if she has any questions. Each time she reports "no." You are scheduled to administer an assessment that you know she has learned in school. You offer her the opportunity to assist with the administration. Alicia turns red and says she is not ready. You have decided to address the matter at the end of the day.

   a. How can you structure the feedback?

   b. How would a briefing-debriefing be different?

3. Jenna is a first-year occupational therapy student and her 1-week Level I fieldwork is scheduled next month. Your interactions with her have been brief, and she has not shared a lot of information about herself. She has let you know she is excited but very nervous.

   a. What are some strategies you can use to structure the fieldwork for Jenna?

   b. What recommendations can you make for Jenna to increase her confidence before fieldwork?

   c. How will you manage the situation if the student discloses she has recently been diagnosed with depression?

REFERENCES

Abdelkader, A. M., El-Aty, N. S. A., & Abdelrahman, S. M. (2021). The relationship between self-confidence in learning and clinical educators' characteristics by nursing students. *International Journal of Nursing Education, 13*(2), 1-10. https://doi.org/10.3705/ijone.v13i2.14614

Accreditation Council for Occupational Therapy Education. (2018). *2018 Accreditation Council for Occupational Therapy Education standards and interpretive guidelines.* https://acoteonline.org/wp-content/uploads/2020/10/2018-ACOTE-Standards.pdf

Almhdawi, K. A., Kanaan, S. F., Khader, Y., Al-Hourani, Z., Almomani, F., & Nazzal, M. (2018). Study-related mental health symptoms and their correlates among allied health professions students. *Work, 61*(3), 391-401. https://doi.org/10.3233/wor-182815

American College Health Association. (2019). *National College Health Assessment II: Reference group executive summary spring 2019.* https://www.acha.org/documents/ncha/NCHA-II_SPRING_2019_US_REFERENCE_GROUP_EXECUTIVE_SUMMARY.pdf

American Occupational Therapy Association. (1997). *Self-assessment tool for fieldwork educator competency.* https://www.aota.org/~/media/Corporate/Files/EducationCareers/Educators/Fieldwork/Supervisor/Forms/Self-Assessment%20Tool%20FW%20Ed%20Competency%20(2009).ashx

American Occupational Therapy Association. (2001). *Fieldwork experience assessment tool (FEAT).* https://www.aota.org/education/fieldwork/-/media/01c63b933e5f41a0b7cce3da3cf8bdba.ashx

American Occupational Therapy Association. (2004) Psychosocial aspects of occupational therapy. *American Journal Occupational Therapy, 58*(6), 669-672. https://doi.org/10.5014/ajot.58.6.669

Andonian, L. (2017). Occupational therapy students' self-efficacy, experience of supervision, and perception of meaningfulness of Level II fieldwork. *Open Journal of Occupational Therapy, 5*(2). https://doi.org/10.15453/2168-6408.1220

Artino, A. R., Jr. (2012). Academic self-efficacy: From educational theory to instructional practice. *Perspectives on Medical Education, 1*(2), 76–85. https://doi.org/10.1007/s40037-012-0012-5

Beiter, R., Nash, R., McCrady, M., Rhoades, D., Linscomb, M., Clarahan, M., & Sammut, S. (2015). The prevalence and correlates of depression, anxiety, and stress in a sample of college students. *Journal of Affective Disorders, 173*, 90-96. https://doi.org/10.1016/j.jad.2014.10.054

Bethea, D. P., Castillo, D. C., & Harvison, N. (2014). Use of simulation in occupational therapy education: Way of the future? *American Journal of Occupational Therapy, 68*(Suppl. 2), S32-S39. https://doi.org/10.5014/ajot.2014.012716

Brown, T., Williams, B., & Etherington, J. (2016). Emotional intelligence and personality traits as predictors of occupational therapy students' practice education performance: A cross-sectional study. *Occupational Therapy International, 23*, 412–424. https://doi.org/10.1002/oti.1443

Case, P. (1981). *Communication styles: A self-assessment exercise "Teaching for the Cross-Cultural Mind".* SIETAR.

Chaffey, L., Unsworth, C. A., & Fossey E. (2012). Relationship between intuition and emotional intelligence in occupational therapists in mental health practice. *American Journal of Occupational Therapy, 66*(1), 88-96. https://doi.org/10.5014/ajot.2012.001693

DeIuliis, E. D., & Saylor, E. (2021). Bridging the gap: Three strategies to optimize professional relationships with Generation Y and Z. *Open Journal of Occupational Therapy, 9*(1), 1-13. https://doi.org/10.15453/2168-6408.1748

Derdall, M., Olson, P., Janzen, W., & Warren, S. (2002). Development of a questionnaire to examine confidence of occupational therapy students during fieldwork experiences. *Canadian Journal of Occupational Therapy, 69*(1), 49–56. https://doi.org/10.1177/000841740206900105

Fleming, N. D. (1995). I'm different; not dumb. Modes of presentation (VARK) in the tertiary classroom. In A. Zelmer (Ed.), *Research and development in higher education, proceedings of the 1995 annual conference of the higher education and research development society of Australasia* (Vol. 18, pp. 308-313).

Gignac, G. E. (2008). *Genos emotional intelligence inventory technical manual.* Genos Press.

Giles, A. K., Carson, N. E., Breland, H. L., Coker-Bolt, P., & Bowman, P. J. (2014). Use of simulated patients and reflective video analysis to assess occupational therapy students' preparedness for fieldwork. *American Journal of Occupational Therapy, 68*(2), S57-S66. https://doi.org/10.5014/ajot.2014.685S03

Grenier, M. L. (2015). Facilitators and barriers to learning in occupational therapy fieldwork education: Student perspectives. *American Journal of Occupational Therapy, 69*(2), 1-9. https://doi.org/10.5014/ajot.2015.015180

Hackenberg, G. R., & Toth-Cohen, S. (2018). Professional behaviors and fieldwork: A curriculum-based model in occupational therapy. *Journal of Occupational Therapy Education, 2*(2). https://doi.org/10.26681/jote.2018.020203

Hashempour, S., & Mehrad, A. (2014). The effect of anxiety and emotional intelligence on students' learning process. *Journal of Education and Social Policy, 1*(2), 115-122.

Haynes, C. J. (2011). Active participation in fieldwork Level I: Fieldwork educator and student perceptions. *Occupational Therapy in Health Care, 25*(4), 257-269. https://doi.org/10.3109/07380577.2011.595477

Houldin, A., McEwen, S. E., Howell, M. W., & Polatajko, H. J. (2018). The cognitive orientation to daily occupational performance approach and transfer: A scoping review. *OTJR: Occupation, Participation and Health, 38*(3), 157-172. https://doi.org/10.1177/1539449217736059

Iliff, S. L., Tool, G., Bowyer, P., Parham, D., Fletcher, T. S., & Freysteinson, W. M. (2019). Occupational therapy student conceptions of self-reflection in Level II fieldwork. *Journal of Occupational Therapy Education, 3*(1). https://doi.org/10.26681/jote.2019.030105

Ingwersen, K., Lyons, N., & Hitch, D. (2017). Perceptions of fieldwork in occupational therapy. *The Clinical Teacher, 14*(1), 55-59. https://doi.org/10.1111/tct.12518

Karp, P. (2020). Occupational therapy student readiness for transition to the fieldwork environment: A pilot case study. *Open Journal of Occupational Therapy, 8*(4), 1-14. https//: doi.org/10.15453/2168-6408.1719

Koenig, K., Johnson, C., Morano, C. K., & Ducette, J. P. (2003). Development and validation of a professional behavior assessment. *Journal of Allied Health, 32*(2), 86-91.

Kolb, D. A. (1976). *The learning style inventory: technical manual.* McBer.

Krabbe, D., Ellbin, S., Nilsson, M., Jonsdottir, H., & Samuelsson, H. (2017). Executive function and attention in patients with stress related exhaustion: perceived fatigue and effect of distraction. *Stress, 20*(4), 333-340. https://doi.org/10.1080/10253890.2017.1336533

Mackenzie, L. (2002). Briefing and debriefing of student fieldwork experiences: Exploring concerns and reflecting on practice. *Australian Occupational Therapy Journal, 49*(2), 82-92. https://doi.org/10.1046/j.1440-1630.2002.00296.x

Mattila, A. M. (2019). Practice-ready skills for the capstone. In E. D. DeIuliis, & J. A. Bednarski (Eds.), *The entry level occupational therapy doctorate capstone: A framework for the experience and project* (pp. 79-91). SLACK Incorporated.

Mattila, A., DeIuliis, E. D., Martin, R. M., & Grogan, J. (2020). Mindfulness in the occupational therapy classroom: Infusing grit, gratitude practice, and a growth mindset into OT education. *Journal of Occupational Therapy Education, 4*(4). https://doi.org/10.26681/jote.2020.040410

Mental Health Foundation. (2021). *Stress.* https://www.mentalhealth.org.uk/a-to-z/s/stress

Mulholland, S., & Derdall, M. (2007). An early fieldwork experience: Student and preceptor perspectives. *Canadian Journal of Occupational Therapy, 74*(3), 161-171. https://doi.org/10.1177/000841740707400304

Naidoo, D., & Van Wyk, J. (2016). Fieldwork practice for learning: Lessons from occupational therapy students and their supervisors. *African Journal of Health Professions Education, 8*(1), 37-40. https://doi-org.ezproxy.umary.edu/10.7196/AJHPE.2016.v8i1.536

Nielsen, S., Jedlicka, J. S., Hanson, D., Fox, L., & Graves, C. (2017). Student perceptions of non-traditional Level I fieldwork. *Journal of Occupational Therapy Education, 1*(2). https://doi.org/10.26681/jote.2017.010206

Øgård-Repål, A., De Presno, Å. K., & Fossum, M. (2018). Simulation with standardized patients to prepare undergraduate nursing students for mental health clinical practice: An integrative literature review. *Nurse Education Today, 66*, 149-157. https://doi-org.ezproxy.umary.edu/10.1016/j.nedt.2018.04.018

Pedrelli, P., Nyer, M., Yeung, A., Zulauf, C., & Wilens, T. (2015). College students: Mental health problems and treatment considerations. *Academic Psychiatry, 39*(5), 503-511. https://doi.org/10.1007/s40596-014-0205-9

Rezaee, M., Rassafiani, M., Khankeh, H., & Hosseini, M. A. (2014). Experiences of occupational therapy students in the first field- work education: A qualitative study. *Medical Journal of the Islamic Republic of Iran, 28*(13), 1-12.

Robertson, L., Smellie, T., Wilson, P., & Cox, L. (2011). Learning styles and fieldwork education: Students' perspectives. *New Zealand Journal of Occupational Therapy, 58*(1), 36-40.

Robinson, O. J., Vytal, K., Cornmell, B. R., & Grillon, C. (2013). The impact of anxiety upon cognition: Perspectives from human threat of shock studies. *Frontiers in Human Neuroscience, 7*, 203. https://doi.org/10.3389/fnhum.2013.00230

Sarkar, S., Menon, V., & Kumar, S. (2020). Reducing stress among medical students: A qualitative study of students' perspectives. *Indian Journal of Psychiatry, 62*(2), 198-201. https://doi.org/10.4103/psychiatry.IndianJPsychiatry_354_19

Sterrett, E. A. (2000). The manager's pocket guide to emotional intelligence. In D. E. Feldman, *The handbook of emotionally intelligent leadership*. HBD Press.

Tran, Q. D., & Hendrickson, R. C. (2015). *Transitioning from academic to clinical practice. Presented at 2015 Association of Counselor Educators and Supervisors Annual Conference*. https://www.counseling.org/docs/default-source/vistas/article_5753f227f16116603abcacff0000bee5e7.pdf?sfvrsn=4

Voyer, S., & Hatala, R. (2015). Debriefing and feedback: Two sides of the same coin? *Simulation in Health Care: The Journal of the Society for Simulation in Health care, 10*(2), 67-68. https://doi.org/10.1097/SIH.0000000000000075

Wegmann, J., Marshall, J., Tsai, C., & Dionne, S. (2020) Health education and changing stress mindsets: The moderating role of personality. *American Journal of Health Education, 51*(4), 244-256. https://doi.org/10.1080/19325037.2020.1767002

Wehrenberg, M. (2008). *Ten best-ever anxiety management techniques*. WW Norton & Company, Inc.

Unit IV

Level I
Fieldwork Assessment

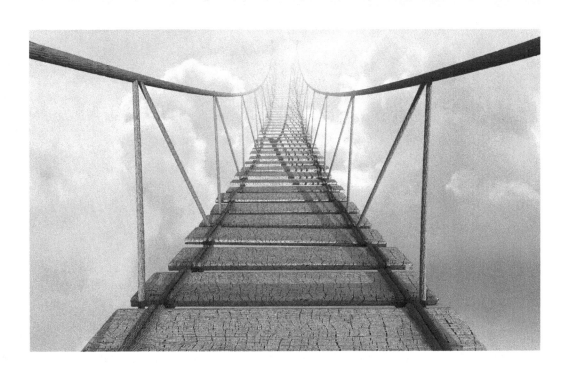

12

Effective Use of Feedback During Level I Fieldwork

Jeanette Koski, OTD, OTR/L

Level I fieldwork provides opportunities for occupational therapy/occupational therapy assistant students to incorporate their academic learning into practical experiences with occupational therapy service delivery. With this in mind, fieldwork educators (FWeds) can enhance student learning by providing opportunities to practice therapeutic skills and demonstrate professional behavior within the context of the practice setting. An important feature of this active learning process is the provision of formative feedback *designed to help students integrate* classroom and fieldwork knowledge and prepare for the demands of Level II fieldwork. The term *designed* was chosen intentionally. Feedback can be an effective learning tool if it is crafted and delivered with individual student learning characteristics in mind. In contrast, feedback that is rote, nonspecific, and/or inauthentic can leave the student in a position of confusion and ultimately unable to meet behavioral expectations. At its fundamental level, feedback is information that helps a learner construct their knowledge and skills, which can be particularly helpful for the struggling student. This chapter will give the Level I FWed tools and techniques to provide feedback in a way that is most likely to yield positive learning outcomes.

Hanson, D., & DeIuliis, E. D. (Eds.).
Fieldwork Educator's Guide to Level I Fieldwork (pp. 339-351).
© 2023 Taylor and Francis Group.

LEARNING OBJECTIVES

By the end of reading this chapter and completing the learning activities, the reader should be able to:

1. Understand the essential considerations underpinning the effective provision of feedback.
2. Develop and implement a culture of feedback within the Level I fieldwork context.
3. Contrast the efficacy of three common feedback models.
4. Implement a feedback format into Level I fieldwork experiences for the benefit of the student and the FWed.

ESSENTIAL CONSIDERATIONS FOR PROVIDING FEEDBACK

The goal of feedback for both the FWed and the student is to ensure that the student is able to successfully integrate academic and clinical learning and be as prepared as possible for Level II fieldwork (Accreditation Council for Occupational Therapy Education, 2018) and eventual occupational therapy practice. Providing useful feedback is not unique to the occupational therapy profession. Many disciplines have studied feedback models, and best practice recommendations are rich in the literature, particularly studies related to feedback for all types of clinical trainees. It is clear from a variety of sources that certain principles apply regardless of the feedback model a FWed might choose to frame information. These principles include situating the feedback in the specific context of the fieldwork experience, creating a culture of feedback, and giving feedback with respect to the personal factors of the learner.

Situated in Context

Feedback is best when it is situated in the learning context (Ajjawi & Boud, 2017) and is relevant to the specific needs of the learner. Level I fieldwork, as an adjunct to classroom instruction, affords a student important access to an experiential learning environment. Feedback given during Level I should be primarily formative, used to prepare students for Level II clinical reasoning and professional behavior. The conditions illustrated in Box 12-1 can assist a FWed in designing their Level I fieldwork program to maximize student learning in this context.

In Box 12-2, an example is provided illustrating how a FWed, in collaboration with the student, can develop a learner-centered goal based on an item from a Level I competency tool. This example is used to illustrate how to situate student learning outcomes relative to professional standards within the context of the experiential learning opportunities at the fieldwork site.

Culture of Feedback

Establishing a culture of feedback (Eva et al., 2011) includes the idea of feedback as an essential, expected, and valued part of the learning process (Henderson et al., 2019), a culture where feedback is related to mutual goals, is given with a spirit of caring and concern, and is supported by a strong relationship between FWed and student (Eva et al., 2011; Gaunt et al., 2017). Feedback grounded in this way is most likely to facilitate a student emerging from the experience with enhanced practical knowledge and also communication skills. Some ideas for how to create a culture of feedback are presented next.

BOX 12-1

FEEDBACK SITUATED IN CONTEXT

- Establish **learner-centered goals** so that the student has clear and meaningful objectives. The more relevant and specific the learning objectives, the more likely the student will be invested in incorporating feedback that will help them meet their goals.
- Align learner-centered goals with **site-specific objectives**, professional standards for **Level I competency** (such as the Level I evaluation form published on the American Occupational Therapy Association website), and/or **Level I objectives** from the academic program (Figure 12-1). Aligning these goals allows feedback about meeting competency expectations to be relevant and meaningful to the student's target growth areas.
- Base **feedback on direct observations** of student performance. In the event that feedback comes from someone other than the FWed, ensure the source is credible (Eva et al., 2011) and unbiased; acknowledge the observer when delivering the feedback.
- Use feedback as an opportunity to **facilitate critical self-reflection** by intentional guidance of student self-assessment (Jug et al., 2019) as demonstrated in the Pendleton Model example later in the chapter. Teach the student to reflect after each session, whether they are leading or not, about what went well, and what could be done differently next time to better serve the clients. Engaging in self-reflection translates directly to best practice and is an important skill for students to develop as early as possible.
- **Model self-reflection** for students. Questions such as "Did I check for student understanding?", "Is there a different way I could teach that technique?", "Did I challenge the student at the right level?", "Can I back up what I am teaching with evidence?" can be used to assess a FWed's student-centered approach to feedback and teaching.

BOX 12-2

DEVELOPING A LEARNER-CENTERED GOAL

Item 10 from the Level I Fieldwork Competency Evaluation for OT and OTA Students (American Occupational Therapy Association, 2017)

Consider student's ability to interact appropriately with individuals, such as eye contact, empathy, limit setting, respectfulness, use of authority, and so forth; degree and quality of verbal interactions; use of body language and nonverbal communication; and exhibition of confidence.

Learner-centered goal developed in collaboration with the FWed and Level I student

By the end of the Level I fieldwork experience, student will demonstrate appropriate therapeutic use of self with a challenging client while leading one treatment session as demonstrated by client participation in treatment activity.

- Explicitly dedicated feedback sessions at regular and expected intervals contribute to retention of information (Korenstein et al., 2012). Informal spontaneous feedback is important as well, but a formal feedback structure has been shown to be more effective in terms of the student integrating what is being taught. Box 12-3 illustrates an example of a way to structure feedback sessions in a formal way.
- Feedback should be constructive, descriptive, nonjudgmental, and based on skill performance. How feedback is constructed and given is as important as the actual feedback. Adcroft (2011)

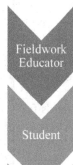

Fieldwork Educator
- Fieldwork educator observes and gives feedback

Student
- Student receives feedback and reflects on performance
- Student requests clarification and is given an opportunity to provide feedback as appropriate

Fieldwork Education
- Fieldwork educator receives feedback and reflects
- Fieldwork educator provides clarification or changes approach as appropriate

Figure 12-1. A model for bidirectional feedback.

Box 12-3
FORMAL FEEDBACK SESSION STRUCTURE

Weekly Meeting: Every Thursday at 3 p.m.
- Student weekly self-reflection: (1) What went well this week? (2) What was unclear this week? (e.g., feedback, concept, patient related)
- FWed feedback on student self-reflection
- Collaborative goal setting

---

noted that a lack of effective feedback delivery can lead to discrepancy between the learner's perceived receipt of feedback and the instructor's perception of the amount of feedback they give. In this study, the students perceived that they were not given useful feedback while the instructor perceived that they were giving a lot of feedback. Use of descriptive terms (primarily nouns and verbs) vs. evaluative words (such as adjectives) will ensure that the feedback is linked to correctable processes and skills (Jug et al., 2019; Table 12-1).

- In order for a student to make a change to their behavior, they must understand the feedback they are given (Eva et al., 2011). A format such as the **teach back method** can be used to have the student articulate or demonstrate their comprehension. Some students come to Level I fieldwork with constructs that may inhibit their ability to incorporate new learning. The teach back method, or a similar technique, can help an educator move a student toward breaking down those constructs and opening the door to new learning (Caplin & Saunders, 2015).

- Contextual factors, such as an increasingly diverse student population and institutional policies and factors that may impact feedback delivery (Evans & Waring, 2011; Price et al., 2011). Institutional factors may include caseload demands, space for private meetings, facility culture supporting (or not supporting) fieldwork students, etc. A FWed would need to ensure that the many barriers to the fieldwork experience were acknowledged or addressed. Teaching to a diverse student population means that a FWed needs to be aware of how cultural, gender identity, religious, generational, and other factors may influence student learning. For example,

TABLE 12-1

COMPARISON OF DESCRIPTIVE AND EVALUATIVE TERMS

DESCRIPTIVE TERM EXAMPLES	EVALUATIVE TERM EXAMPLES
Demonstrate	Inferior
Reason	Amazing
Implement	Substandard
Distinguish	Perfect
Prioritize	Lamentable
Articulate	Pleasant
Develop	Disappointing

BOX 12-4

BIDIRECTIONAL FEEDBACK PROCESS

"Is there a way that I can give you feedback in a session so that you feel supported and get the immediate information you need?"

"At what point during this week did you feel most supported?"

BOX 12-5

GUIDED QUESTIONS FOR ELICITING STUDENT FEEDBACK

"Help me understand your choice of [insert intervention approach]"

"I hear you say [observation of client performance], does that mean [interpretation of student observation]?"

for a student who is transgender, a FWed can use the student's correct pronouns in all communication and when introducing the student to staff and clients in the setting. Consideration for a student's personal context can ensure that the feedback relationship is based on mutual respect and trust.

A culture of feedback ensures that information is flowing both directions, (i.e., learners should be an active part of the feedback process; Henderson et al., 2019). Bidirectional feedback (Jug et al., 2019) has the potential to enhance the FWed's teaching skills (given that the FWed incorporates useful feedback) and allow for modeling professionalism in terms of being a receiver of feedback. A model for bidirectional feedback is provided in Figure 12-1. Illustrations of bidirectional feedback are provided in Boxes 12-4 through 12-6.

Bidirectional feedback often involves using guided questions to help the student structure their feedback to be constructive, descriptive, and nonjudgmental (see Box 12-4). It is important that the student tie their feedback to the FWed's goals, using active listening techniques and asking clarifying questions (see Box 12-5). Modeling of self-reflection techniques is helpful to the student, as well as demonstrating for the student how to respond to and implement the feedback that is provided. Box 12-6 gives a contrast of two feedback examples in terms of being constructive,

---

Box 12-6

SAMPLE DESTRUCTIVE VERSUS CONSTRUCTIVE FEEDBACK

Example 1: Script from the FWed: *"Your treatment plan shows poor understanding of activity analysis. You need to figure out how to break tasks down or you will not be a successful student."*

Example 2: Script from the FWed: *"Tell me about your choice of activity and how it addresses the client factors you and the client are working on."* [Student explains reasoning behind treatment design]. *"You were able to identify an occupation-based activity that does address the client factor, well done. Did you notice that the client still had a difficult time completing the activity? How could you grade the task next time so that the client is challenged at an appropriate level?"* [Student gives answer but needs additional guidance]. *"You are on the right track. I would like you to review what you learned about activity analysis in your classes and come tomorrow with a treatment plan integrating what you learned in the classroom with what you learned from today's experience."*

---

descriptive, nonjudgmental, and based on skill performance. Consider which example would be more effective in developing a culture of feedback during the Level I fieldwork experience.

Personal Factors of the Learner

The feedback delivery itself is important, however, personal factors such as fear, confidence, experiences, and biases can impact the degree to which feedback is integrated. Therefore, it is important to consider how feedback is received and interpreted by the student (Eva et al., 2011). Students' desire to become skilled occupational therapy practitioners exists at the same time as they fear making mistakes and "doing it wrong." Lack of confidence may make it harder to receive constructive feedback, while a reasonable amount of confidence can set a student up for being able to be more realistic about areas for growth (Eva et al., 2011). Experience is directly linked to an increase in confidence, and students value feedback given in a way that increases confidence through experience. Utilizing a bidirectional feedback model, such as the One-Minute Preceptor or the Pendleton Method (which will be further discussed later in this chapter), will allow a student to demonstrate what they have learned in the fieldwork experience and allow the FWed to facilitate further learning with less risk of negatively impacting student confidence.

Timing and Complexity

Additional considerations when giving feedback to a Level I fieldwork student include timing and complexity of feedback (Hattie & Timperley, 2007). In terms of timing, the FWed should assess the student's skill development in relation to their didactic learning. For example, what is the timing of the Level I fieldwork in relation to the scope of the whole academic curriculum? Is this the student's first Level I? What types, if any, of experiential learning has the student engaged in? Another aspect of timing is determining when the feedback will be delivered. Is it best for the learner to get the feedback in situ or after a session? When does the student seem most ready to engage in the feedback process? Are they better at the beginning of the day? The end of the day? Throughout the day? Additionally, are there environmental factors that impact timing of feedback that should be considered (e.g., environmental distractions, space considerations, time limitations, workplace demands)?

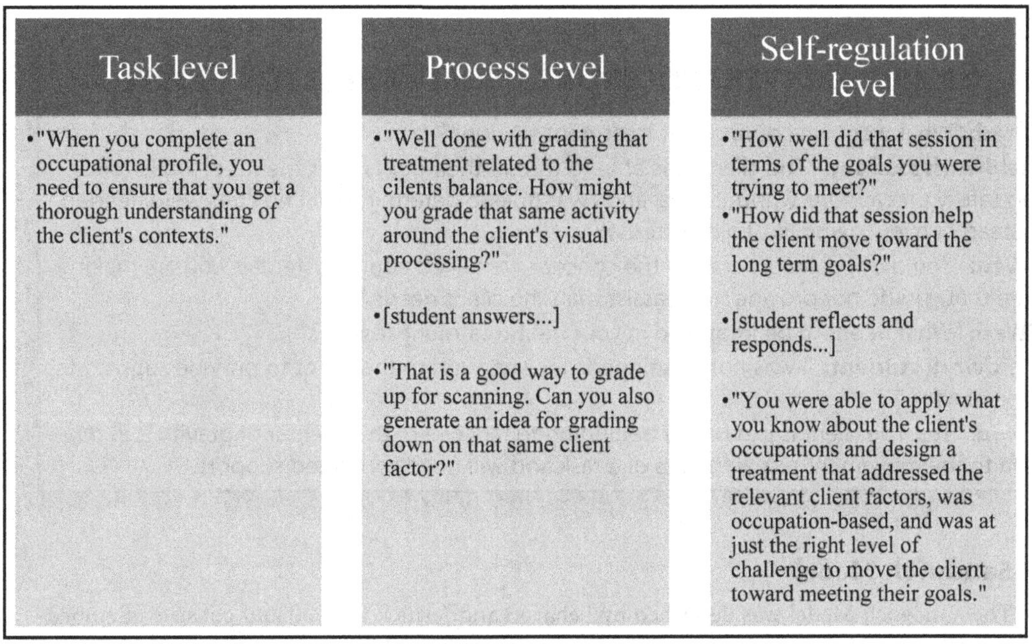

Task level	Process level	Self-regulation level
• "When you complete an occupational profile, you need to ensure that you get a thorough understanding of the client's contexts."	• "Well done with grading that treatment related to the cilents balance. How might you grade that same activity around the client's visual processing?" • [student answers...] • "That is a good way to grade up for scanning. Can you also generate an idea for grading down on that same client factor?"	• "How well did that session in terms of the goals you were trying to meet?" • "How did that session help the client move toward the long term goals?" • [student reflects and responds...] • "You were able to apply what you know about the client's occupations and design a treatment that addressed the relevant client factors, was occupation-based, and was at just the right level of challenge to move the client toward meeting their goals."

Figure 12-2. Modulating the cognitive complexity of feedback.

Box 12-7

SAMPLE SANDWICH MODEL FEEDBACK STRUCTURE

"You were prepared with all of the materials for the assessment, well done *(positive)*. For next time, ensure you practice the wording for this standardized assessment to improve the patient understanding *(negative)*. You did a great job of building rapport during your part of the assessment *(positive)*."

The complexity of the feedback should also be considered. Modulating the cognitive complexity of feedback (Hattie & Timperley, 2007) can be done at three levels as illustrated in Figure 12-2:

- **Task level:** Feedback about content and facts
- **Process level:** Feedback about strategies or clinical reasoning
- **Self-regulation level:** Feedback at the level of metacognition (i.e., strategies to self-evaluate clinical reasoning)

A feedback session could incorporate feedback in all three of these areas. Conversely, the FWed can select one particular level in which to provide feedback in order to ensure that the student does not get overwhelmed.

Feedback Models

In this chapter, three feedback models will be described: Sandwich, Pendleton, and the One-Minute Preceptor, which is also known as *the five micro-skills for one-on-one teaching*. Feedback models provide a structure for FWeds in which to frame their instruction and reinforce or correct student learning. All of the principles discussed in this chapter should be incorporated into feedback sessions regardless of the model used to deliver that feedback.

Box 12-8

SAMPLE CONVERSATION ONE USING PENDLETON MODEL

FWed: "What went well during that treatment session?"

Fieldwork student: "The client was able to thread their pants over their feet while following safety precautions without cues, and I was able to determine that no cues were needed, instead of over-cueing like I did yesterday."

FWed: "You did well incorporating the concept we talked about yesterday. You are making sure that you do not provide more assist than the client needs."

FWed: "What needs to be improved in your next treatment session?"

Fieldwork student: "I was not positioned close enough to the client to provide support in case of a fall."

FWed: "Yes. The client is just barely beginning to feel where their center of gravity is in relation to the movement requirements of a task and will need continued support."

Sandwich Model

The Sandwich Model was described by Lebaron and Jernick in 2000 and consists of embedding negative feedback in between two layers of positive. Box 12-7 provides an example of what a FWed might say to a student.

The Sandwich is a simple model to understand and deploy; however, there are some drawbacks in terms of how this feedback is structured and received. A really good sandwich has a balance of ingredients (e.g., the bread has to be able to support the meat). There is a potential, when giving feedback, to go slim on the positive "bread" and then overload the negative "meat" in the sandwich. Care must be given to create this balance to ensure that the student does not get overwhelmed by the negative and subsequently reject feedback. Refer back to the Essential Considerations for Providing Feedback section of this chapter to review the impact negative feedback has on confidence and the concept of the learner rejecting negative feedback.

Another drawback to using this model includes the terminology *positive* and *negative*. The problem with the phrase *negative feedback* is the implication that an improvement is not necessarily expected. Contrast the term *negative feedback* with *constructive feedback*. While negative feedback implies that there is a lack of performance, the term constructive leaves room for growth or constructing new learning with the knowledge gained about performance from the feedback. Negative feedback can have an impact on motivation and self-efficacy if it is controlling, destructive, and/or uninformative (Ryan & Deci, 2000). In addition to the other drawbacks, in the sandwich format the feedback is unidirectional (i.e., information goes from the FWed to the student). Therefore, this model does not inherently set a student up for any kind of self-reflection or problem solving related to their learning needs nor the ability to participate actively in the feedback process.

Pendleton Model

In the Pendleton Model (Pendleton et al., 2003), the instructor facilitates a structured bidirectional dialogue where the learner is asked to describe what went well and what needs to be improved, in that order. The method is intended to help the learner engage in self-reflection and analysis of their own learning and understanding. Box 12-8 is an example of how this dialogue might go.

In the Box 12-8 sample conversation, the FWed asks guided questions formulated to lead the student to self-assess a specific aspect of their learning. The student is then held responsible for reflecting on their performance in terms of behaviors to continue and behaviors that need to be

---

Box 12-9

SAMPLE CONVERSATION TWO USING PENDLETON MODEL

FWed: "What went well during that treatment session?"

Fieldwork student: "The client was able to thread their pants over their feet while following safety precautions without cues."

FWed: "What went better than yesterday's activities of daily living session in terms of your role in that treatment session?"

Fieldwork student: "I was able to provide greater physical assistance and guarding during the activity."

FWed: "You did well incorporating the concept we talked about yesterday. You want to be making sure that you do not provide more assistance than the client needs."

FWed: "What needs to be improved in your next treatment session?"

Fieldwork student: "I can be more aware of the use of manual contacts during moving and handling to provide the just-right amount of assistance."

FWed: "Right on!"

Box 12-10

SAMPLE STRUCTURING OF FACILITATION QUESTIONS

Designing questions to facilitate clinical reasoning and student ability to reflect on their performance.

Too vague: "What problem did the client have with that laundry activity?"

Too specific: "Were you targeting balance with that activity?"

Just-right: "What client factor were you targeting when you had the client reach into the lower cabinet?"

---

changed in order to make progress toward their learning goals. In the example in Box 12-8, the student came to the conclusions that the FWed was guiding them toward. What happens if a student does not understand their own performance at the expected level? Box 12-9 provides another example of the Pendleton Model.

As seen in the question and response in Box 12-9, if the student does not identify what the FWed is trying to get them to see, the FWed phrases the next question in a way that provides even more guidance. The FWed may need to continue honing the guidance as needed to ensure that the student is able to understand the concept. A challenge with this method is that the FWed needs to learn to ask the guiding questions in a way that facilitates the student reflection on the targeted skills. If the FWed asks questions that are too vague, the student may not know what specific target the question is designed to get them to consider. If the FWed asks a question that is too specific, the answer may already be in the question, and the student could just parrot the answer back to the instructor. Therefore, effective use of this method requires practice on the part of the FWed. An example of considerations in designing questions is provided in Box 12-10.

BOX 12-11

FIVE STEPS OF THE ONE-MINUTE PRECEPTOR

Step 1: Get a commitment: The instructor asks the learner to state something definitive about their observation or experience in a clinical situation, with the goal of gaining an understanding of the learner's clinical reasoning.

Step 2: Probe for supporting evidence: In this step, the instructor asks the learner to provide rationale for their reasoning in the previous step. Not only are these first two steps important during the clinical training period, but they also mirror the clinical reasoning process that professionals use every day in their practice. Having a student engage in this process as they are on fieldwork will likely provide them with tools that they will use on their own during Level II and as future practitioners. This step will also help the instructor determine if the student is able to support their choice or if the student got the right answer in Step 1 with a lucky guess.

Step 3: Reinforce what was done well: The instructor reinforces specific student behavior and reasoning, increasing the likelihood that the student will retain the skill.

Step 4: Give guidance about errors and omissions: In this step, as in all of the others, the focus is on behavior/skills and should be free of value judgement. The guidance can come from the instructor or can be the instructor facilitating the learner to identify errors or omissions themselves. This step can also include the instructor/learner identifying possible consequences of continued errors or omissions.

Step 5: Teach a general principle: The instructor helps the learner generalize what they have learned from the previous steps to other clinical situations.

One-Minute Preceptor

Developed by Neher et al. in 1992 to frame teaching in a clinical setting, the One-Minute Preceptor Model is made up of five steps or micro-skills. This model has been studied in relation to clinical training for students of many disciplines and has been shown to be an effective tool for the provision of feedback that directly and positively impacts a student's clinical reasoning (Gatewood & De Gagne, 2019). The Gatewood and De Gagne (2019) meta-analysis showed that the One-Minute Preceptor feedback format was preferred over other models by both the students and the preceptors. According to a meta-analysis done by Wisniewski et al. (2020), students learn best when they understand what they need to correct, why they need to correct it, and how they can do better in the future. The One-Minute Preceptor Model allows for this type of feedback processing— the instructor guiding the learner with direct questions and relevant behavioral feedback. The steps for this model are illustrated in Box 12-11.

To be confident in the use of the One-Minute Preceptor method, it takes practice. The learning activities provided at the end of the chapter involve the application of the One-Minute Preceptor Model in case examples to give the FWed an opportunity to implement a feedback format into Level I fieldwork case example.

SUMMARY

The intentional incorporation of the essential considerations for giving feedback can ensure the most effective use of any feedback model. These considerations include situating the learning in the fieldwork context and facilitating a culture of feedback—specifically, the development of student-centered and professionally relevant learning objectives, facilitation of student and FWed self-reflection, and provision of bidirectional, explicit, understandable, constructive, and non-judgmental feedback. The essential considerations presented in this chapter can impact how well feedback is understood and integrated by a Level I fieldwork student and may ultimately impact how well a student performs on future academic and clinical competencies. A FWed can embed the essential considerations for giving feedback into a feedback structure or model, such as the Sandwich Model, the Pendleton Model, or the One-Minute Preceptor Model. As a FWed becomes proficient with the use of one or more of the feedback models described in this chapter, the process of educating Level I students can be enhanced and maximized for both the student and instructor.

LEARNING ACTIVITIES

In this section, two case studies will be presented along with a sample dialogue demonstrating an application of the One-Minute Preceptor Model in practice.

Review of the five steps of the One-Minute Preceptor Model:

Step 1: Get a commitment

Step 2: Probe for supporting evidence

Step 3: Reinforce what was done well

Step 4: Give guidance about errors and omissions

Step 5: Teach a general principle

CASE 1: TEACHING FUNCTIONAL TRANSFER TECHNIQUES

FWed: "I have had multiple Level I students whose transfer techniques were ineffective. The students were not using good body mechanics. I wanted to help them learn to evaluate their own techniques so that in the future they could effectively assess their own performance. I knew the academic curriculum well enough to know that therapist body mechanics during transfers had been covered in classes, so I used that information to set up the feedback session for each of these students. In the case of one particular student, I knew that they did better when they were able to observe a skill before trying it themself."

Case 1: Application Activity

- Using the five steps of the One-Minute Preceptor Model from the beginning of section, develop your side of the feedback session between you and the student in the Case 1.
- Check your response with how the FWed in this case applied the One-Minute Preceptor Model:

- Step 1: "Observe as I transfer this patient from bed to wheelchair. What are the basic principles of good body mechanics during transfers? And how do those apply to this particular transfer situation?"

- Step 2: "Show me how you would apply those principles by transferring this patient from bed to wheelchair. I will be here to assist as needed."

- Step 3: "What went well in terms of your body mechanics with that transfer?" (After asking this question, I gave the student time to respond and then supplemented with additional reinforcement.)"

- Step 4: "What would you do differently next time to improve your own body mechanics?" (After asking this question, I gave the student time to respond and then supplemented with additional areas for growth.)"

- Step 5: "You have 3 days left of this fieldwork, and I would like you to perform three more bed-to-wheelchair transfers of patients with different mobility needs. How will you apply what you learned about body mechanics during your observation and this transfer to the next client's transfer?"

CASE 2: TEACHING PROFESSIONAL BEHAVIOR

FWed: "A few years ago, I was in a situation where I needed to teach a Level I student to set appropriate boundaries with clients. One day, we were treating a patient who swore a lot and was verbally inappropriate with the student and other staff. The student had no idea how to handle the situation, and they got very quiet. On that day, I stepped in and had to tell the patient to be appropriate and improve their behavior. After the treatment session, the student and I discussed my approach to managing this situation with the client including the tone of voice and the words I chose to firmly and respectfully convey my message to the client. We discussed how the student could develop the skill within their own therapeutic use of self. After this conversation, the student started to stand up for themselves and even developed a good relationship with the patient for the rest of their Level I."

Case 2: Application Activity

- Using the five steps of the One-Minute Preceptor Model from the beginning of this section, develop your side of the feedback session between you and the student in Case 2.

- Check your response with how the FWed in this case applied the One-Minute Preceptor Model:

  - Step 1: "How would you define professional behavior in terms of delivery of occupational therapy services? Describe the interactions you just observed between the patient and me as it relates to your definition of professional behavior."

  - Step 2: "Describe how you might achieve the same result that I did in terms of setting boundaries and ensuring mutual respect with this patient. Keep in mind that though you are working toward the same outcome as I am, you will have your own style in communicating with your patients."

  - Step 3: "When you stated, 'I want to ensure you are getting the best occupational therapy experience possible and to achieve that I believe that mutual respect should be part of our interactions,' the client clearly felt reassured that you cared about them."

- ◦ Step 4: "It seemed like you might have been fearful of having this conversation, evident by the waver in your voice and a tone that might have been interpreted as self-righteous. I know that this was not your intent."

- ◦ Step 5: "Think about the concept of mutual respect and therapeutic use of self. Think about the ways in which you can modulate your tone of voice as a means of nonverbally communicating mutual respect. How would that sound? How could you convey that same nonverbal message in your interactions with a patient who is vocal about their political views during therapy that are different from your political views?"

REFERENCES

Accreditation Council for Occupational Therapy Education. (2018). *Standards and interpretative guide* [PDF]. https://www.aota.org/~/media/Corporate/Files/EducationCareers/Accredit/StandardsReview/2018-ACOTE-Standards-Interpretive-Guide.pdf

Adcroft, A. (2011). The mythology of feedback. *Higher Education Research and Development, 30*(4), 405-419. https://doi.org/10.1080/07294360.2010.526096

Ajjawi, R., & Boud, D. (2017). Researching feedback dialogue: An interactional analysis approach. *Assessment & Evaluation in Higher Education, 42*(2), 252-265. https://doi.org/10.1080/02602938.2015.1102863

American Occupational Therapy Association. (2017). *Level I fieldwork competency evaluation for OT and OTA students.* https://www.aota.org/-/media/Corporate/Files/EducationCareers/Educators/Fieldwork/LevelI/Level-I-Fieldwork-Competency-Evaluation-for-ot-and-ota-students.pdf

Eva, K. W., Armson, H., Holmboe, E., Lockyer, J., Loney, E., Mann, K., & Sargeant, J. (2011). Factors influencing responsiveness to feedback: On the interplay between fear, confidence, and reasoning processes. *Advances in Health Sciences Education, 17*(1), 15-26. https://doi.org/10.1007/s10459-011-9290-7

Evans, C., & Waring, M. (2011). Exploring students' perceptions of feedback in relation to cognitive styles and culture. *Research Papers in Education, 26*(2), 171-190. https://doi.org/10.1080/02671522.2011.561976

Caplin, M., & Saunders, T. (2015). Utilizing teach-back to reinforce patient education: A step-by-step approach. *Orthopedic Nursing, 34*(6), 365-368. https://doi.org/ 10.1097/NOR.0000000000000197

Gatewood, E., & De Gagne, J. C. (2019). The one-minute preceptor model: A systematic review. *Journal of the American Association of Nurse Practitioners, 31*(1), 46-57. https://doi.org/10.1097/JXX.0000000000000099

Gaunt, A., Patel, A., Fallis, S., Rusius, V., Mylvaganam, S., Royle, T. J., Almond, M., Markham, D. H., & Pawlikowska, T. R. B. (2017). Surgical trainee feedback-seeking behavior in the context of workplace-based assessment in clinical settings. *Academic Medicine, 92*(6), 827-834. https://doi.org/10.1097/ACM.00000000001523

Hattie, J., & Timperley, H. (2007). The power of feedback. *Review of Educational Research, 77*(1), 81-112. https://doi.org/10.3102/003465430298487

Henderson, M., Phillips, M., Ryan, T., Boud, D., Dawson, P., Molloy, E., & Mahoney, P. (2019) Conditions that enable effective feedback. *Higher Education Research & Development, 38*(7), 1401-1416. https://doi.org/10.1080/07294360.2019.165780

Jug, R., Jiang, S., & Bean, S. M. (2019). Giving and receiving effective feedback: A review article and how-to guide. *Archives of Pathology and Laboratory Medicine, 143*(2), 244-250. https://doi.org/10.5858/arpa.2018-0058-RA

LeBaron, S. W., & Jernick, J. (2000). Evaluation as a dynamic process. *Family Medicine, 32*(1), 13-14.

Neher, J. O., Gordon, K. C., Meyer, B., & Stevens, N. (1992). A five-step "microskills" model of clinical teaching. *Journal of the American Board Family Practice, 5*(4), 419-424.

Pendleton, D., Schofield, T., Tate, P., & Havelock, P. (2003). *The new consultation: Developing doctor–patient communication* (2nd ed.). Oxford University Press.

Price, M., Carroll, J., O'Donovan, B., & Rust, C. (2011). If I was going there I wouldn't start from here: A critical commentary on current assessment practice. *Assessment & Evaluation in Higher Education, 36*(4), 479-492. https://doi.org/10.1080/02602930903512883

Ryan, R. M., & Deci, E. L. (2000). Intrinsic and extrinsic motivations: Classic definitions and new directions. *Contemporary Educational Psychology, 25*(1), 54-67. https://doi.org/10.1006/ceps.1999.1020

Wisniewski, B., Zierer, K., & Hattie, J. (2020). The power of feedback revisited: A meta-analysis of educational feedback research. *Frontiers in Psychology, 22.* https://doi.org/10.3389/fpsyg.2019.03087

13

Assessment of Student Learning During Level I Fieldwork

Jayson Zeigler, DHSc, MS, OTR

As each previous chapter of this book has pointed out, Level I fieldwork is a very important component of an occupational therapy students' learning and professional transformation. Evaluation of student performance is an essential component in experiential learning. Not only is an evaluation mechanism a requirement set by the Accreditation Council for Occupational Therapy Education (ACOTE) in the United States, but the evaluation criteria outline the outcomes to be achieved by the experience and the evaluation process provides the student and fieldwork educator (FWed) the opportunity for reflection and feedback, which promotes personal and professional growth. Evaluation is a process that can occur informally and formally. Self-assessment conducted in combination with evaluation offers students the opportunity to reflect and become more self-aware. FWeds should be mindful that the evaluation process for Level I differs from Level II.

In the context of the Level I fieldwork placement, students can receive feedback on their performance and skill development from someone traditionally outside of the occupational therapy faculty who deliver their didactic coursework. Feedback and earned performance scores received from FWeds during early, introductory experiential learning experience such as Level I are essential to the continued growth and development of fieldwork students, particularly as they prepare for more rigorous clinical learning such as Level II fieldwork. The evaluation process is more than just inserting ratings and comments on an evaluation form at the conclusion of the Level I

Hanson, D., & DeIuliis, E. D. (Eds.).
Fieldwork Educator's Guide to Level I Fieldwork (pp. 353-387).
© 2023 Taylor and Francis Group.

fieldwork experience. There are best practices that might be applied to the evaluation process to facilitate your fieldwork student's growth and development. This chapter will guide the Level I FWed through the evaluation process for Level I fieldwork student performance.

KEY WORDS

- **Evaluation:** A means by which to collect information about student performance related to their didactic knowledge, clinical skill, and professional behavior skill acquisition (University of Michigan Center for Research on Learning and Teaching, 2021).
- **Formative evaluation:** Information collected about a student to improve curriculum design of an academic institution, or the educator is collecting information on teaching a particular skill set to a student with immediate evaluation of performance conducted to assess instruction efficacy (University of Michigan Center for Research on Learning and Teaching, 2021; Wiggins, 1998).
- **Summative evaluation:** Information collected on the student's demonstration and competence for translation of knowledge from classroom to clinic at various points of time in a student's curriculum (University of Michigan Center for Research on Learning and Teaching, 2021; Wiggins, 1998).

LEARNING OBJECTIVES

By the end of reading this chapter and completing the learning activities, the reader should be able to:

1. Understand the relationship between curriculum design and Level I fieldwork assessment.
2. Explain differences between formative and summative assessment processes.
3. Explore differences in scope and focus of Level I assessment tools.
4. Review best practices for introducing and delivering assessment expectations and outcomes to students.
5. Identify common pitfalls in student assessment and how to avoid them as a Level I FWed.
6. Understand the value of the student assessment of the Level I fieldwork experience and explore resources to build FWed competency.

THE RELATIONSHIP BETWEEN CURRICULUM DESIGN AND LEVEL I FIELDWORK ASSESSMENT

Occupational therapy programs (across all degree levels) are required to have some sort of mechanism in place to evaluate Level I fieldwork in the United States. ACOTE (2018) standard C.1.19 stipulates a requirement that there is formal evaluation of student performance in Level I fieldwork. Because there is more latitude within occupational therapy programs to design and deliver Level I fieldwork using different instructional methods, the evaluation mechanisms among occupational therapy programs will look different. An important aspect of the fieldwork experience is that it reflects the sequence and scope of content in the curriculum design. Understanding the program's curriculum design is an important step in developing an understanding of the evaluation expectations of the Level I fieldwork. For example, is the Level I fieldwork experience embedded in a course or is it a stand-alone course? Is the Level I fieldwork to occur via the dose placement model (over the course of a semester) or in blocked format, 1 or 2 weeks at a time? How does the curriculum design inform the Level I fieldwork objectives? For example, do the objectives have a focal point on professional behavior development? Specific technical skill exposure? And how does the evaluation tool relate back to the curriculum design and fieldwork objectives? Is the evaluation tool to be used as a summative or formative assessment? These are all important questions that should arise and be addressed as you embark on the role of a Level I FWed.

At its core, evaluation is a process that involves observation, collecting and appraising information, and making a judgment about something. In the role of FWed, evaluation is the process of collecting information regarding student performance and providing feedback in a manner that introduces the student to the profession and to the role of professional based on their observed performance during Level I fieldwork. As a process, evaluation is not just a formality that should occur at the culmination of the fieldwork experience. There are important steps that should occur before, during, and after the fieldwork experience. Box 13-1 provides a breakdown of suggested actions steps for the Level I FWed.

When an academic program initiates the process to assign a Level I fieldwork student, the academic program will provide you with a Level I fieldwork evaluation form (evaluation mechanism) that is intended for you to provide feedback regarding the student's performance in the areas of clinical skill acquisition within the occupational therapy process and related to their ongoing professional development (ACOTE, 2018). The American Occupational Therapy Association (AOTA, 2017) has put forward the following recommendations for *Level I Fieldwork Competency Evaluation for OT and OTA Students*:

1. Fundamentals of practice

2. Foundations of occupational therapy

3. Professional behaviors

4. Screening and evaluation skills

5. Intervention skills

Because Level I fieldwork is designed to "enrich didactic coursework" and provide the fieldwork student opportunity for "directed observation and participation in selected aspects of the occupational therapy process" (ACOTE, 2018, p. 41), most Level I fieldwork evaluation forms will ask you to critique student performance in similar categories such as those stated previously. An important mindset to have as a FWed is to not view evaluation as a critical or punitive process. Instead, it is important to approach the evaluation in partnership with your student. It is in the best interest of the student to understand their personal strengths and weaknesses as they influence client care to become a competent therapist. The FWed represents the interests of the clients served who also deserve quality care. The FWed, in partnership with the student, provides evaluation feedback that will help the student perform well and provide quality services to the profession. Keep in mind that your evaluation should not only provide a critique on areas needing improvement, but also identify strengths that will be an asset to the student in the field of occupational therapy. Remember that students completing a Level I experience are often looking for validation that they are in the right profession (Honey & Penman, 2020). As you evaluate students, be sure that you provide this confirmation when warranted. Honey and Penman (2020) also found in their focus group research that occupational therapy students value getting feedback on their skills and being challenged to think analytically and reflectively about their own performance. Through the evaluation process, students are able to critically reflect on their performance and the impact they might have on client care. It is also in the best interest of the profession and of the student to receive honest objective feedback early in the professional career, so the feedback can be built upon in

> ### Box 13-1
> ## PREPARATIONS FOR ASSESSING LEVEL I FIELDWORK STUDENTS
>
> Steps that the FWed should consider taking **BEFORE** student's Level I fieldwork experience include:
> 1. Define evaluation for your student's performance (Figure 13-1)
> 2. Review the evaluation mechanism received from student's program
> 3. Differentiate if the mechanism is a formative or summative assessment tool
> 4. Attempt to better understand the student's curriculum design and Level I fieldwork objectives
>
> Steps that the FWed should consider taking **DURING** the student's Level I fieldwork experience include:
> 1. Review the Level I assessment tool with the student and identify the behaviors expected in response to the learning experiences provided
> 2. Observe the student's performance
> 3. Score the student's performance in compliance with program's expectations
> 4. Provide feedback to the student based on observed performance and student's response to feedback
>
> Steps that the FWed should consider taking **AFTER** the student's Level I fieldwork experience include:
> 1. Reflect on your role as educator to determine strengths and weaknesses
> 2. Review and respond to feedback received from the Level I fieldwork student on their experience

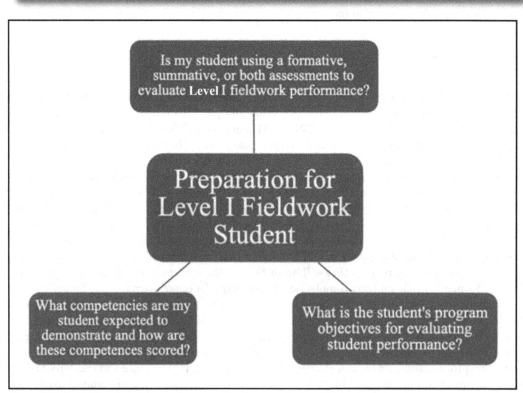

Figure 13-1. Student-centered approach to preparing for assessing Level I student performance.

Box 13-2

Examples of Summative Evaluation

Other examples of summative evaluation following didactic course work participation during Level I fieldwork assessing student performance include:

- Assessment of evaluation skills within occupational therapy specialty settings (oncology, pediatric specialty clinics, psychosocial settings, etc.)
- Assessment of student performance for advanced intervention skills, such as casting to facilitate constraint, induced movement therapy, or wound care within a burn unit, after the student's participation in an elective occupational therapy graduate course
- Assessment of acquired intrinsic and extrinsic qualities of professionalism throughout a curriculum
- Assessment of interprofessional collaboration skills within an intensive care unit after student's participate in advance acute care best practices graduate course

---

subsequent learning experiences. Embodying a more strength-based mindset will allow the FWed and, ultimately, the fieldwork student to view the evaluation process as an essential step in their growth and development. An understanding of one's strengths and weaknesses is essential for success in Level II fieldwork and subsequent entry-level practice. There are different approaches and forms of evaluation. For instance, evaluation can be *summative* or *formative*.

FORMATIVE AND SUMMATIVE ASSESSMENT

In the process of reviewing the information provided by the academic program, the FWed will need to understand if the student's program provided evaluation mechanism is intended to be used and facilitated in a formative fashion or summative or potentially both. This step may require communication with the student's academic fieldwork coordinator (AFWC) if the type of evaluation format is not easily determined. *Summative* Level I fieldwork forms are designed to determine at a particular point in time what occupational therapy students know and do not know in the clinic environment. The student's academic program operationally defines what the student is to know and do during the Level I fieldwork experience, which is often referred to as program objectives (Costa, 2015). For example, a student's early and first Level I fieldwork experience may take place in a pediatric clinical setting. Following a semester of didactic coursework focused on the pediatric population, the student may need to have a FWed summatively assess their knowledge of the pediatric population in the clinic environment over 1-week or intermittently after didactic sections during embedded pediatric Level I fieldwork experiences over the course of a semester. See Box 13-2 for more examples of summative evaluation for Level I fieldwork skills.

In contrast, and less routinely used, *formative assessment* is when the FWed is utilizing an instructional role to teach in the clinic environment a particular clinical skill within the occupational therapy process for a particular practice setting and population. Then, the FWed formally assesses the student's ability to do what is taught in the clinical setting. Two distinctions exist that will inform the FWed that formative vs. summative assessment is expected in a Level I fieldwork experience. Formative assessment is taking place if the student's academic institution refers to clinical practice or that the student should be also engaging in evaluation of themself after gaining knowledge and practice in the clinical setting for a particular competency. For example, a later Level I fieldwork may be sequenced in an academic program's curriculum that focuses on student skill acquisition and practice for orthotic fabrication and hand therapy interventions following supervision from a certified hand therapist over 1 or 2 weeks. Therefore, the hand therapist is

---

Box 13-3
EXAMPLES OF FORMATIVE EVALUATION

Other examples of formative evaluation following didactic course work participation during Level I fieldwork assessing student performance include:

- The student is taught how to coban upper extremity digits within a burn unit and provided ample practice time to understand and demonstrate the skill for which they are later assessed for the performance to initiate and complete the skill.
- The student learns from the educator the proper steps for interprofessional communication related to patient handoffs and at midterm of a semester-long experience is assessed for competency in this skill.
- The student learns and practices how to perform screening on a patient and completing a chart review using the site's electronic medical record platform to be later assessed for competency in this skill.

Box 13-4
QUESTIONS FOR FWEDS TO CONSIDER WHEN PREPARING FOR ASSESSING LEVEL I STUDENT PERFORMANCE

1. What program objectives are being measured by the Level I evaluation tool?
2. Based on these objectives, is my student's Level I fieldwork performance being evaluated using a routine summative assessment process or is formative assessment also expected of me?
3. What competencies must the student demonstrate, and how are these competencies scored?

---

expected to be in an instructor's role to teach orthotic fabrication for different hand-related injuries and associated interventions. The FWed then provides time for the student to practice and utilize the knowledge gained while in this clinical environment. Following this practice time, the student is formatively evaluated and assessed for what they know and can do in this practice setting. Box 13-3 provides more examples of formative assessment during Level I fieldwork experiences.

Formative assessment usually occurs across multiple points in the learning experience. The first assessment early in the experience develops a baseline, whereas subsequent assessments occur as the student has opportunity to practice a skill. An advantage of formative assessment is that students can actively work on problem areas over the Level I experience rather than find out on the last day that they displayed a problem in the first day of the experience that was not brought to their attention. Not only is the student more engaged in their learning, but the FWed can more easily employ a strengths-based mindset. When a formative assessment process is used, the FWed should become familiar with the Level I assessment tool early in the experience and use it throughout the experience as a reference point for the skills to be developed during the experience.

Once the evaluation format is understood by the FWed, it is then time for the educator to gain a deeper understanding of the competencies expected in relation to the program objectives of the Level I fieldwork experience. Box 13-4 provides the FWed with a checklist to determine a student-centered approach to evaluating and assessing their student's performance subjective to the student's curriculum design.

For the FWed to be able to appropriately answer the last two questions in the checklist mentioned in Box 13-4, they need to know the detailed objectives of the Level I fieldwork experience for the student and how the program operationally defines the expected competencies to be scored

---

Box 13-5

Example Level I Fieldwork Objectives Provided by the Student's Program

1. The student will demonstrate direct clinical observation skills by asking at least two to three questions related to an observed pediatric patient or client evaluation, intervention, or discharge session.
2. The student will demonstrate appropriate screening skills by completing a thorough chart review of a pediatric patient or client and reporting their findings to you using professional terminology.
3. The student will complete and present at least one intervention for a pediatric patient/client during this Level I fieldwork experience.
4. The student will verbalize to you at least two to three discharge considerations for one pediatric patient/client during the Level I fieldwork experience.
5. The student will demonstrate intrinsic and extrinsic qualities of professionalism and be able to verbally reflect on strengths and weakness of their ongoing professional development after receiving feedback at the end of this Level I fieldwork experience.

---

by the Level I FWed for their student's performance and the rating scale for scores applied. Box 13-5 provides a list of specific objectives that the FWed may receive if the student is completing a pediatric Level I fieldwork experience that requires summative assessment within the occupational therapy process.

Once the FWed has a clear understanding of expected objectives, a knowledge of defined competencies and how they will be scored is needed. Table 13-1 provides examples of expected competencies and sample score rating scales that may be assigned in the formative or summative assessment of Level I fieldwork student performance.

When scoring a student, it is important that you avoid a *response set*, such as scoring all students at a middle rating so that they know they still have more to learn or scoring students as though they were experienced therapists and not Level I students. The way to avoid a response set is to clarify competency expectations with the academic program if needed and to score each competency separately.

In summary, a student's curriculum design and the Level I fieldwork sequence developed by the program might determine if a summative or formative assessment is to be completed by the FWed. With thorough understanding of assessment type, program objectives, and understanding for scoring application for defined competencies, the FWed can better complete the evaluation process for Level I fieldwork student performance. Next, the FWed should consider variations in design of Level I fieldwork assessment tools.

DIFFERENCES IN SCOPE AND FOCUS OF LEVEL I ASSESSMENT TOOLS

The scope and focus of the Level I fieldwork assessment tool from the student's academic institution is completely dependent on the student's curriculum design, which includes the sequence and duration of Level I fieldwork experiences. Keep in mind, Level I fieldwork is the student's *introduction to learning* in the clinical environment and their opportunity to construct from their existing knowledge and transform actively their assumptions of what has been learned in the past (Costa, 2015). The FWed should use the Level I fieldwork evaluation tool provided by the student's

TABLE 13-1

LEVEL I FIELDWORK COMPETENCIES
AND SCORING OPPORTUNITIES

LEVEL I FIELDWORK SKILL COMPETENCIES	POTENTIAL SCORING
Clinical observation skills: Please apply a score based on the rating scale provided for the depth of the questions asked by the student based on their direct clinical observations in your pediatric practice setting.	3- or 5-point Likert Scale (unacceptable, below standards, poor, fair, good, excellent, exceeds standards, and outstanding; Costa, 2015; Deluliis, 2017).
Screening and evaluation skills: Please apply a score based on the rating scale provided regarding the student's performance to complete a thorough chart review of a pediatric patient/client and report their findings to you.	3- or 5-point Likert Scale (unacceptable, below standards, poor, fair, good, excellent, exceeds standards, and outstanding; Costa, 2015; Deluliis, 2017).
Intervention skills: Please apply a score based on the rating scale provided regarding the student's performance ability to complete a thorough intervention plan for a pediatric patient/client.	3- or 5-point Likert Scale (unacceptable, below standards, poor, fair, good, excellent, exceeds standards, and outstanding; Costa, 2015; Deluliis, 2017).
Discontinuation of services (discharge): Please apply a score based on the rating scale provided regarding the student's performance to verbalize two to three discharge considerations for one pediatric patient/client during the Level I fieldwork experience.	3- or 5-point Likert Scale (unacceptable, below standards, poor, fair, good, excellent, exceeds standards, and outstanding; Costa, 2015; Deluliis, 2017).
Intrinsic (student's mindset and knowledge) and **extrinsic qualities** (observable behavior of professionalism [Deluliis, 2017]): Please apply a score based on the rating scale provided regarding the student's demonstration of appropriate (at the discretion of the FWed and site expectations) extrinsic (time management, professional appearance, communication skills, etc.) and intrinsic (self-management, problem-solving or critical reasoning skills, integrity and honesty, dependability, and generational and cultural sensitivity) qualities of professionalism while participating in the occupational therapy process for this Level I fieldwork experience (Deluliis, 2017).	3- or 5-point Likert Scale (unacceptable, below standards, poor, fair, good, excellent, exceeds standards, and outstanding; Costa, 2015; Deluliis, 2017).

program to reflect on how the student acts and responds in any given situation while supervised. The FWed is frequently seeking opportunities to evaluate student performance based on what is known of the focus and type of assessment tool provided by the student's school.

For instance, assume you are a Level I FWed who works in an acute care setting, and you are assessing a student's performance at culmination of their second Level I fieldwork experience. You see that the focus of the assessment tool is to evaluate how the student engages in the evaluation, intervention, and discharge process of acute care patients. In understanding the curriculum sequence of the program, you are aware that the fieldwork student has already completed a physical rehabilitation clinical intervention course and completed an elective course on acute care practice. Therefore, based on the scope of the student's knowledge acquisition, as the FWed, you are evaluating their performance skills based on their ability to build on their current knowledge of acute care and rating their ability to generalize past knowledge based on other experiences to acute care practice (Costa, 2015).

Another example of scope and focus for Level I fieldwork assessment tools is when clinical skills learning is needed for a specific skill acquisition for students to demonstrate. For example, a community practitioner, who works with the geriatric population, might be asked to serve as a FWed to summatively assess functional transfers from many types of surfaces during a Level I fieldwork simulation event at an academic institution. Assume that it has been determined by the academic program that in semester three of year two, students in a Level I fieldwork clinical education environment will demonstrate the ability to perform functional transfers safely through hands-on practice with standardized patients after having formative practice all semester in didactic coursework. Therefore, the expected focus when completing this Level I fieldwork assessment tool is summative evaluation of the student's performance in regard to ability to demonstrate different types of functional transfers.

Appendices A through C show examples of Level I fieldwork assessment tools that you may encounter as a Level I FWed. Appendix A provides an example of a summative assessment tool used to evaluate student performance after completing fundamental occupational therapy didactic courses and participating in a community student outreach center serving a marginalized population of individuals in Indianapolis, Indiana. Appendix B is an example of a summative evaluation tool for student performance with a focus on psychosocial factors (ACOTE standard C.1.7) experienced and introduced to the student during a traditional one-on-one supervised fieldwork placement (ACOTE, 2018). Finally, in Appendix C, the FWed can review an example of a summative evaluation tool that encompasses and bridges all didactic coursework to traditional one-on-one supervised clinical sites in which students are expected to demonstrate all competencies learned at this point in their curriculum. The examples provided are limited, demonstrating only a few different Level I fieldwork assessment tool types and focus. Many other options exist, as other academic programs may choose to focus on other elements of performance, such as how students are constructing their learning, reflecting within practice, applying clinical skills learning, engaging in problem-based learning, collaborating with others, and acquisition of professional behaviors in the practice environments.

Depending on the purpose and sequence of Level I in the curriculum, the focus of Level I fieldwork may be more general and broad. For example, assume you have agreed to host a Level I fieldwork student at the end of their first academic year. Their program would like to broadly assess their learning skills thus far in the program by using the *Level I Fieldwork Competency Evaluation for OT and OTA Students* presented earlier in this chapter (AOTA, 2017); refer to Box 13-6 for more information.

Occasionally, you may encounter a situation where the student's occupational therapy program in a specific geographic area participates in a fieldwork consortium that mandates the use of a standardized Level I fieldwork assessment tool for FWeds to evaluate student performance. This is typically another broad focused and general type of Level I fieldwork assessment tool. For example, assume you are a FWed in Eastern Pennsylvania and have agreed to host an occupational therapy student from Philadelphia who is completing their first Level I fieldwork experience in an outpatient adult therapy setting. The program will provide you with the Philadelphia Region Fieldwork Consortium (2018) designed tool, *Philadelphia Region Fieldwork Consortium Level I Student Evaluation, Second Edition*, found at the following webpage, http://www.philaotfwconsortium.org/resources. Therefore, as the FWed, you will need to know what didactic courses have been completed by the student in their program-specific curriculum and what broad and generally focused competencies you should score using the standardized Level I fieldwork evaluation tool provided.

Box 13-6

DID YOU KNOW?

The *Level I Fieldwork Competency Evaluation for OT and OTA Students* (AOTA, 2017) is a great place for a FWed to start to prepare for engaging in the summative assessment process for student performance because it provides an example of clear competencies that the student is expected to learn and introduced during Level I fieldwork experiences. This tool also provides the educator within a clear scoring criterion. It is advised to review this endorsed AOTA (2017) Level I fieldwork student competency tool in prep for your student's performance summative assessment. It could also be used as a tool used for role playing with colleagues and practice for providing feedback on these basic student competencies prior to hosting your first Level I fieldwork student. Academic FWeds can find a usable copy (for evaluation of student performance purposes only) of the *Level I Fieldwork Competency Evaluation for OT and OTA Students* (AOTA, 2017) at: https://www.aota.org/~/media/Corporate/Files/EducationCareers/Educators/Fieldwork/LevelI/Level-I- Fieldwork-Competency-Evaluation-for-ot-and-ota-students.pdf.

In summary, fieldwork experience duration and sequence of a Level I fieldwork experience for a student, as well as the type and focus of a Level I fieldwork assessment tool should guide how the FWed evaluates (summatively or formatively) the student's performance. With foundational knowledge addressed, it is time for a discussion of the evaluation process, and best practices that set the stage for clear and respectful communication between the FWed and the student.

INTRODUCING AND DELIVERING ASSESSMENT EXPECTATIONS AND OUTCOMES TO STUDENTS

In general, students appreciate assessment that is objectively conducted according to performance standards and based on objective information (Koski et al., 2013). It is important that the FWed is attentive to both the process for assessment as well as the information that is delivered. Best practices in assessment occur prior to the student's arrival, when the student arrives onsite, and culminate at the completion of the experience. See Box 13-7 for an overview of best practices in introducing and delivering assessment expectations and outcomes.

As is evident in Box 13-7, preparation prior to the student's arrival sets the stage for a successful assessment process. Many of these best practices were already discussed in Chapter 8. As discussed, the Level I fieldwork assessment tool is designed to be a measurement of learning objectives, and the learning activities are designed to provide the context for the FWed to measure student competency. Regarding competency measurement, it is important to note that students appreciate assessment feedback that is based on direct observation of behavior, in-person discussion with the FWed, review of student documentation, and, lastly, observation by others (Koski et al., 2013). Using the assessment tool as a reference, the FWed can ensure that the student is receiving adequate opportunities to practice a skill (which is especially important when the fieldwork serves a formative function) and that the student has multiple opportunities to demonstrate competency on a given assessment competency.

Early review of the assessment tool with the student and discussion regarding assessment expectations is critical to an objective evaluation process. Students appreciate upfront information about expectations, as well as prompt, direct, specific, and constructive feedback throughout the

---

Box 13-7
Best Practices for Introducing and Delivering Assessment Expectations and Outcomes

Best practices for preparation are to review the assessment tool **prior to the student's arrival** to:

1. Understand where Level I fieldwork experience fits in the sequence of the curriculum for the student and the curricular design of the program.
2. Understand the student's program expectations for competency.
3. Plan learning activities that correlate with the expectations of the program.

Best practices for when the student **arrives onsite** are to:

1. Review early the Level I assessment tool with the student to communicate all expectations for performance.
2. Refer often to the assessment tool throughout the students learning process. Use it as a reference point to ensure that the student has adequate opportunity to both learn (if formative) and demonstrate skills (for summative assessment).
3. Set aside adequate time for summative Level I assessment, at least 30 minutes, in order to provide opportunity for communication exchange between you and the student. Hit and run exchanges are discouraged and not optimal for student learning during the Level I assessment process.

Best practices for scoring student Level I fieldwork performance **at completion of experience**:

1. Complete assessment review with the student in a private environment for implications related to Family Educational Rights and Privacy Act (FERPA).
2. Give the student time to review scores.
3. Explain your scores in a positive and constructive manner.
4. Explore student's response to feedback regarding scores (their reaction, feelings, thoughts, etc.).
5. Discuss scores with student relative to their experiences in their curriculum to put the experience in perspective.
6. Suggest areas of improvement and provide examples of strategies to help the student construct better clinical and professional behavior skills.

---

fieldwork experience. They desire an evaluation process that advises and guides them regarding their strengths and opportunities for growth based onsite-specific objectives (Koski et al., 2013). In preparation for the cumulative assessment, it is helpful for the FWed to identify specific behaviors that validate the assessment scoring; there is typically a comment section in most assessment tools for this purpose. Taking time for this provides the student tangible evidence for the ratings given and a clearer opportunity to see patterns in their behavior and skills. It also makes it easier for the FWed to explain or justify the ratings given. Although time for FWed and student discussion is often limited during fieldwork placement (Hanson, 2011; Varland et al., 2017), it is important that at least a half-hour time period is given for communication of the summative assessment scores.

It is important that the final assessment be conducted in a private environment and that the results of the assessment are not communicated to anyone not directly involved in the assessment, as these are federal guidelines outlined in FERPA (U.S. Department of Education, 2018). Specific guidelines related to FERPA are outlined more carefully in Chapter 10. Giving the student time to review the scores provides opportunity for the student to take in the information so that your explanation of the scores can be more readily received. Having objective examples of specific behaviors noted and skills evident will be helpful to you in reviewing the scores in a positive and constructive manner. In doing so, you might have both positive and constructive examples to share with the student for a given item to show the student that beginning competency might be evident in some areas but missing in others. By using a variety of examples, you will be better able to justify examples based on the need for consistency in performance. Although you do not need to explore the student's response to each evaluation item, opportunity to reflect on the evaluation scores will help you to discern whether, or to what degree, the student is ready or open to advisement regarding their strengths and opportunities for growth based onsite-specific objectives (Koski et al., 2013).

When exploring with the student factors that influenced their performance, it is helpful to begin by putting performance in the context of learning experiences available in the curriculum. For example, if the student received lower scores in the area of assessment administration but explained that classroom experiences to date had been focused on administering assessments to peers rather than clients, you can help the student to put the assessment score into perspective by discussing the broader continuum of assessment administration skills with clients. It is important to help students to put the assessment scores into perspective so that they do not have unrealistic expectations of themselves and understand the Level I fieldwork as part of a continuum of learning. At times, the student may identify psychosocial issues that have impacted performance, such as transitional stress, developmental/life issues, and mental health issues, which are discussed in more detail in Chapter 11. When this is the case, it is important to listen carefully, validate the student's perceptions, and help them to put their experience in perspective of the need for healthy self-care to build a foundation for success in the occupational therapy profession and in life. Conclude the assessment process by suggesting broad areas of improvement, considering any discussion that has occurred. For example, if the student has identified issues with anxiety, and you have given a low assessment rating on the competency of explaining occupational therapy to others, you might suggest strategies for addressing anxiety along with strategies for altering explanations of occupational therapy for a variety of populations and situations. Discussion and examples of specific strategies for clinical and professional growth will be helpful to the student as it is often difficult for students to translate feedback into action and take initiative for their own learning (Mattila, 2019; Mattila et al., 2020). Use of a guided discovery approach, discussed in Chapter 11, might also include helping students to identify individuals and resources within their community and professional program that might be helpful in building skills and professional growth.

AVOIDING COMMON ASSESSMENT PITFALLS

Two common pitfalls for FWeds to consider avoiding are evaluating student performance based on experienced practices, personal wisdom at your site, and the failure to fail a student who demonstrated actions that constituted the need for failure based on outlined criteria provided by the student's academic program.

First, as a FWed who is an active employee in your practice setting, you may grow accustomed to certain organizational norms and knowledge sharing at your site regarding occupational therapy practices, which represents *tacit knowledge*. However, during Level I fieldwork, the student is being introduced to experiential learning and simultaneously navigating the real world employer–employee relationship. The Level I fieldwork student is dependent on their didactic coursework thus far in their curriculum and most likely is unaware of any subjective practices that you or your colleagues engage in that may deviate away from expected *explicit knowledge* acquisition. Understanding differences in tacit vs. explicit knowledge is helpful to the evaluation process. Tacit knowledge is also understood as personal wisdom and insight, is often abstract and complex, and is very difficult to communicate to someone via oral language. This type of knowledge can be

---

Box 13-8

CLINICAL VIGNETTE OF COMMON PITFALL ONE

A student is expected to accomplish the following objectives during a Level I fieldwork:

1. Administer a sensory integration standardized assessment
2. Demonstrate the skill to facilitate a sensory integration intervention, such as Wilbarger's Brushing Protocol

As the FWed, you are expected to score the student's performance on both of these objectives. You begin by auditing the student's performance based on your organizational practice knowledge for both administration of the standardized assessment and intervention for sensory integration practice. For example, you score the student 3 out of 5 for facilitating the brushing protocol based on number of strokes applied to each upper limb vs. time brushing applied to the limbs. Moreover, your work setting modifies one part of the instructions for a certain test procedure on the sensory integration standardized assessment used for which the student was unaware, and you reported a score of 2 out of 5 for this observed performance action by the student.

How could the objectives for these scoring items have been observed and scores applied differently by the FWed during this Level I fieldwork experience?

---

challenging for students to acquire in introductory experiential learning such as Level I fieldwork (Carrier et al., 2010). In apprenticeship learning, which is evident in many Level I fieldwork programs, occupational therapy students can acquire tacit knowledge by observation and imitation of their FWed and via direct practice. For example, you may demonstrate tacit knowledge when, before you enter a client's room, you subconsciously go to the supply closet and gather some extra items, such as nonskid socks, oral hygiene items, and an extra hospital gown. After a fieldwork student observes the routine of their FWed doing this, day in and day out, they start to demonstrate it. In contrast, explicit knowledge refers to knowledge that is directly gained through and can be retrieved and accessed from books, procedural manuals, and other tangible resources. Understanding the fire emergency protocol of a fieldwork site via reading and remembering the health and safety manual is an example of explicit knowledge. In order to effectively and accurately evaluate performance, FWeds need to be mindful of how the fieldwork student's knowledge base has been acquired and if the culture or historical practice at the site varies. If performance expectations or site-specific knowledge has not been directly articulated or taught, is the student responsible for it? See Box 13-8 for a scenario illustrating conflicts that might occur during the evaluation process based on tacit knowledge acquisition.

Another common pitfall in student evaluation is the FWed reluctance to fail a Level I student due to feelings of fear and discomfort. This phenomenon is so common that 26% of FWeds in one survey indicated that they should have failed a student during a fieldwork experience (Cardell et al., 2017). In this study, the FWeds who were surveyed decided not to fail the student due to lack of evidence, vague program objective descriptions, and feelings of discomfort (Cardell et al., 2017). Varland et al. (2019) identified fear of failing a student as one of the top five reasons FWeds surveyed would not serve as a FWed. However, when students are not given the specific feedback and summative evaluation that shows the need to correct their behaviors, they are more likely to experience difficulty on their Level II fieldwork, where the stakes are higher. FWeds can avoid this phenomenon (*failure to fail*) from occurring by gaining a detailed understanding of the information previously mentioned for the program's objectives, expected competencies that the student is responsible to have learned and demonstrated, and understanding the scoring criteria for student performance defined by their program (Cardell et al., 2017). The FWed should also consider logging all objective and subjective findings when observing student performance and interacting often with the student about program expectations. It is important that the FWed record times and dates when the student was provided with feedback and their response to the feedback. The student's response to feedback will be an aspect of consideration for the open-ended comment section of the form, and this information will be very helpful to the program and to the student who needs to further develop skills in professional communication. For example, did the student demonstrate a defensive or unprofessional response to feedback, such as rolling their eyes, or did they demonstrate positive active listening, such as good eye contact and open body postures? When provided feedback, did the student make an attempt later in the experience to act on the feedback provided?

To avoid this *failing to fail* pitfall, the FWed should review the evaluation tool early in the placement, with and without the student present, and then refer back to the tool as a reference point to providing the student feedback on various elements of taught clinical or professional skills throughout the experience. By doing so consistently, the scores provided at the conclusion of the experience should not be surprising to the student. In addition, by providing the student feedback all along, the student is consistently aware of expectations and has more opportunity to improve performance. In contrast, the FWed who notices unprofessional behavior or difficulty with various aspects of the occupational therapy process but does not bring it up to the student until the final day of the experience is even more likely to avoid failing the student due to personal discomfort. When the FWed and the student are held to the expectations of the Level I fieldwork program-specific objectives to score student performance throughout the experience, there is less likelihood the educator would fail to fail the student unless false positive scoring is applied when rating the student's competencies. Box 13-9 provides an example of how this pitfall may occur when evaluating Level I fieldwork student performance. Please also note that it is important to contact the AFWC of the associated program should you have concerns about student performance at any time during the Level I placement, and especially if you believe failure may be imminent. It is important that both the academic program and the student are informed of problems before a failure occurs, unless the student behavior is a threat to the immediate safety of clients requiring immediate suspension of the fieldwork placement.

EVALUATOR AND REFLECTIVE PRACTICE

While the evaluation process during Level I fieldwork does provide the student with specific feedback and an appraisal of the student's performance, it should also be a meaningful activity in the overall ongoing professional development of the Level I FWed. Outside of the FWed evaluating the student, occupational therapy academic programs might also require the student to complete an evaluation on the FWed and/or the Level I fieldwork experience. Common components of a Student Evaluation of Level I Fieldwork form consist of:

- Site characteristics

- General fieldwork preparation and FWed concerns if any

- Supervision model used and any concerns reported with supervision type facility by FWed

- Student's observation of how curriculum threads were facilitated by educator reported

- Student's opportunity to be provided general feedback onsite, FWed, and any other concerns

Appendix D provides an example of a program developed Student Evaluation of Level I Fieldwork tool that details the components listed previously. In addition to engaging in active reflection on the feedback received from the Level I fieldwork student, there are other tools designed to support service competency in the FWed role, specific to evaluation. Self-reflection as a Level I FWed engaging in the assessment process of student performance can begin with the AOTA (2009) tool called the Self-Assessment Tool for FWed Competency. Specifically, the FWed will want to analyze their competencies in the evaluation category to best prepare and model for the student to entry-level practice while keeping in mind that the student is not expected to be at

---

Box 13-9

CLINICAL VIGNETTE OF COMMON PITFALL TWO

You are supervising a Level I fieldwork student who has completed 75% of their didactic coursework and is now participating in their last Level I fieldwork experience prior to starting their Level II fieldwork rotations and Doctoral Capstone Experience and courses. This Level I fieldwork is a 2-week experience assigned by the academic program with focus on safety and ethical practice within a general physical dysfunction practice setting. The FWed is to instruct on safe functional transfer execution using a gait belt with ample time provided by the FWed for the student to practice prior to applying scoring on the assessment tool provided by the student's program.

The FWed provides instruction on proper site procedures related to using the gait belt, provides patient and rehabilitation technician instructions as needed, and reviews body mechanics for both a stand pivot and a squat pivot transfer in an inpatient rehabilitation setting.

The student is provided 5 days of practice and told that their performance skills related to safety and ethical practice during transfers will be scored during the last 4 days of the 2-week experience. During the practice days, the FWed provides frequent verbal prompts for the student to use the gait belt prior to the patient standing or squatting during the functional transfer. The FWed also asks the student why they feel the gait belt is not needed with the noted reply from student being, "I am strong enough to catch them if they fall, and they seem perfectly capable without one." During the practice days, the student is provided with documented mock scores for their performance and a summary of feedback provided. The FWed observes no response to feedback by the student during the remaining practice days. These behaviors continue during the official scoring days instructed by the educator to the student at the beginning of the rotation.

The FWed then begins to review the academic program's issued resources regarding failure of the focused content during this Level I fieldwork experience. The educator is made aware that if safety and ethics are scored below a 2 out of 5, it will result in automatic failure for the student. The student scored 1 out of 5 during the practice days and continues to earn these scores during the official scoring days indicated by the FWed. The FWed has overheard the student excitedly talking with other practitioners about this being their last Level I fieldwork rotation prior to starting their Level II fieldwork rotations. The educator begins to feel guilty about considering the failure of the student for this Level I fieldwork experience. However, it is clear based on the student's objectives and scoring criterion (determined by objective evidence gathered during rotation by educator) provided by the school that this student's performance should result in the failure of this rotation.

What actions could the FWed have taken to avoid the phenomena of failure to fail the student in this fieldwork education situation due to feelings of guilt (Cardel et al., 2017)?

---

entry level during Level I fieldwork experiences. For example, using the scenario depicted in Box 13-9, it would be confusing for the student if the Level I FWed were consistently providing feedback to the student that they did not utilize a gait belt during transfers, yet during their own moving and handling, the Level I FWed was inconsistent in their gait belt use. Should a situation like this be brought to the attention of the Level I FWed in the student evaluation of the fieldwork, the FWed could use the feedback for their professional development, as well as further development of the Level I experience. For example, the FWed might set a professional development goal to better model and teach safe practices related to gait belt use within the clinical setting during future Level I fieldwork experiences. For the development of future Level I experiences, the FWed might review the learning experiences provided to the student to ensure that both tacit and explicit knowledge was represented in the learning plan.

Given that the role of Level I FWed is often the stepping stone to the role of Level II educator, what skills can the FWed learn to better prepare for the Level II FWed role? Several studies have indicated that the ability to communicate in a professional and supportive manner is highly valued by students (Koski et al., 2013; Rodger et al., 2014). Koski et al. (2013) found that students highly valued the role of the FWed in serving as a role model, teacher, and provider of feedback. The Level I FWed might carefully reflect on the student's feedback to identify whether there were areas of growth identified in any of those categories that might be addressed.

A next step following self-reflection is to seek out learning resources to enhance skills in fieldwork education. Several mechanisms for continuing education have been identified in the literature (Provident et al., 2009). In-services or trainings are often offered to FWeds through academic institutions seeking to meet fieldwork accreditation requirements. Online coursework may be available through professional occupational therapy associations, such as the preceptor education training offered through www.preceptor.ca by Kinsella et al. (2016). More recently, journal clubs have been used as a mechanism for FWeds to interact with one another while developing competency in the FWed role (Ellington & Janes, 2020). In addition, enhancement of FWed skills may be accomplished by direct contact with AFWCs who are equipped to provide educational resources as a part of their professional role (Evenson et al., 2015).

SUMMARY

Evaluation is an important part of the teaching-learning paradigm, and in clinical learning models, such as fieldwork, this can occur in different ways. Because occupational therapy programs have latitude to design how their Level I fieldwork program will be evaluated, FWeds need to take the initiative to review and understand the evaluation tools used by all affiliating academic programs. Evaluations might differ based upon the type of fieldwork, the curriculum design of the program, and the sequence of learning expected in relation to the competencies measured. The rating scales used to measure learning competencies are also unique to the academic program. Adequate preparation to serve as a FWed includes reviewing the tool prior to the start of the experience, reviewing the tool with the student at the start of the experience, and reference to the evaluation tool during regular feedback sessions throughout the duration of the experience. Providing accurate ratings and clear comments on the evaluation tool is very helpful to the growth and development of the student. FWeds also need to be mindful of the overall process for conducting evaluations and the alignment of the process with role modeling and the learning activities provided.

The FWed is privileged to aid in the early development of future practitioners through the evaluation process and to have a voice in contributing to the curriculum design of the academic program. Yet we know that this privilege and responsibility does not come without challenges. Evaluation of the student is the method by which the academic program is accountable for the clinical and professional skill training provided. When the student performs well, the FWed can celebrate good performance with the student and confirm with the student their aptitude for the occupational therapy practitioner role. When poor student performance occurs, the FWed must be prepared to address the challenges presented and to provide both the student and the program feedback on student performance, which can be used to inform future planning for the individual student and the academic program. Through the strategies and resources provided in this chapter, the FWed has been provided an overview of the assessment process, exemplars of best practices in assessment, and considerations for future professional development in the FWed role. The desired outcome is that FWeds will neither be fearful nor reluctant to assume the evaluation role but will welcome the opportunity to provide objective, meaningful, and useful assessment information to both the student and the academic program.

LEARNING ACTIVITIES

1. You have agreed to host your first Level I fieldwork student as an educator in your career. You know that the student's 1-week experience is following the completion of an occupational performance course on geriatric practice standards, and you were asked to host the student because you are an occupational therapist working at a local skilled nursing facility. You are to instruct the student and provide practice time for skill acquisition when facilitating evaluation, intervention, and discharge practices within this type of practice setting for the geriatric population. First, what type of assessment are you expected to complete based on the description provided for evaluating student performance? Second, using the information provided in this chapter, what detailed questions could you ask to ensure that you collect accurate evaluative information about your student's performance based on their curricular design?

2. What sequence of steps can you take as a future Level I FWed to best prepare for assessing Level I fieldwork student performance within your practice setting? Consider that you wish to provide the student with a positive and constructive experience while also respecting their educational rights.

3. Reflect on and list examples of tacit knowledge practices that may occur at your site. What are some actions you could take to transfer this tacit knowledge to explicit knowledge expectations at your clinical site?

4. Consider the phenomena *failure to fail* and list personal attributes that you may consider improving, suppressing, or maintaining to avoid objectively failing a student based on acquired evidence and compliance with program objectives and expectations (Cardell et al., 2017). Refer to Boxes 13-8 and 13-9 for practice examples that may help to initiate reflection and facilitate better the completion of this learning activity.

5. Following a Level I fieldwork experience, the student provides you with feedback that they perceived your comments to them during the experience were often negative and unconstructive. How would you plan to reflect on this feedback and make changes to your teaching style during future Level I fieldwork experiences?

REFERENCES

Accreditation Council for Occupational Therapy Education. (2018). 2018 Accreditation Council for Occupational Therapy Education standards and interpretive guide. *American Journal of Occupational Therapy, 72*(Suppl. 2), 7212410005p1-7212410005p83. https;//doi.org/10.5014/ajot.2018.72S217

American Occupational Therapy Association. (2009). *Self-assessment tool for fieldwork educator competency.* https://www.aota.org/-/media/Corporate/Files/EducationCareers/Educators/Fieldwork/Supervisor/Forms/Self-Assessment%20Tool%20FW%20Ed%20Competency%20(2009).pdf

American Occupational Therapy Association. (2017). *Level I fieldwork competency evaluation for OT and OTA students.* https://www.aota.org/-/media/Corporate/Files/EducationCareers/Educators/Fieldwork/LevelI/Level-I-Fieldwork-Competency-Evaluation-for-ot-and-ota-students.pdf

Cardell, B., Koski, J., Wahl, J., Rock, W., & Kirby, A. (2017). Underperforming students: Factors and decision-making in occupational therapy programs. *Journal of Occupational Therapy Education, 1*(3), 1-21. https://doi.org/10.26681/jote.2017.010301

Carrier, A., Levasseur, M., Bedard, D., & Desrosiers, J. (2010). Community occupational therpists' clinical reasoning: Identifying tacit knowledge. *Australian Journal of Occupational Therapy, 57*(6), 1-10. https://doi.org/10.1111/j.1440-1630.2010.00875.x

Costa, D. M. (2015). *The essential guide to occupational therapy fieldwork education: Resources for today's educators and practitioners.* AOTA Press.

DeIuliis, E. D. (2017). Definitions in professionalism. In E. D. DeIuliis (Ed.), *Professionalism across occupational therapy practice* (pp. 3-42). SLACK Incorporated.

Ellington, A, & Janes, W. E. (2020). Online journal clubs to enhance fieldwork educator competency in support of student experiential learning. *American Journal of Occupational Therapy, 74*(3), 7403205150p1-7403205150p9. https://doi.org/10.5014/ajot.2020.035733. PMID: 32365321.

Evenson, M. E., Roberts, M., Kaldenberg, J., Barnes M. A., & Ozelie, R. (2015). National survey of fieldwork educators: Implications for occupational therapy education. *American Journal of Occupational Therapy, 69*(Suppl. 2), 6912350020. https://doi.org/10.5014/ajot.2015.019265

Hanson, D. J. (2011). The perspectives of fieldwork educators regarding Level II fieldwork students. *Occupational Therapy in Health Care, 25*(2-3), 164–177. https://doi.org/103109/07380577.2011.561420

Honey, A., & Penman, M. (2020). "You actually see what occupational therapists do in real life": Outcomes and critical features of first-year practice education placements. *British Journal of Occupational Therapy, 83*(10), 638-647. https://doi.org/10.1177/0308022620920535

Kinsella, E. A., Bossers, A., Ferguson, K., Jenkins, K., Bezzina, M. B., MacPhail, A., Moosa, T., Schurr, S., Whitehead, J., & Hobson, S. (2016). *Preceptor education program for health professionals and students.* The University of Western Ontario.

Koski, J. K., Simon, R. L., & Dooley, N. R. (2013). Valuable occupational therapy fieldwork educator behaviors. *Work, 44*, 307-315. https://doi.org/10.3233/WOR-121507

Mattila, A. M. (2019). Practice-ready skills for the capstone. In E. D. DeIuliis & J. A. Bednarski (Eds.), *The entry level occupational therapy doctorate capstone: A framework for the experience and project* (pp. 79-91). SLACK Incorporated.

Mattila, A., DeIuliis, E. D., Martin, R. M., & Grogan, J. (2020). Mindfulness in the occupational therapy classroom: Infusing grit, gratitude practice, and a growth mindset into OT education. *Journal of Occupational Therapy Education, 4*(4). https://doi.org/10.26681/jote.2020.040410

Philadelphia Region Fieldwork Consortium. (2018). *Philadelphia region fieldwork consortium Level I student evaluation* (2nd ed.).

Provident, I. M., Leibold, M. L., Dohli, C., & Jeffcoat, J. (2009). Becoming a fieldwork "educator" enhancing your teaching skills. *OT Practice, 14*(19), CE-1–CE-8.

Rodger, S., Thomas, Y., Greber, C., Broadbridge, J., Edwards, A., Newton, J., & Lyons, M. (2014). Attributes of excellence in practice educators: The perspectives of Australian occupational therapy students. *Australian Occupational Therapy Journal, 61*, 159-167. https://doi.org/10.1111/1440-1630.12096

U.S. Department of Education. (2018). *Family educational rights and privacy act (FERPA).* https://www2.ed.gov/policy/gen/guid/fpco/ferpa/index.html

University of Michigan Center for Research on Learning and Teaching. (2021). *Summative and formative evaluation.* https://crlt.umich.edu/tstrategies/tsfse

Varland, J., Cardell, E., Koski, J., & McFadden, M. (2017). Factors influencing occupational therapists' decision to supervise fieldwork students. *Occupational Therapy in Health Care, 31*(3), 238-254. https://doi.org/10.1080/07380577.2017.1328631

Wiggins, G. P. (1998). *Educative assessment: Designing assessments to inform and improve student performance.* Jossey-Bass.

APPENDIX A

Sample Level I Fieldwork Summative Assessment Tool
(Introduction to Community Practice at a Student Outreach Clinic)

Indiana University School of Health & Human Sciences
Department of Occupational Therapy
Fieldwork Level I: Student Evaluation Form—T590 FW I-A

Student Name _____

Date _____

Facility Name _____

Dates of Placement _____

Number of Hours Completed _____

GENERAL FIELDWORK I OBJECTIVES INCLUDE:

1. Satisfactorily demonstrates professional communication skills (oral/written, interpersonal) during participation in a Level I fieldwork experience

2. Satisfactorily demonstrates professional skills related to process of occupational therapy practice (e.g., evaluation, intervention) during participation in a Level I fieldwork experience

3. Satisfactorily demonstrates professional behaviors (e.g., safety, confidentiality, promptness, appearance, etc.) during participation in a Level I fieldwork experience

INSTRUCTIONS:

- **Fieldwork educator(s) please respond to items 1-23 by placing a checkmark in the satisfactory (S), needs improvement (NI), or unsatisfactory (U) columns.**

- **Designate NA in the comment section if the item is not applicable.**

- **Please add clarifying statements and/or examples in the comment column.**

OBJECTIVE	S	NI	U	COMMENTS: REQUIRED FOR NI AND U RATINGS
Professional Communication				
1. Completes three professional interviews with an Indiana University Student Outreach Clinic partner services and explains how occupational therapy can interprofessionally collaborate with partner(s) at this clinic				
2. Participates in the interprofessional health screening process and can indicate when a referral to occupational therapy may be indicated				
3. Introduces self professionally to a client and provides an understandable description of scope of occupational therapy practice				
4. Sought, accepted, and provided feedback from/to clients, their families, FWed, and other staff and documents experiences in an essay reflecting on content and provided alternatives for approaching situation in the future				
5. Modified behavior according to feedback received				
6. Compose a minimum of two progress notes including long- and short-term occupation-based intervention goals				
Screening, Evaluation, and Intervention				
7. Oriented self to fieldwork site including mission/philosophy, population served, disciplines, physical space, etc.				
8. Completed electronic record reviews to obtain background information and incorporates into professional communication				
9. Observed client after review of record in at least one treatment session and discussed with FWed				

10. Suggested appropriate intervention plans for at least two clients			
11. Developed at least one appropriate individual intervention with a rationale to discuss with FWed			
12. (If possible) Implemented the intervention with the respective client and discussed outcome with the FWed			
Professional Behaviors			
13. Identified safety and confidentiality rules of the fieldwork site			
14. Maintained the confidentiality of the fieldwork site, staff, clients, and family members			
15. Punctual for fieldwork experience and other scheduled meetings			
16. Adapted to the pace of the fieldwork site using time effectively			
17. Submitted all assignments on or before date due			
18. Projected self-confidence appropriate to Level of training			
19. Demonstrated appropriate personal and professional appearance during fieldwork			
20. Articulated to clients, family members, FWed, or other staff member the meaning of occupation to the occupational therapy profession and the value to the client			
21. Completed a self-assessment of personal assets and limitations and reviewed it with FWed (create own form)			
22. Researched unfamiliar diagnoses and shared findings			
23. At the end of the Level I fieldwork experience, completed and submitted a **Student Feedback Form** to the FWed			

COMMENTS *(When completing this section, you may include diagnoses, age ranges, optional experiences, remediated problems, strengths, and weaknesses. Please use back of form if needed)*:

STRENGTHS *(Must document)*:

PROFESSIONAL SKILLS AND BEHAVIORS TO IMPROVE *(Must document)*:

RECOMMENDED OVERALL RATING *(Please circle only one rating and do not add 0.5)*:

Exceptional				Inadequate*
4	3	2	1	0

*For a 0 or 1 to be circled, at least six of the 29 items should be checked as unsatisfactory. A 0 or 1 rating may require special intervention or more extensive fieldwork Level I experience for the student.

_____   _____

Fieldwork Educator   Student
Signature & Date   Signature & Date

_____   _____

Fieldwork Educator Printed Name   Fieldwork Educator Email Address

Objectives adapted from American Occupational Therapy Association. (2002). *Fieldwork performance evaluation for the occupational therapy student.* AOTA Press

Reproduced with permission from Indiana University Purdue University Indianapolis.

APPENDIX B

Level I Summative Evaluation Form (Introduction to Traditional One-on-One Supervised Fieldwork With Psychosocial Focus)

Indiana University School of Health & Human Sciences
Department of Occupational Therapy
T591 Fieldwork Level I: Student Evaluation Form

Student Name _____

Date _____

Facility Name _____

Facility Address _____

Dates of Placement _____

Number of Hours Completed _____

GENERAL FIELDWORK I OBJECTIVES INCLUDE:

1. Satisfactorily demonstrates professional communication skills (oral/written, interpersonal) during participation in a Level I fieldwork experience

2. Satisfactorily demonstrates professional skills related to process of occupational therapy practice (e.g., evaluation, intervention) during participation in a Level I fieldwork experience

3. Satisfactorily demonstrates professional behaviors (safety, confidentiality, promptness, appearance, etc.) during participation in a Level I fieldwork experience

INSTRUCTIONS:

- **Fieldwork educator(s) please respond to items 1 to 27 by placing a checkmark in the satisfactory (S), needs improvement (NI), or unsatisfactory (U) columns.**

- **Designate not applicable (NA) in the comment section if the item is not applicable.**

- **Please add clarifying statements and/or examples in the comment column.**

OBJECTIVE	S	NI	U	COMMENTS: REQUIRED FOR NI AND U RATINGS
Professional Communication Skills				
1. Interacted with client and members of their support system and documented in a journal their fieldwork experiences reflecting on content and quality **ONE JOURNAL ENTRY MUST FOCUS ON THE OBSERVED AND DISCUSSED PSYCHOSOCIAL AND SOCIAL FACTORS THAT INFLUENCE ENGAGEMENT IN OCCUPATIONS WITH FWed** (ACOTE C.1.7)	Two journal entries are required and must be completed by the end of the fieldwork rotation. AFWC will review. **Students: Please upload your journals on Canvas.**			
2. Sought, accepted, and provided feedback from/to clients, their families, FWed, and other staff and documented experiences in a journal reflecting on content and provided alternatives for approaching situation in the future				
3. Completed at least one interview with a client and/or family member using AOTA occupational profile or site-specific document				
4. Presented an informal oral report on a patient/client interview, treatment progress, or group summary to FWed or other professional staff				
5. Completed a minimum of three documentation notes. Examples include interview summaries, progress notes, SOAP notes, group notes/summaries, and/or observation worksheets/summaries on clients using fieldwork site documentation format and submitted to FWed for feedback *For emerging fieldwork setting: Student will complete a minimum of one agency summary, four structured observation summaries, and one to two interview summaries*				

Professional Clinical Skills			
6. Completed at least one client therapy record review (if possible) and discussed relevant findings with FWed to understand contextual factors that may impact assessment and intervention planning			
7. Identifies relevant psychosocial and social factors that influence patient/client engagement in occupations			
8. Compared and contrasted information gathered (performance skills, patterns, contexts, and client factors) on client to normal development and reviewed with FWed *Emerging fieldwork setting: Compare and contrast agency services with other similar community programs*			
9. Listed at least two potential affected areas of occupation and reviewed with FWed *Emerging fieldwork setting: List and discuss two areas where occupational therapy services could be implemented to enhance the current agency programming*			
10. Developed at least one long-term goal for two clients using fieldwork site documentation format and submitted to the FWed for feedback *Emerging fieldwork setting: Develop at least one long-term goal for the agency*			
11. Developed at least two short-term goals for each long-term goal using fieldwork site documentation format and submitted to the FWed for feedback *Emerging fieldwork setting: Develop at least two programming ideas for the agency*			

12. Suggested appropriate occupation-based interventions suitable to incorporate among two clients *Emerging fieldwork setting: Develop at least two programming ideas for at least two clients*				
13. Developed at least one appropriate individual or group intervention/activity with a rationale and submitted it to the FWed for approval				
14. Implemented the intervention with the respective client or group and discussed it with the FWed				
Professional Behaviors				
15. Oriented self to fieldwork site including mission/philosophy, population served, disciplines, forms of reimbursement, physical space, and materials				
16. Identified safety and confidentiality rules of the fieldwork site				
17. Maintained the confidentiality of the fieldwork site, staff, clients, and family members				
18. Punctual for fieldwork experience and other scheduled meetings				
19. Adapted to the pace of the fieldwork site using time effectively				
20. Submitted all assignments on or before date due				
21. Projected self-confidence appropriate to level of training				
22. Demonstrated appropriate personal and professional appearance during fieldwork				
23. Articulated to clients, family members, FWed, or other staff member the meaning of occupation to the occupational therapy profession and the value to the client				
24. Completed a self-assessment of personal assets and limitations and reviewed it with FWed (student creates a list or site-specific form)				

25. Researched unfamiliar diagnoses and shared findings			
26. In cooperation with the FWed, identified additional learning experiences			
27. At the end of the Level I fieldwork experience, completed and reviewed **Fieldwork I to B Student Feedback Form** with the primary FWed			

COMMENTS *(When completing this section, you may include diagnoses, age ranges, optional experiences, remediated problems, strengths, and weaknesses. Please use back of form if needed)*:

FIELDWORK PERFORMANCE STRENGTHS *(Must document)*:

PROFESSIONAL SKILLS AND BEHAVIORS TO IMPROVE *(Must document)*:

RECOMMENDED OVERALL RATING *(Please circle only one rating and do not add 0.5)*:

Exceptional				Inadequate*
4	3	2	1	0

*For a 0 or 1 to be circled, at least six of the 27 items should be checked as unsatisfactory. A 0 or 1 rating may require special intervention or more extensive fieldwork Level I experience for the student.

_____

Fieldwork Educator
Signature & Credentials

_____

Student
Signature & Date

_____

Fieldwork Educator Printed Name

_____

Fieldwork Educator
Preferred Email Address

Objectives adapted from American Occupational Therapy Association. (2002). *Fieldwork performance evaluation for the occupational therapy student.* AOTA Press

APPENDIX C

Level I Summative Evaluation Form
(Final Level I Fieldwork Summative Evaluation of Student Performance in Traditional One-on-One Supervised Setting)

Indiana University School of Health & Human Sciences
Department of Occupational Therapy
T690 Fieldwork Level I-C: Student Evaluation Form

Student Name _____

Date _____

Facility Name _____

Facility Address _____

Dates of Placement _____

Number of Hours Completed _____

GENERAL FIELDWORK I OBJECTIVES INCLUDE:

1. Satisfactorily demonstrates professional communication skills (oral/written, interpersonal) during participation in a Level I fieldwork experience

2. Satisfactorily demonstrates professional skills related to process of occupational therapy practice (e.g. evaluation, intervention) during participation in a Level I fieldwork experience

3. Satisfactorily demonstrates professional behaviors (safety, confidentiality, promptness, appearance, etc.) during participation in a Level I fieldwork experience

INSTRUCTIONS:

- **Fieldwork educator(s) please respond to items 1 to 27 by placing a checkmark in the satisfactory (S), needs improvement (NI), or unsatisfactory (U) columns.**

- **Designate not applicable (NA) in the comment section if the item is not applicable.**

- **Please add clarifying statements and/or examples in the comment column.**

OBJECTIVE	S	NI	U	COMMENTS: REQUIRED FOR NI AND U RATINGS
Professional Communication Skills				
1. Interacted with client and members of their support system and documented appropriately any significant interactions within the site's documentation system	Two journal entries are required and must be completed by the end of the fieldwork rotation. AFWC will review. **Students: Please upload your journals on Canvas.**			
2. Sought, accepted, and provided feedback from/to clients, their families, FWed, and other staff and documented experiences in a journal reflecting on content and provided alternatives for approaching situation in the future				
3. Completed at least one interview with a client and/or family member using AOTA occupational profile or site-specific document				
4. Presented an informal oral report on a patient/client interview, treatment progress, or group summary to FWed or other professional staff				
5. Completed a minimum of three documentation notes. Examples include interview summaries, progress notes, SOAP notes, group notes/summaries, and/or observation worksheets/summaries on clients using fieldwork site documentation format and submitted to FWed for feedback *For emerging fieldwork setting: Student will complete a minimum of one agency summary, four structured observation summaries, and one to two interview summaries*				

Professional Clinical Skills				
6. Completed at least one client therapy record review (if possible) and discussed relevant findings with FWed to understand contextual factors that may impact assessment and intervention planning				
7. Identifies relevant psychosocial and social factors that influence patient/client engagement in occupations				
8. Compared and contrasted information gathered (performance skills, patterns, contexts, and client factors) on client to normal development and reviewed with FWed *Emerging fieldwork setting: Compare and contrast agency services with other similar community programs*				
9. Listed at least two potential affected areas of occupation and reviewed with FWed *Emerging fieldwork setting: List and discuss two areas where occupational therapy services could be implemented to enhance the current agency programming*				
10. Developed at least one long-term goal for two clients using fieldwork site documentation format and submitted to the FWed for feedback *Emerging fieldwork setting: Develop at least one long-term goal for the agency*				
11. Developed at least two short-term goals for each long-term goal using fieldwork site documentation format and submitted to the FWed for feedback *Emerging fieldwork setting: Develop at least two programming ideas for the agency*				

12. Suggested appropriate occupation-based interventions suitable to incorporate among two clients *Emerging fieldwork setting: Develop at least two programming ideas for at least two clients*			
13. Developed at least one appropriate individual or group intervention/activity with a rationale and submitted it to the FWed for approval			
14. Implemented the intervention with the respective client or group and discussed it with the FWed			
Professional Behaviors			
15. Oriented self to fieldwork site including mission/philosophy, population served, disciplines, forms of reimbursement, physical space, and materials			
16. Identified safety and confidentiality rules of the fieldwork site			
17. Maintained the confidentiality of the fieldwork site, staff, clients, and family members			
18. Punctual for fieldwork experience and other scheduled meetings			
19. Adapted to the pace of the fieldwork site using time effectively			
20. Submitted all assignments on or before date due			
21. Projected self-confidence appropriate to level of training			
22. Demonstrated appropriate personal and professional appearance during fieldwork			
23. Articulated to clients, family members, FWed, or other staff member the meaning of occupation to the occupational therapy profession and the value to the client			
24. Completed a self-assessment of personal assets and limitations and reviewed it with FWed (student creates a list or site-specific form)			

25. Researched unfamiliar diagnoses and shared findings				
26. In cooperation with the FWed, identi-fied additional learning experiences				
27. At the end of the Level I fieldwork experience, completed and reviewed **Fieldwork I – B Student Feedback Form** with the primary FWed				

COMMENTS *(When completing this section, you may include diagnoses, age ranges, optional experiences, remediated problems, strengths, and weaknesses. Please use back of form if needed)*:

FIELDWORK PERFORMANCE STRENGTHS *(Must document)*:

PROFESSIONAL SKILLS AND BEHAVIORS TO IMPROVE *(Must document)*:

RECOMMENDED OVERALL RATING *(Please circle only one rating and do not add 0.5)*:

Exceptional				Inadequate*
4	3	2	1	0

*For a 0 or 1 to be circled, at least six of the 27 items should be checked as unsatisfactory. A 0 or 1 rating may require special intervention or more extensive fieldwork Level I experience for the student.

Fieldwork Educator
Signature & Credentials

Student
Signature & Date

Fieldwork Educator Printed Name

Fieldwork Educator
Preferred Email Address

Objectives adapted from American Occupational Therapy Association. (2002). *Fieldwork performance evaluation for the occupational therapy student.* AOTA Press

Reproduced with permission from Indiana University Purdue University Indianapolis.

APPENDIX D

Example Level I Fieldwork Student Evaluation of Fieldwork Experience Form

Indiana University

Student _____

Fieldwork Educator _____

Site _____

Date _____

Level I Fieldwork Student Evaluation of Fieldwork Experience

Site/Setting Characteristics
Please describe all site characteristics (practice population with age range, adult physical dysfunction [18 to 80], adult neuro, pediatric oncology, etc.) and the practice setting (adult acute rehab, outpatient, school-based, etc., also indicate if practice setting was simulated or onsite). **Question Comments: *Comment Required**
General Fieldwork and FWed Considerations
Did you feel prepared for this Level I fieldwork experience? If no, please explain. **Question Comments: *Comment Required**
What resources would have improved your general Level I fieldwork experience? **Question Comments: *Comment Required**
Did you feel that the Level I fieldwork environment was a suitable learning environment? If not, please explain. **Question Comments: *Comment Required**

What are the credentials of your FWed?
What supervision model was used for this Level I fieldwork experience?
If the collaborative model was used, what is your feedback in the use of this supervision model? **Question Comments:**
Please describe how observation and active (hands-on) engagement enhanced your Level I fieldwork learning experience? **Question Comments: *Comment Required**
Did your FWed contribute to your development for the fundamentals of practice? If not, please explain. **Question Comments: *Comment Required**
Did your FWed communicate and provide opportunities to communicate the foundations of the occupational therapy profession? If not, please explain. **Question Comments: *Comment Required**
How did your FWed's feedback promote the development of your professional behaviors? **Question Comments: *Comment Required**
How did interactions with your FWed develop your screening, evaluation, and intervention skills? **Question Comments: *Comment Required**

Curriculum Threads
What course threads were observed in the Level I fieldwork experience based on your course participation and didactic coursework in the semester in which this experience took place? Please select all options that may apply to this Level I fieldwork experience from the drop box below. Then, provide a reflective statement on why you feel this curricular thread was present in this experience.

Required

1. Foundations of Human Occupation and Participation

2. Optimizing Occupation and Facilitating Participation

3. Critical Inquiry and Reflective Practice

4. Leadership and Advocacy

5. Socially Responsive Health Care

Question Comments: *Comment Required

What areas of improvement could you identify to better thread curricular content from this semester or bridge classroom to clinic for this Level I fieldwork experience?

Question Comments: *Comment Required

General Feedback

Please provide any general feedback (positive or negative) regarding your Level I fieldwork experience that may not have been included in the criterion listed above.

Question Comments: *Comment Required

FINANCIAL DISCLOSURES

Dr. Becki Cohill has no financial or proprietary interest in the materials presented herein.

Dr. Elizabeth D. DeIuliis has no financial or proprietary interest in the materials presented herein.

Dr. Marsena W. Devoto has no financial or proprietary interest in the materials presented herein.

Dr. Anna Domina has no financial or proprietary interest in the materials presented herein.

Dr. Nancy R. Dooley has no financial or proprietary interest in the materials presented herein.

Dr. Cherie Graves has no financial or proprietary interest in the materials presented herein.

Dr. Debra Hanson has no financial or proprietary interest in the materials presented herein.

Dr. Jeanette Koski has no financial or proprietary interest in the materials presented herein.

Dr. Angela M. Lampe has no financial or proprietary interest in the materials presented herein.

Dr. Jason C. Lawson has no financial or proprietary interest in the materials presented herein.

Dr. Amy Mattila has no financial or proprietary interest in the materials presented herein.

Dr. Hannah Oldenburg has no financial or proprietary interest in the materials presented herein.

Dr. Julia Shin has no financial or proprietary interest in the materials presented herein.

Dr. Rebecca L. Simon has no financial or proprietary interest in the materials presented herein.

Dr. Lacey Spark has no financial or proprietary interest in the materials presented herein.

Dr. Jaynee Taguchi Meyer has no financial or proprietary interest in the materials presented herein.

Dr. Joscelyn Varland has no financial or proprietary interest in the materials presented herein.

Dr. Jayson Zeigler has no financial or proprietary interest in the materials presented herein.

INDEX

Printed in the United States
by Baker & Taylor Publisher Services